COUNSELING AND INTERVIEWING

IN SPEECH-LANGUAGE PATHOLOGY AND AUDIOLOGY

A Therapy Resource

Cari M. Tellis, PhD, CCC-SLP
Associate Professor
Misericordia University

Orlando R. Barone, MA
Executive Leadership Coach
Wharton School of Business, University of Pennsylvania

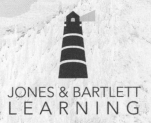

JONES & BARTLETT
LEARNING

World Headquarters
Jones & Bartlett Learning
5 Wall Street
Burlington, MA 01803
978-443-5000
info@jblearning.com
www.jblearning.com

Jones & Bartlett Learning books and products are available through most bookstores and online booksellers. To contact Jones & Bartlett Learning directly, call 800-832-0034, fax 978-443-8000, or visit our website, www.jblearning.com.

Substantial discounts on bulk quantities of Jones & Bartlett Learning publications are available to corporations, professional associations, and other qualified organizations. For details and specific discount information, contact the special sales department at Jones & Bartlett Learning via the above contact information or send an email to specialsales@jblearning.com.

11287-0

Production Credits

VP, Executive Publisher: David D. Cella
Executive Editor: Matt Kane
Acquisitions Editor: Laura Pagluica
Editorial Assistant: Mary Menzemer
Vendor Manager: Sara Kelly
Associate Marketing Manager: Alianna Ortu
VP, Manufacturing and Inventory Control:
    Therese Connell
Composition and Project Management:
    Cenveo Publisher Services
Cover Design: Kristin E. Parker
Rights & Media Specialist: Jamey O'Quinn
Media Development Editor: Troy Liston
Cover Image: © tusharkoley/Shutterstock
Printing and Binding: RR Donnelley
Cover Printing: RR Donnelley

Library of Congress Cataloging-in-Publication Data

Names: Tellis, Cari M., author. | Barone, Orlando R., author.
Title: Counseling and interviewing in speech-language pathology and audiology
  : a therapy resource / Cari M. Tellis and Orlando R. Barone.
Description: First edition. | Burlington, MA : Jones & Bartlett Learning,
  [2018] | Includes bibliographical references and index.
Identifiers: LCCN 2016026383 | ISBN 9781284112870 (paperback : alk. paper)
Subjects: | MESH: Communication Disorders—therapy | Counseling—methods |
  Interview, Psychological—methods | Speech-Language Pathology—methods
Classification: LCC RC423 | NLM WL 340.2 | DDC 616.85/5—dc23 LC record available at https://lccn.loc.gov/2016026383

6048

Printed in the United States of America
20 19 18 17 16   10 9 8 7 6 5 4 3 2 1

CONTENTS

INTRODUCTION

Imagine a Kansas farmhouse swirling in a hectic cyclone. You see it spin higher and higher, recede from the black and white comfort of all that is familiar. Then, with a crunch, it alights in an outlandish Technicolor world filled with Munchkins and witches, a straw man without brains, a tin man without a heart, and a kingly lion lacking courage. The tale's heroine, a child named Dorothy, misses home.

In *The Wizard of Oz*, the four main characters initiate a quest to discover the important thing that each of them lacks. The Scarecrow wants brains, the Tin Man a heart, the Lion courage. Dorothy wants only to find her way home. As a speech-language pathologist or audiologist, you also require similar "important things" to achieve success in treating your clients: an intelligent procedure, an emotional connection, a courageous determination, and an ultimate goal. Dorothy's quest for home is the overarching theme of the tale. For your clients, too, home is the end point of the journey. Home is the ultimate goal of therapy.

To reach that goal, your clients, like Dorothy, also need the assets brought by the Scarecrow, the Tin Man, and the Lion. Clients must move into uncharted territory to find their way home, just as Dorothy did by making her way through Oz. With your help, they will proceed along a well-thought-out path as they develop a new understanding and move closer to their goals. Your clients will cultivate an open and honest relationship with you, a relationship that can overcome obstacles and help to maintain motivation throughout the course of therapy. Counseling is a key factor driving this process, propelling clients on their journey home.

Oz, of course, becomes a parable for the journey you undertake with your clients. This therapy journey consists of treatment within which counseling is an indispensable component. Employing the tools described in this book, you will define success in terms of the goals you set with your clients. If success is your journey's end, the starting point is determining what you and your clients will be working on to get there.

Once an issue, problem, or disorder has been identified, you, the speech-language pathologist or audiologist, will begin the process of developing a treatment plan. This plan will be tailored to each client's disorder and can include compensatory strategies and practical techniques for improving the client's quality of life or the client's situation. The development and implementation of this treatment plan is central to the therapy process.

The treatment plan will begin with the establishment of goals for improving speech, language, swallowing, or hearing problems. Examples of these goals include the correct tongue placement for the /s/ phoneme or the adjustment of the frequency bandwidth on a hearing aid. Where such improvement is not the aim, as with clients with mid-stage dementia, goals will address maintenance of your clients' abilities as well as caregiver training and education.

Charles Van Riper, a pioneer in the field of speech-language pathology, stated, "It is not enough to know the kind of disorder a person has, one must know the kind of person who has the disorder" (Riley, 2002, p. 6). From the moment you and each of your clients begin your journey together, you are required to focus not only on the disorder but also on the person who has the disorder. You are required to render the caring support we call counseling. When you counsel clients, you target the feelings, thoughts, and behaviors that may be obstructing the treatment plan. With counseling, clients can remove those obstacles and get back on track.

Often counseling seems quite distinct from the treatment plan and can even be the primary activity within a planned session. Just as often, you will find yourself shifting from a disorder-specific technique to counseling and back in a brief period of time. These shifts will depend on your judgment about what your clients need at a given moment. This book will address your planned counseling events along with those that arise spontaneously during treatment.

Getting to know yourself is as important as getting to know your clients. Employing an approach that best fits your own unique personality, values, and beliefs will lead to the most effective outcomes in counseling and treatment (Riley, 2002). The American Speech-Language-Hearing Association clearly defines counseling as an integral and necessary component of preferred professional practice within speech-language pathology and audiology (ASHA, 2007). Limited research, however, exists on counseling issues directly related to speech-language pathology and audiology (Kaderavek, Laux, & Mills, 2004; Parkinson & Rae, 1996; Phillips & Mendel, 2008), despite clinicians' widely accepted view of its importance to the therapy process (Culpepper, Mendel, & McCarthy, 1994; Luterman, 2001; Riley, 2002; Simmons-Mackie & Damico, 2011).

This book offers our counseling methodology in speech-language pathology and audiology with a basis in a solution-focused approach (Berg & Miller, 1992; Berg & Steiner, 2003; de Shazer, 1985; O'Hanlon & Weiner-Davis, 1989; Selekman, 1997; Walter & Peller, 1992), while gleaning important aspects from historical and more recent counseling and psychotherapy approaches (Egan, 2007; Ellis, 1984; Rogers, 1951, 1961; Skinner, 1953). The goals of our approach to counseling are to instill in clients a solution-centered outlook on treatment; facilitate motivation within clients based on the concepts of purpose, growth, and ownership; and leave clients believing that they have the tools and skills to maintain their abilities once treatment has ended. Some of the models depicted in the book have been developed to help the novice student organize and understand how concepts behind our approach can be utilized in counseling within the therapy process.

The Flow of this Book

The book has been designed to be used as a text for courses that focus on counseling people with communication disorders and is suitable for speech-language pathology or audiology courses which include units devoted to counseling. After laying the groundwork for counseling in communication science and disorders, the text details the framework for effective counseling and then covers appropriate interviewing and counseling techniques at each point in the therapy process. Every technique is enhanced with case studies and opportunities for significant practice through targeted exercises.

Layout

There are three main organizing principles of the textbook:

1. The Solution Cycle
2. The Five Intentions
3. Solution-focused theoretical framework

The Solution Cycle provides a model for understanding the therapy process and elucidates the four phases of the process. The Five Intentions clarify the reasons we communicate. These intentions are used in the book to indicate interactive techniques and skills necessary for effective counseling. A solution-focused philosophy offers specific guidance for clinicians as they set goals and help their clients work toward a preferred future.

We will address the four phases of The Solution Cycle and discuss what should happen during each phase and what skills and techniques are most useful. We will discuss the appropriate use of specific techniques and practices from historical counseling theories, as well as elements derived from psychotherapy. Practice scenarios are weaved into the text, and exercises follow each chapter.

Videos have been created to reinforce concepts that we believe are better understood through dramatized, recorded examples. There are videos that refer to each section of the book, and videos are titled according to their content. Some of the videos provide examples of errors that can be made in counseling. The preferred employment of these strategies is also included. Instructors can use the videos during lectures, and students can refer to the videos while reading the text.

Other useful pedagogical models appear throughout the book. These include responsive listening, advanced counseling skills, "repatterning" a behavior, motivation, the counseling integration matrix, stages of grief, and dealing with negative emotions. Diagrams and figures are provided in many instances to illustrate the conceptual framework of the model.

Throughout the book the text features embedded scenarios and case studies taken from real-life clinical settings. These scenarios illustrate a wide variety of speech, communication, swallowing, and hearing disorders, along with relevant counseling techniques. The scenarios are deliberately concise and serve to represent the main concept being presented. A lengthy but important case study may appear, but it will be broken down into a set of manageable scenarios.

The glossary at the end of the book contains keywords and concepts from the text. All these words and concepts appear in boldface color when first mentioned in the text.

Following each chapter is a bulleted review of key ideas from the chapter and a number of practical exercises that provide simulations and real-life applications. The exercises present brief case studies, individual and small group learning tasks, and issues for discussion and possible resolution. The exercises in one chapter may include applications of concepts from other chapters to enrich and reinforce important learnings. These final sections allow you and your instructor to revisit the main concepts in the chapter and pose relevant questions for classroom discussion.

The instructor resources accompanying this text include additional resources that are helpful during course planning and teaching. Fully prepared, ready-to-use, digital lecture files are provided that follow the content in each chapter. Slides in the lecture files include figures and tables from the chapters. Instructors can spend more time preparing how they will present the material rather than constructing their lecture slides for presentation. Instructors are also given possible answers to the exercises at the end of each chapter. These answers provide a guide for instructors to use during in-class discussions or when grading homework assignments.

The Logic of This Book

The solution-focused approach utilized in this book offers you a goal-centered framework for achieving success in treating individuals with speech, language, swallowing, and hearing disorders. An advantage of this approach is its emphasis on the emotions, attitudes, and motivations of the individual client and the incorporation of counseling to determine what is possible and what is changeable in the life of the client (Cook, 2012). This approach shifts the emphasis from the disorder being treated to the goals or changes the client wants to achieve during treatment.

Solution-focus, correctly understood, does not replace classic counseling theories but places counseling into a framework that is always connected to and driven by the goals of treatment (de Shazer, 1985; Egan, 2007; Sklare, 2005). This approach enables you to choose from among both classic and more current counseling theories and methods as you and your clients maintain a goal-centered framework. Descriptions, figures, and clinical scenarios throughout the book will clarify the application and use of a variety of counseling methodologies.

The value of a solution-focused approach has been well established in a broad range of settings (Berg & Miller, 1992; Berg & Steiner, 2003; de Shazer, 1985; Egan, 2007; O'Hanlon & Weiner-Davis, 1989; Selekman, 1997; Walter & Peller, 1992). DeJong and Berg (1998) found that when using a solution-focused model, over 80% of clients 18 years or younger met all or part of their counseling aims in fewer than 9 months. Similar results with adults have been reported (Mireau & Inch, 2009). Botterill and Cook (2010) have even found successful applications of the solution-focused approach in treating people who stutter. We have also seen successful applications of this approach in our own clinical practice, although more research is needed on this and other counseling methodologies in communication science and disorders (Kaderavek, Laux, & Mills, 2004; Parkinson & Rae, 1997; Phillips & Mendel, 2008).

The solution-focused framework also has been found to be effective with individuals from a variety of backgrounds. Sklare (2005) highlighted that "many characteristics of the solution-focused approach make it an ideal counseling approach with diverse populations" (p. 8). For over 25 years, the American Speech-Language-Hearing Association has emphasized the value of multicultural professionalism in both speech-language pathology and audiology clinical practice (ASHA, 1987). The solution-focused approach, therefore, has the dual advantage of being effective in a multicultural setting and being consistent with the aims of the American Speech-Language-Hearing Association.

The Solution Cycle is a model we developed in part from Egan's The Skilled-Helper Model (Egan, 2007) and Weisbord's Future Search Model (Weisbord, 2004; Weisbord & Janoff, 2010). The cycle illuminates the solution-focused method as a process with four identifiable phases. These phases can assist you in planning the therapy journey and evaluating what needs to happen at important junctures along the way. The Solution Cycle is not a static or linear model; the information gathering begun in Phase One does not end in Phase Two or even Phase Four. The Cycle does, however, serve as a guide for you and helps answer three questions: (1) Where are we now? (2) Where do we go from here? (3) How do we get there?

Unlike Dorothy from *The Wizard of Oz*, you won't get there by simply clicking your heels. Like the Scarecrow, the Tin Man, and the Lion, you will need brains, heart, and courage. You will need a well-researched and rational process, an enduring emotional connection with your client, and the courage to take the therapy journey to a successful culmination. Effective counseling will remove obstacles and smooth your path. The ultimate result is enhancement, insofar as is possible, of your client's quality of life.

That is a goal worthy of your best efforts as you embark on the therapy journey. That is the goal we have had in mind in each chapter, each page, of this book.

Acknowledgments

A comprehensive, state-of-the art textbook like *Counseling and Interviewing in Speech-Language Pathology and Audiology: A Therapy Resource* requires the dedicated efforts of many talented individuals contributing in a variety of ways. Without their unreserved commitment and perseverance as deadlines approached, the superior quality of the final product could not have been attained.

Maida Barone and Glen Tellis, your patience and encouragement through this lengthy process, your good counsel, and many words of wisdom have elevated every passage and infused each with humanity and heart.

We authors are deeply indebted to award winning students and graduates of Misericordia University for their dedication, tireless work, and commitment throughout the writing and production of the book and videos. Tia Spagnuolo, MS, Erin Roberts, MS, Danielle Spagnuolo, Allison McCallister, Tori Flormann, MS, CCC-SLP, Amanda Barone, MS, CCC-SLP, and Nicholas Barone, PhD, CCC-SLP, many thanks to all of you.

Thanks are due also to the many students who, during the past few years, have utilized this text in their counseling courses and have provided the invaluable feedback that has served to infuse this book with a style and approach that is accessible and relevant to those pursuing their bachelor's and advanced degrees in speech-language pathology and audiology.

This text would not be possible without the many clients who over the years have entrusted their care in us. Their stories have given life to the fictionalized characters seen in the dialogues throughout the text. Our counseling method has become real and actualized through experience and practice. Our clients' journeys make this book more than a method; they have made it a human interaction and a human connection filled with compassion, love, and support.

Last, we would like to thank the reviewers of the manuscript, for their valuable feedback and advice:

Adrienne McElroy-Bratcher
Eastern New Mexico University

Rebecca L. Nelson Crowell
St. Cloud State University

Lynn E. Fox
Portland State University

Susan M. Moore
University of Colorado—Boulder

Debra Schober-Peterson
Georgia State University

Diane Constantino
Boston University

Stacey Wallen
Georgia State University

REFERENCES

American Speech-Language-Hearing Association. (2007). *Scope of practice in speech-language pathology* [Scope of practice]. Rockville, MD: Author. Retrieved from www.asha.org/policy

ASHA Committee on the Status of Racial Minorities. (1987). *Multicultural professional education in communication disorders: Curriculum approaches.* Rockville, MD: American Speech-Language-Hearing Association.

Berg, I., & Miller, S. D. (1992). *Working with the problem drinker: A solution-focused approach.* New York, NY: Norton.

Berg, I. K., & Steiner, T. (2003). *Children's solution work.* New York, NY: Norton.

Cook, F. (2012). Solution-focused brief therapy: What is going well? And what else? And what else? Retrieved from: http://www.stutteringhelp.org/solution-focused-brief-therapy

Culpepper, B., Mendel, L., & McCarthy, P. (1994). Counseling experience and training offered by ESB-accredited programs. *ASHA, 36,* 55–58.

de Shazer, S. (1985). *Keys to solution in brief therapy.* New York, NY: Norton.

DeJong, P., & Berg, I. K. (1998). *Learner's workbook for interviewing for solutions.* Pacific Grove, CA: Brooks/Cole.

Egan, G. (2007). *The skilled helper* (8th ed.). Belmont, CA: Thomson Brooks/Cole.

Ellis, A. (1984). The essence of RET—1984. *Journal of Rational-Emotive & Cognitive-Behavior Therapy, 2*(1), 19–25.

Kaderavek, J. N., Laux, J. M., & Mills, N. H. (2004). A counseling training module for students in speech-language pathology training programs. *Contemporary Issues in Communication Science and Disorders, 31,* 153–161.

Luterman, D. M. (2001). *Counseling persons with communication disorders and their families* (5th ed.). Austin, TX: Pro-Ed.

Mireau, R., & Inch, R. (2009). Brief solution-focused counseling: a practical effective strategy for dealing with wait lists in community-based mental health services. *Social Work, 54*(1), 63–70.

O'Hanlon, W. H., & Weiner-Davis, M. (1989). *In search of solutions: A new direction in psychotherapy.* New York, NY: Guilford Press.

Parkinson, K., & Rae, J. P. (1996). The understanding and use of counseling by speech language therapists at different levels of experience. *European Journal of Disorders of Communication, 31,* 140–152.

Phillips, D.T., & Mendel, L.L. (2008). Counseling training in communication disorders: A survey of clinical fellows. *Contemporary Issues in Communication Science and Disorders, 35,* 44–53.

Riley, J. (2002). Counseling: An approach for speech-language pathologists. *Contemporary Issues in Communication Science and Disorders, 29,* 6–16.

Rogers, C. R. (1951). *Client-centered therapy: Its current practice, implications and theory.* Boston, MA: Houghton Mifflin.

Rogers, C. R. (1961). *On becoming a person.* Boston, MA: Houghton Mifflin.

Selekman, M. D. (1997). *Solution-focused therapy with children: Harnessing family strengths for system change.* New York, NY: Guilford Press.

Simmons-Mackie, N., & Damico, J. S. (2011). Counseling and aphasia treatment. *Topics in Language Disorders, 31*(4), 336–351.

Skinner, B. F. (1953). *Science and human behavior.* New York, NY: Macmillan.

Sklare, G. B. (2005). *Brief counseling that works: A solution-focused approach for school counselors and administrators.* Thousand Oaks, CA: Corwin Press.

The Stuttering Foundation. (2010). *Tools for Success: A Solution-Focused Brief Therapy Taster* (DVD). United States: The Stuttering Foundation.

Walter, J. L., & Peller, J. E. (1992). *Becoming solution-focused in brief therapy.* New York, NY: Brunner/Mazel Publishers.

Weisbord, M. R. (2004). *Productive workplaces revisited: Dignity, meaning, and community in the 21st century.* San Francisco, CA: Jossey-Bass.

Weisbord, M. R., & Janoff, S. (2010). *Future search: Getting the whole system in the room for vision, commitment, and action.* (3rd ed.). San Francisco, CA: Berrett-Koehler Publishers.

SECTION I

Groundwork for Interviewing and Counseling in Communication Science and Disorders

Section One focuses on setting the groundwork and establishing the framework for effective interviewing and counseling in communication science and disorders. In the Introduction, "The Wizard of Oz" provides an analogy of what is necessary to execute a successful relationship between you and your clients. The Scarecrow, Tin Man, Cowardly Lion, and Dorothy point to the four requisites: a workable plan, an emotional connection, a courageous determination, and an ultimate goal. That goal is usually established first. It is the reason treatment is taking place. The other three components are often required for a person with a speech, language, swallowing, or hearing disorder to reach the goal. Counseling is an essential means of formulating an acceptable and compelling path to that goal, making an emotional connection along the way, and enhancing your client's courage and determination to succeed. Chapters 1 and 2 discuss the definition of counseling, the Solution Cycle, the Counseling-Integration Matrix, and the Five Intentions of Communication.

CHAPTER 1

The Role of Counseling in Communication Science and Disorders

KEY TERMS

- Client advocates
- Counseling
- Ego impedance
- Obstacle dominance

LEARNING OBJECTIVES

After reading this chapter, you will be able to:

- Define counseling as it relates to speech-language pathology and audiology
- Identify the individuals who may receive counseling during the clinical process
- Explain why it is important to integrate counseling and treatment to promote client success
- List and describe the benefits and limitations of historical counseling theories to a solution-focused counseling approach

The Speech-Language Pathologist and Audiologist as Counseling Professionals

The Counseling Mandate

Counseling is defined as caring support in the form of information, guidance, or assistance provided to clients, families, caretakers, and advocates so that clients can use such insight to pursue realistic and clearly understood goals, as well as attain a more fulfilling quality of life (Gustad, 1953; Riley, 2002). Counseling achieves its purpose when that support either bolsters clients' motivation to succeed in treatment or reduces attitudinal, behavioral, or emotional barriers to progress in treatment (Figure 1-1). Although counseling individuals with communication disorders is similar to counseling in other fields, the type of counseling speech-language pathologists and audiologists conduct is not psychotherapy. The psychological and behavioral therapy designed to treat clients who are diagnosed with emotional or mental disorders is best left to licensed psychologists, psychiatrists, or psychotherapists (Crowe, 1997; Kaderavek, Laux, & Mills, 2004; Riley, 2002). Speech-language pathologists and

Counseling:
Caring support in the form of information, guidance, or assistance provided to clients, families, caretakers, and advocates; clients can use such insight to pursue realistic and clearly understood goals and attain a more fulfilling quality of life. Counseling achieves its purpose when that support either bolsters clients' motivation to succeed in treatment or reduces attitudinal, behavioral, or emotional barriers to progress in treatment.

3

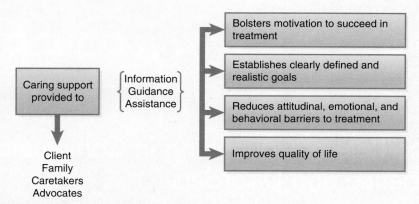

FIGURE 1-1 Counseling. This figure provides a visual representation of the definition, action, and recipients of counseling during the therapy process.

audiologists do, however, utilize similar counseling tools derived from some of these therapy approaches to help clients deal with the feelings, thoughts, and behaviors that are related to their communication disorder or that have impeded their progress in treatment.

Counseling, then, is not merely a helpful tool in the clinician's repertoire of competencies; it is integral to the therapy process itself (Conture, 1990; Phillips & Mendel, 2008; Wolter, DiLollo, & Apel, 2006; Zebrowski & Schum, 1993). If you are involved in speech-language pathology or audiology treatment, you will inevitably engage in counseling. It is critical that the counseling be deliberate, intentional, and skillful.

Counseling may be of primary importance in some situations. For instance, there are times when clients are no longer responsive to disorder-specific treatment. For these clients, acceptance of their current status is the only viable option. June, despite many years working on fluency-enhancing techniques, is still negatively affected by her stuttering. Ricardo, who has received a cochlear implant, may not be achieving significant improvement in decoding auditory signals. For June and Ricardo, counseling to achieve peace of mind, a higher level of social engagement, or better family relationships related to their communication disorder may be seen as a legitimate description of success.

In such cases, structuring treatment primarily around counseling goals is not unjustified. This orientation is compassionate, and most experienced speech-language pathologists and audiologists have had more than one occasion to consider it. The decision to forgo, even temporarily, disorder-specific goals is a serious matter. Clinicians must take many factors into account before taking such a step. They should also be competent and comfortable in applying effective counseling strategies in these circumstances so that, if necessary, treatment-specific goals can be reintroduced as soon as possible.

Overview of Skills and Techniques Specific to Counseling

Speech-language pathologists and audiologists may use a variety of counseling methodologies in the therapy process (Cook, 2012; Kaderavek et al., 2004; Manning, 2000;

Riley, 2002; Wolter et al., 2006). Whichever methodology you choose to employ, you will rely on similar counseling skills to be effective. Chief among these counseling competencies are human interaction or interpersonal skills, probing, observation, information gathering, listening, responding, paraphrasing, and summarizing (Ivey, D'Andrea, Ivey, & Simek-Morgan, 2002). As a clinician, you learn to select the techniques that will propel your clients along the path of improvement or work to remove obstacles blocking the path.

In the solution-focused approach detailed in this book, core techniques include planning, decision making, goal setting, alliance building, empathetic interaction, and encouragement. Other important factors to address are issues related to ethics, willingness to change, backsliding, and end-of-life considerations. Some of these techniques and issues require advanced communication skills such as challenging, dealing with resistance, trusting intuition, using leverage, and maintaining motivation. You will learn how to apply these strategies and techniques to a variety of different clients and communication disorders.

The Speech-Language Pathologist and Audiologist in a World Without Counseling

Acquiring the skill set necessary to apply counseling techniques is a learning process. Applying the techniques in an effective and appropriate fashion is likewise learned over time. Be patient with yourself while you are learning these skills and techniques. You must be willing to try these techniques in the clinical setting and face the possibility that you may not always succeed. Even the most highly skilled clinicians may resist learning and applying counseling strategies to the clinical setting.

Rasheela is an example of a clinician who rarely uses counseling in her sessions. She is an energetic, well-trained audiologist. Once she diagnoses a disorder or an issue, she is eager to get started with disorder-specific treatment. She is not nearly as confident about her ability to provide counseling. Learning how to counsel clients takes time and Rasheela believes she can get more accomplished if she does not bother with her clients' emotions and feelings. Rasheela cannot be blamed for wanting to conduct treatment in a clinical setting that does not include counseling. Working toward a treatment-specific end should propel clients toward their goals, making time in treatment shorter and goal attainment faster.

Well, the good news is that sometimes treatment can be conducted with little or no counseling. Rasheela might make her diagnosis, lay out the plan of treatment, and go to work. Her clients progress step by step and achieve the desired result in textbook fashion—a textbook with not a single chapter on counseling.

There is more than a little bad news, though, in the world without counseling. Rasheela will experience such smooth sailing infrequently. Soon enough, she will come across a client who requires help in gaining the self-confidence needed to make progress. She will encounter another client who refuses to go along with treatment because of a lack of trust in Rasheela or in the therapy process. She will meet clients afraid of trying, angry at the world's unfairness and cruelty, seemingly satisfied with things as they are, or discouraged by the low expectations of family and peers. She will also have clients who relapse and return to her office unsure of why they did not maintain their therapy strategies.

Without recourse to counseling, Rasheela applies her treatment techniques in these cases and is confronted with passivity, resistance, reluctance, and sometimes downright defiance. Solidarity fractures into hostility on the client's part and utter frustration for Rasheela. Her single remaining strategy is to trade one ineffective treatment technique for another, persevere with a process that goes nowhere, or simply dismiss the client.

The world without counseling may become a series of dead-ends, an unproductive environment where success is rare and failure a constant companion. Counseling presents a welcome choice of options and opens a multitude of new pathways to progress. While it may take time for Rasheela to learn, apply, and tailor counseling strategies to her treatment sessions; it will be time well spent.

Limits of the Clinician's Role in Counseling

Empowering as skilled counseling can be, there are limitations for even the most competent speech-language pathologists or audiologists. The first limitation is the one that defines the speech-language pathologist's or audiologist's role when including counseling within treatment. Once Rasheela learns and adopts counseling strategies into her treatment sessions, she does not become a counselor simply because she includes counseling in her therapy approach. She is, in fact, an audiologist who incorporates counseling strategies to reach her main objective. This main objective is to resolve or reduce a hearing issue or disorder or to lessen the impact the disorder has on her clients' quality of life. Rasheela's mission is not to address emotional issues unrelated to her clients' hearing disorders.

There are boundaries to what Rasheela can counsel her clients about in her treatment sessions. Knowing these boundaries and adhering to the speech-language pathologist's and audiologist's scope of practice regarding counseling are essential competencies of a skilled clinician. When appropriate, speech-language pathologists and audiologists should refer clients to the appropriate mental health professional so that clients receive needed counseling in areas that are beyond their scope of practice.

Another limit to the clinician's role in counseling in speech-language pathology and audiology is related to some of the aspects of the communication disorders they treat. Individuals with emotional lability due to a brain injury or dementia may have unpredictable mood swings and changes, laugh and cry involuntarily, and perseverate on an emotion or situation that caused a certain emotion. Acute counseling may not be appropriate during these moments. When emotional lability is recognized as an issue, many times the best recourse is to ignore the emotional response until it has passed. Steps can be taken in treatment to work on identification, awareness, and management of the emotional lability or perseveration to reduce the impact they have on treatment sessions and in the client's life.

The last limitation to the clinician's role in counseling relates to clients' personal preferences about treatment. There are clients who simply reject counseling. These clients have come to therapy for the sole purpose of treatment related to reducing or eliminating their communication issues and believe that any discussion about feelings, thoughts, and emotions is not needed. Clinicians should respect their client's personal preferences about treatment but work to build a stable, trusting relationship so that if counseling is warranted later in the therapy process, clients are more willing to give it a try.

Who Gets Counseled?

Clients with speech, language, swallowing, or hearing disorders are the primary focus of your clinical efforts. Clinicians often give parents and other client advocates instructions, even training, so they can assist clients in achieving progress outside of treatment. The advocates are not themselves directly receiving treatment specific to the disorder but are becoming party to the mission of improving clients' communication issues.

Some aspects of counseling by their nature are different from disorder-related treatment. The areas that counseling addresses suit the needs not only of clients but also of those around the clients. As clients work and practice to improve, the people close to them adapt and grow and encounter emotions that are responsive to effective counseling.

The Client

The client and the client's needs are foremost. This principle is illustrated by June, an individual who stutters. If it turns out that treatment begins to work for her, she may still continue to require counseling at any point in the process and for a host of reasons. Counseling may consist of a planned set of sessions or portions of sessions. Counseling may be unplanned; it may be a tactic dictated by the emergence of an issue that requires it. The clinician will often initiate counseling, but June, too, is empowered to seek it. She may detect the need for the kind of support available from counseling and let her clinician know about it.

The shift from disorder-specific treatment to counseling can be subtle and brief. June might need words of encouragement, gentle reminders of her commitment, or time to share feelings and doubts. As clinicians gain skill and experience, they will engage in counseling seamlessly and instinctually. The shift will be deliberate and intentional, but not necessarily conscious. The apt clinician often moves into counseling mode without saying explicitly, "I am now counseling as opposed to doing treatment specific to the disorder." This maneuver can become as instinctive as choosing to accelerate the treatment plan when a client exhibits mastery.

The Client Advocates

Depending on June's age and circumstances, counseling may be appropriate for those who are influential in her life. We will call these individuals client advocates, a term that identifies them as coconspirators in the mission to help June reach her treatment goals. Counseling will be designed to help the client advocates grapple with their own feelings as June improves, and the advocates will become a more and more positive factor in June's journey.

Client advocates: People influential in a client's life. They tend to be assertive in their commitment to what they see as beneficial to the client. They can be helpful in the therapy process, but they may, under certain circumstances, become adversarial.

Again, you can plan counseling for client advocates to take place at key stages in the process, or make adjustments to the treatment plan as the need arises. The "Circle of Power," or client support system, considers the importance of client advocates and details what client advocates need to know as treatment proceeds.

The Client's Social and Professional Networks

Everyone associated with the client can potentially be a client advocate. Some individuals may be obvious advocates such as parents, spouses, and significant others. A wider net should be cast to consider other places where advocates might be found, including social groups like June's sports teams as well as her friends on social media. June could be working with a psychologist or school counselor. She may be under a physician's care or getting additional speech therapy services elsewhere. She could be a professional herself or an employee with a circle of colleagues she sees regularly.

All of these contacts have the potential to support or hinder your clients' attainment of treatment goals. You must maintain an awareness of obvious and potential advocates throughout treatment. How you enlist these networks into your clients' treatment will be important to consider at any stage in the process.

Integrating Counseling and Treatment

Ramsey is a sixth-grade boy with a lateral emission lisp. His speech is otherwise typical for his age, and assessments have confirmed that there is no organic, anatomic, or physiological reason he does not produce /s/ correctly. Still, the lisp was significant enough to qualify Ramsey for treatment sessions with the school speech-language pathologist. During the first session, the speech-language pathologist became aware of noticeable barriers to the effectiveness of the usual treatment techniques. Despite what may have been apparent to his clinician, Ramsey seemed quite certain that he was physically incapable of producing a correct /s/ phoneme. He exhibited very little confidence in his ability to improve.

Other issues soon became apparent. Believing his articulation disorder would subject him to ridicule from his peers, he rarely initiated conversations. He was an excellent singer in the school choir but turned down several opportunities to perform solos because he "would ruin everything." He claimed that his parents, especially his father, were very disappointed that he "can't talk right and will never talk right."

Internal Barriers: Obstacle Dominance and Ego Impedance

The speech-language pathologist's primary goal remained the correction of the lisp, but the path to that goal was being obstructed, and those obstructions had to be removed first and foremost. Obstructions can come in the form of ego impedance and obstacle dominance (Rosenzweig, 2002). These are two core indicators of the need to integrate counseling into treatment. Both of these obstructions were rooted in Ramsey's perceptions about himself and his perceptions about the obstacles he was encountering.

Ego impedance is defined as an aspect of clients' self-perception that prevents them from achieving a goal because of a negative attitude about themselves, their skills, or their abilities. Ego impedance was developed from Rosenzweig's (1945) concept of ego defense, which is described as one reaction to frustration. Clients exhibiting ego impedance might say, "I just can't do it" or "I know I'm the type of person who won't see this through."

Another reaction to frustration is obstacle dominance. This reaction is defined as an aspect of the outer world perceived by clients as creating a barrier so great that access to the goal is unachievable. Clients exhibiting obstacle dominance may lose sight of the goal altogether; they may say things like, "I feel like I'm banging my head against a brick wall" or "I'll never make progress with *that* standing in my way."

Both ego impedance and obstacle dominance are internal barriers—they originate in the beliefs and attitudes of clients. Ego impedance is a negative self-perception created by clients about their ability. Obstacle dominance is a negative self-perception the client has that is related to something external to the client. Nonetheless, clients experience them as real and powerful blocks to improvement (**Figure 1-2**).

Ramsey's case study provides a clarifying example of ego impedance and obstacle dominance. Ramsey's belief that he could not produce the /s/ phoneme because of a deficit in his physical ability is an illustration of ego impedance. His perception of his deficient ability will inhibit his progress in therapy. An example of obstacle dominance is Ramsey's conviction that his father's assertions were correct, that he would "never talk right." The obstacle, Ramsey's belief in his father's assertions, is the seemingly insurmountable barrier between Ramsey and his goal. In both cases, Ramsey's issues center on his negative perceptions.

Obstacle dominance can come in many different forms. Clients may blame their attendance issues in therapy on an inability to travel to treatment sessions because of distance or lack of transportation. They may associate their lack of improvement in therapy with reservations they have about their clinician. Clients may also indicate that

> **Ego impedance:** An aspect of clients' self-perception that prevents them from achieving a goal because of a negative attitude about themselves, their skills, or their abilities. Ego impedance is a negative self-perception created by clients about their ability.

> **Obstacle dominance:** An aspect of the outer world perceived by clients as creating a barrier so great that access to the goal is unachievable. Obstacle dominance is a negative self-perception the client has that is related to something external to the client.

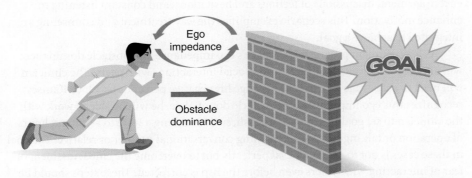

FIGURE 1-2 Ego Impedance and Obstacle Dominance. Both of these blocks occur within the client and can affect progress toward therapy goals. Ego impedance is a maladaptive perception the client generates about his or her own abilities that is in response to the client's own perceptions. Obstacle dominance is a maladaptive perception the client generates about his or her own abilities that is influenced by outside perceptions.

they are unable to find time to practice techniques because their schedule is too busy. Obstacle dominance can hinder clients' progress in therapy and must be addressed in treatment to decrease its effect on the achievement of clients' goals.

Before Ramsey can make meaningful progress toward the long-term goal of removing his lisp and generalizing that correct production to his everyday speech, his speech-language pathologist must use short-term counseling goals to tackle both Ramsey's ego impedance and his obstacle dominance. One of the goals might focus on Ramsey's ego impedance by challenging his conviction that he is simply incapable of making the /s/ sound correctly. To address Ramsey's obstacle dominance, the clinician might set a goal that helps him realize that his father's pessimism about his capabilities is not a final judgment on his potential.

This "layering" of goals, the incremental process of moving to an ultimate goal by setting and achieving intermediate goals, is at the heart of the solution-focused approach. Once you have set your long-term goals, you should ask yourself two questions repeatedly throughout the process: What are the short-term treatment and counseling goals? Do these goals relate to the long-term goals?

A solution-focused approach can be effective because it shifts the emphasis from the disorder being treated to the goals clients want to achieve in treatment. In essence, once the problem is defined, clinicians help their clients by building on the things clients do right, not by focusing on what they do wrong. In a solution-focused approach, the primary goal for clients like Ramsey is not to extinguish the misarticulation of the phoneme /s/ but rather to incorporate the correct production of /s/ into his speech. As the example reveals, this long-term goal will almost always generate intermediate counseling and treatment goals.

A first step to the correct production of a sibilant sound may be learning to place the tongue appropriately for /s/. There is a second step and then a third, and several more, until Ramsey finally reaches his long-term goal, the ability to produce /s/ and transfer it into his speech. The speech-language pathologist does a great deal of counseling as Ramsey meets his treatment goals. The counseling occurs in moments of encouragement, discussions of feelings and hesitations, and constant listening to enhance motivation. This scenario exemplifies the way treatment and counseling are integrated to achieve a goal.

As his treatment progresses, Ramsey's ego impedance and obstacle dominance will almost certainly cause him to avoid social interactions with peers. The clinician will need to encourage him to acknowledge his negative perceptions. Once Ramsey recognizes this ego impedance and obstacle dominance, he will be able to work with the clinician to set goals he can accomplish, such as calling a store to ask about hours of operation or talking to a nonthreatening conversational partner or relative. The goal in these cases is not to pronounce /s/ perfectly but to overcome the embarrassment or fear of interacting with others even before the lisp is corrected. These steps should be planned counseling objectives and should take place while Ramsey is learning to make the correct /s/ sound.

Eventually, Ramsey will participate more freely in discussions with his peers, and before long he will reach the point in treatment where he can produce the

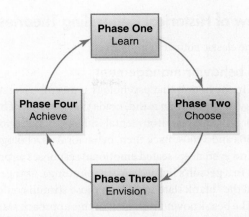

FIGURE 1-3 The Solution Cycle. There are four nonlinear phases of the Solution Cycle: Learn, Choose, Envision, and Achieve.

correct /s/ phoneme. He will be ready to begin incorporating /s/ into his everyday speech. He will practice alone, of course, but he will be able to begin using his /s/ phoneme with his peers. The treatment goal of generalizing the correct production of /s/ into his speech is reached using a step-by-step method that includes counseling integrated into the treatment plan. The counseling goals that foster more open and frequent interaction with peers are achieved during treatment and make Ramsey less hesitant to generalize the corrected /s/ phoneme into his conversations with peers and others.

To guide you through this often complex integration of counseling with treatment, this book offers a leadership model of an inclusive interviewing and counseling process. It is a practical, four-step, nonlinear process called the "Solution Cycle" (**Figure 1-3**) (Egan, 2006; Weisbord, 2004). Phase One of the Solution Cycle is the learning stage, which involves observation, study, and listening. Phase Two is the development of an alliance base or "Circle of Power." Phase Three is the description of a vision of success and associated goals. Phase Four encompasses the achievement of the goals.

As each of the four phases is examined in the text, the evolving intentions of the clinician–client interactions are enumerated, and techniques for effectiveness are described and illustrated. In any interaction one or more of five intentions are present. These are self-affirmation, small talk, information sharing, persuasion/direction, and feeling (Barone & Tellis, 2008). Specific applications of each of the "Five Intentions of Communication" are represented in each step of the process.

Solution-focused counseling, then, is framed by the Solution Cycle, which represents the entire counseling–therapy process from the initial interview to the successful conclusion of treatment. Far from displacing other theories of counseling, the Solution Cycle benefits from the use of different modes of counseling. These historical theories can all be useful at various points in the interviewing and counseling processes. Behaviorism, humanistic psychology, cognitive behavioral therapy, and existentialism exemplify the range of approaches and techniques open to clinicians who employ the Solution Cycle.

A Brief Overview of Historical Counseling Theories

Figure 1-4 shows the classic counseling theories.

Behaviorism and behavior management

Behaviorism, rooted in the notion that psychology is an empirical science concerned with observable behavior rather than mind, holds that patterns of behavior are impressed upon an organism by environmental influences. Behaviorism gained wide popularity in the 1950s and 1960s. Back then, behavioral psychology viewed human habits, preferences, and even deep-seated emotional responses as products of the conditioning stimuli in a person's immediate surroundings. Our genes and natural endowment provided the "blank slate" on which those stimuli could shape our routines and practices. The best-known proponent of this approach was B. F. Skinner, who used the term operant conditioning to characterize the way organisms interact with their surroundings to develop their behaviors and habits (Skinner, 1953).

Skinner distinguished operant conditioning from classical conditioning, known to most people through the work of Ivan Pavlov, a Russian scientist. While studying digestion in dogs, Pavlov became aware that a dog salivated whenever meat was presented. This "unconditioned" reflex did not surprise Pavlov. What surprised him was the fact the dog would also secrete saliva when a bell was rung, so long as the dog was "conditioned" to do so by repeatedly hearing the bell shortly after meat was presented.

The conditioned reflex, as it was called, sharpened psychology's focus on discrete behaviors and how these behaviors come about. Skinner emphasized organisms' active participation in the process; conditioning takes place as organisms "operate" on their

	Behaviorist	Cognitive	Humanistic	Existentialist
Proponent	B. F. Skinner	Albert Ellis	Carl Rogers	Søren Kierkegaard
Basic Tenet	Environment impresses behavior patterns.	Rational beliefs cause healthy behavior; irrational cause dysfunctional.	People are good and can solve own problems with caring therapy.	People are free to choose and are totally responsible.
Approach	Change behavior by conditioning, reinforcing desired practices.	Foster rational, not irrational, beliefs and goals to live a happier life.	Use power of choice to opt for treatment goals and redefine oneself.	Non-judgmental, rooted in listening; client defines issues and success.
Limitations	Lab might not duplicate reality; best when correcting discrete behaviors.	Emotive reality might not be considered. Rational way not always chosen.	Not a developed treatment method; may reinforce pessimistic attitude.	Unstructured process; clinician is not to define issues to be addressed.

FIGURE 1-4 Classic Counseling Theories. Many of the classic counseling approaches are still used in current counseling practices. Modern counseling approaches can find their roots in one or more of the five classic approaches detailed in this figure.

	Reinforcement Increase likelihood of behavior	Punishment Decrease likelihood of behavior
Positive Presentation of stimulus	Present stimulus when client performs intended target (e.g., token system—present token for targeted behavior)	Present stimulus to decrease client's behavior (e.g., reprimand client for undesired behavior)
Negative Removal of stimulus	Remove stimulus when client performs intended target (e.g., seatbelt alarm turns off when seatbelt is buckled)	Remove stimulus to decrease client's behavior (e.g., token system—remove token when client performs undesired behavior)

FIGURE 1-5 Operant Conditioning. Basic tenets of operant conditioning consist of both positive and negative forms of reinforcement and punishment.

surroundings and react to stimuli that are presented in their environment. Behavior is made more likely by reinforcement, which can be positive or negative. Behavior is made less likely by punishment, which can also be positive or negative. *Positive* always refers to the presentation of a stimulus, and *negative* refers to the removal of a stimulus (**Figure 1-5**).

With positive reinforcement, the environment "rewards" a given behavior by providing a reinforcing result whenever the organism emits the behavior. If that happens often enough, the new behavior is elicited every time the reinforcing stimulus is produced. With the use of highly targeted positive reinforcement, an organism can acquire complex patterns of behavior incrementally when intermediate steps to the final pattern are reinforced. These steps are called successive approximations (Skinner, 1959).

If Ramsey was given a reward, perhaps a token, every time he positioned his tongue a certain way, he might soon learn that behavior. By giving him a token according to a schedule as he masters the steps to producing a correct /s/ sound, Ramsey might progress, by successive approximations, to the point when he easily produces the /s/ phoneme.

The clinician can also change the environment to increase the likelihood of a behavior. In the event that a client screams and yells (i.e., behavior to be extinguished) when exposed to loud noises or bright lights, the clinician may provide these stimuli until the second screaming or yelling stops. When the behavior momentarily ceases, perhaps even for the client to take a breath, the clinician removes the negative stimulus (i.e., bright lights). The intention is to increase the likelihood that the behavior will stop (reinforcement) by removing a negative stimulus when the desired behavior is observed. This is negative reinforcement.

Car makers also use negative reinforcement to get drivers to wear their seatbelts. The annoying, repeated beeping noise a car emits is the undesired stimulus that is removed once the seatbelt is secured. Drivers are more inclined to buckle up if they know the beeping will not begin if they fasten their seatbelts in time, and certainly will buckle up to get the beeping to stop before the sound escalates.

Positive punishment is used to decrease the likelihood of a behavior by providing an unpleasant stimulus. The undesired behavior becomes "maladaptive" because it results in something perceived as unpleasant. If the maladaptive behavior is positively punished often enough, that behavior might eventually stop altogether; the subject will cease performing it. Sending a "pink slip" or bad report home with your client because of disruptive behavior during the therapy session is an example of positive punishment.

Police officers also use positive punishment to deter drivers from speeding. Drivers who get a ticket for speeding should be less inclined to speed the next time they are on the road. Problematic behavior may be reduced or erased by applications of well-targeted punishment, although a solution-focused approach tends to build on success as opposed to eliminating problems (Murphy, 1997). If police officers really want drivers to stop speeding, they should work with car manufacturers to create a way that dollar bills spew from the steering wheel when drivers obey the speed limit (i.e., positive reinforcement).

Negative punishment reduces the likelihood of a behavior by removing something that is liked or desirable. If Ramsey has one of his tokens taken away every time he misarticulates the /s/ phoneme, he is being negatively punished. Usually negative punishment is linked to positive reinforcement as Ramsey's clinician will also give him tokens for correct productions. In clinical practice, speech-language pathologists and audiologists primarily use positive reinforcement and negative punishment.

To be most effective, clinicians should be cognizant of the type of conditioning they are using, be consistent in its application, and plan the presentation or removal of the stimulus to reflect the desired outcome. First ask yourself, "What do I want to accomplish, increase the behavior (reinforcement) or decrease the behavior (punishment)?" Then you ask yourself, "How do I want to accomplish the goal, present a stimulus (positive) or remove a stimulus (negative)?" Through this process you will identify the type of conditioning you want to target in treatment.

Another way to reduce a behavior's likelihood is to arrange that nothing happens when the behavior is exhibited. In terms of operant conditioning, this is called extinction. If a light switch is flicked and nothing ever happens, the individual flicking the switch will be less and less likely to exhibit the behavior of flicking the light switch. That behavior will be extinguished.

The use of positive and negative reinforcement, punishment and extinction, successive approximation, and related techniques was eventually assigned the catchall term "behavior modification," often nicknamed "behavior mod." In 2007 classic behaviorism became officially known as "behavior analysis" (Twyman, 2007). Applications to speech-language pathology and audiology range from developmental disabilities to autism spectrum disorder to language and cognition (Hayes, Barnes-Holmes, & Roche, 2001; Hernandez & Ikkanda, 2011).

Ramsey's lateral emission lisp, for example, is presumably corrected by a series of observable behaviors, including placing the tongue correctly, focusing the passage of air appropriately, and aligning the lips and jaw. Any one of these behaviors can be seen as an "approximation" of the right way to make an /s/ phoneme. Successive approximations could lead finally to the accomplishment of a correct /s/; further such practice could result in the transfer of /s/ into daily speech.

A similar process could assist clients with cochlear implants in reaching the goal of correctly processing audible language. Aural habilitation in training auditory and speech perception is among the treatments used by clients beginning to acquire auditory-based spoken language, particularly beyond early childhood. Cochlear implants and other hearing aid devices help define the successive approximations essential to a successful behavior management regimen. Solution-focused therapy might characterize these successive approximations as intermediate goals along the path of acquisition and improvement.

There are, in the environment, both positive and negative reinforcers of behaviors that cannot be controlled by the clinician. Behavior management techniques do not necessarily account for these reinforcers. Reinforcing undesirable behaviors can lead to high drop-out rates and relapse after treatment has ended because introduction and use of behavior management in the clinical setting do not guarantee generalization of the behavior change in clients' everyday environment (Bothe, Davidow, Bramlett, & Ingham, 2006; Perkins, 1992; Prins & Ingham, 2009). Clients must learn to generalize in places where the reinforcement schedule used in treatment does not exist. Behavior-ism itself then predicts this limitation of behaviorism!

If behavior analysis is not the whole answer, however, it can be part of the solution in many cases. When successful, the technique empowers Ramsey to say with demon-strable certainty, "I can make an /s/." That is no small step. In the Solution Cycle that ability is a clear goal along the way to achieving Ramsey's vision of a world in which this phoneme is correctly produced.

Cognitive and cognitive behavior therapy

Throughout a long career, Albert Ellis had an immense impact on the way counsel-ing therapy is thought about and done. He began with a healthy skepticism about psychoanalysis along with an equally healthy skepticism about behaviorism's rejec-tion of mind as a focus of therapy. He was able to solve therapy problems by adopt-ing the clearly useful techniques of behavior management and applying them in a world where thinking matters and can be rational or irrational. In fact, Ellis called his approach *rational emotive behavior therapy* (REBT), a term that aptly embodies his openness to the best features of existing methodologies (Ellis & Dryden, 2007).

In Ellis's view, rational (healthy) beliefs are distinguished from irrational beliefs in two powerful ways. First, rational beliefs are provisional, expressed with words like "I want," "I prefer," and "I like." Irrational beliefs are absolute, spoken of as "shoulds" and "musts." People with healthy beliefs experience happiness when they obtain their desires and sadness when they do not. People with irrational beliefs experience bad feelings that actually get in the way of the attainment of their wants and desires. These negative feelings include anger, anxiety, guilt, and depression. They cause dysfunc-tional behavior like substance abuse and procrastination (Ellis & Dryden, 2007; Ellis & Knaus, 1977).

REBT posits that humans are biologically predisposed to think irrationally and therefore dysfunctionally. There would be no hope for us except that we have a competing biological tendency to exercise choice when a constructive way of thinking is counterposed. Clients can take three steps to the ultimate goal of healthy thinking: (1) to be able to observe that their irrational evaluations are harmful to them; (2) to become convinced that they are capable of thinking differently; and (3) to use REBT methods to make progress in changing their thinking in a healthy direction (Ellis & Dryden, 2007).

"Humans are happiest," says Ellis, "when they establish important life goals and purposes and actively strive to attain these" (Ellis & Dryden, 2007, p. 4). Solution-focused counseling, of course, does just that when it sets goals that clients perceive will make their lives happier. There are specific applications of REBT to the practice of treating people with communication disorders (Andersson, Porsaeus, Wiklund, Kaldo, & Larsen, 2005; Blomgren, Roy, Callister, & Merrill, 2005; Menzies, Onslow, Packman, & O'Brian, 2009; Riley, 2002), and these applications are frequently germane to a solution-focused approach.

In Ellis's perspective, Ramsey, the client with the lateral emission lisp, exhibited an irrational evaluation of his situation with a classic "can't." He did not believe himself capable of producing a correct /s/ phoneme. He might even have possessed evidence, like an enlarged tongue, that further convinced him his ego impedance was justified. REBT techniques can assist Ramsey in identifying the roadblock, not as a physical incapacity but as a dysfunctional way of thinking. REBT can help him realize he can think differently about his lisp and move toward that new, rational way of thinking.

Ellis tried to explain this therapy process with what he called the "ABCs of REBT." Ellis himself admitted he was being simplistic when he scoped them out (Ellis & Dryden, 2007). The ABCs are helpful, however, in an overview like this one. *A* stands for an *activating event*, a behavior or thought that either eases the solution focus or proposes a roadblock to solution focus. For Ramsey, a positive activating event might be proper tongue placement, which could lead to a more optimistic *B*, or *belief*, about his ultimate ability to make an /s/ phoneme. *C* encompasses the *behavioral consequences* of A and B. In this case, the C for Ramsey could be a willingness to practice proper tongue placement until it becomes habitual.

Using REBT Ramsey could move from irrational beliefs like "I should always speak correctly" to "I want to speak correctly" and "I will use proper tongue placement when I speak." The guilt and depression he may feel at not being able to attain the "should" is replaced by enthusiasm at progress toward an attainable goal. These results not only are beneficial to the client but also are very much in sync with a solution focus.

The limitations of REBT must be faced even as the clinician makes use of its valuable insights. Clinicians wedded to this "rational emotive" approach need to give full weight to both the rational and the emotive components of their clients' cognitions and behaviors. Sometimes clinicians stress the rational part excessively and give short shrift to the emotive. This imbalance is understandable; always in the back of the clinician's mind is the push to replace the irrational with the rational. After all, that is the goal of cognitive therapy—to reorder the client's thinking.

The reality is that emotions, strong emotions, are frequently an entrenched feature of the situation faced by the clinician, their clients, and those close to the clients. These emotions need expression, validation, discussion, and appreciation, or else the therapy process might be stopped in its tracks. This is an example of a common roadblock.

REBT can also come into conflict with a solution-focused approach's insistence that both goals and progress toward the goals occur at the clients' initiative. The primary skill along the Solution Cycle is listening—on the part of the counselor—to enable clinicians and clients to make progress at the clients' pace. REBT practitioners would argue that they concur with this requirement of strong client involvement, but cognitive therapy can easily take on prescriptive overtones, especially at the point when the counselor recognizes what the clients "should" be thinking.

When, for example, Ramsey indicates to the speech-language pathologist that he "cannot possibly produce an /s/ phoneme," the REBT clinician is certain that Ramsey is expressing an irrational thought. This information is important, but for the solution-focused clinician it is not a signal to "change the client's thinking." It is a signal to explore Ramsey's attitude and help Ramsey take initiative toward improvement. REBT is of immense value in proposing to Ramsey a likely reason for his ego impedance, an aspect of his self-concept that may be impeding progress toward the correction of the lisp. The ego impedance is removed when Ramsey recognizes it as ego impedance and sets goals to remove it.

Humanistic psychology

An approach that always puts the client and the client's emotions first is the humanistic approach, most frequently associated with the hugely influential psychotherapist Carl Rogers. His breakthrough book, *On Becoming a Person* (1961), laid out his philosophy in language that captivated not only a big segment of academia but also an enormous mass audience. Rogers, along with well-known scholars of his day like Abraham Maslow (Maslow, 1968) and Rollo May, were proponents of "Third Force" psychology (Gable, 1970), which stressed personhood and self-actualization rather than observable behavior (First Force) or unconscious states (Second Force). "People are essentially trustworthy (as cited in Corey, 2009, p. 166)," claimed Rogers. They "have a vast potential for understanding themselves and resolving their own problems without direct intervention on the therapist's part....They are capable of self-directed growth if they are involved in a specific kind of therapeutic relationship" (p. 166).

The same optimism about our species was shared by Maslow, who wrote that our inner nature "seems not to be intrinsically or primarily or necessarily evil" (Maslow, 1968, 1999, p. 5). The humanists propose a model of psychological "health" reminiscent of Ellis's "healthy" or rational cognition. This favorable view of people is the impetus behind Rogers's insistence that the therapist maintain what he called unconditional positive regard (Corey, 2009) for clients. What Rogers meant by *positive regard* was a commitment by the therapist to understand clients on their own terms. "I have found it of enormous value when I can permit myself to understand another person" (Rogers, 1995, p. 18). This sentence highlights the difficulty of truly listening to clients; as a clinician, Rogers felt it necessary to literally give himself permission to do it!

Otherwise, says Rogers, "our tendency will be to judge the utterances of the client, to say 'that's right,' or 'that's stupid,' or 'that's incorrect'" (Rogers, 1995, p. 18). Understanding is "risky," because it opens the clinician to change. Rogers uses this understanding and acceptance of the client's world to foster the client's self-understanding and self-acceptance. He does not yield on this stance, even when probing the thoughts and minds of individuals with psychosis (Rogers, 1995). A solution-focused approach is very much client centered, and Rogers's insights are profoundly relevant to this approach.

When the clinician uses the Solution Cycle to help Ramsey envision the world he wants, a world in which he speaks using a correct production of the /s/ phoneme, the clinician is adopting a humanistic orientation that Carl Rogers would recognize. Ramsey must own the vision, and he must own the goals that will help him realize his vision.

It is true that, like all our classical theories, humanism has real limitations. The humanistic approach, including that of Carl Rogers, requires that clients define the issues that will be addressed and the goals that will be set. The solution-focused approach tends to be more structured than Rogers's methods would allow. Ramsey is, after all, being helped to improve a speech problem. He is not meeting the clinician to discuss all his hopes and fears open-endedly. To address his communication disorder, goals will be set, and solutions will be sought.

What Rogers and the humanistic psychologists offer is the constant reminder that the pace is set by the clients and that addressing the client's thoughts and feelings related to the communication disorder is crucial to therapy progress (Kaderavek et al., 2004; Riley, 2002). Humanists would also agree that responsive listening is the core skill of the clinician and that no progress can be made without deep understanding and broad acceptance of clients as they are. These valuable insights are applied throughout the Solution Cycle.

Existentialism

The brilliant, passionate Søren Kierkegaard (1813–1855) conceived many of the key concepts that drove the philosophy of existentialism, one of the most important intellectual movements of the past 200 years and a powerful validation of those who adopt the solution-focused approach to counseling. The concepts that are especially helpful include individual freedom, responsibility, and angst along with the "here and now," the absurd, and, finally, commitment.

Kierkegaard said, "Anxiety is the dizziness of freedom" (Kierkegaard, 1981). Once we realize that we are perfectly free to choose any path and are therefore fully responsible for every step we take, we experience a kind of extreme vertigo, an angst or anxiety. This angst derives from the sheer loneliness of our predicament: we choose our lives, our ethics, even our faith, entirely on our own. As Kierkegaard wrote, "To dare is to lose one's footing momentarily; not to dare is to lose oneself" (Kierkegaard, 1992).

When you utilize the solution-focused approach with your clients, you challenge them to choose their goals. Clients decide what they will become. They remain actively involved in every step of the process. A later existentialist, Albert Camus, believed that our freedom saves us from a meaningless and indifferent universe, because our choices could support our own dignity and that of others (Camus, 1956). The existentialist tells individuals with a speech, language, swallowing, or hearing disorder that they do not have to be defined by their disorder or by the reactions of others to their disorder (Cooper, 1990; Spillers, 2007).

Kierkegaard said, "There is nothing with which every man is so afraid as getting to know how enormously much he is capable of doing and becoming." Camus put it succinctly: "Freedom is nothing but the chance to be better" (Camus, 1961). The key is to use one's freedom bravely, and that is done by making commitments. The existentialists are strong proponents of commitment as a crucial element of "being better."

Yes, existentialists understand and even empathize with the anxiety caused by clients' ability to choose their goals and to define their lives. Understanding the angst, however, does not mean letting clients off the hook. Quite the opposite. Jean-Paul Sartre, an existentialist particularly adamant about our radical freedom, wrote, "Acting is happy agony." He meant that, although we will experience great anxiety when we take on responsibility, we cannot gain real happiness unless we do so. "As far as men go," Sartre claimed, "it is not what they are that interests me, but what they can become."

Existentialism is more a way of thinking than a systematic theory of treatment or counseling like REBT. You will search the existentialists in vain for workable treatment techniques to employ as a clinician. What this philosophy provides is a compelling perspective on the clinician's and the client's role in treatment. "Commitment is an act, not a word," Sartre said. Again: "Freedom is what you do with what's been done to you" (Sartre, 1944).

As the name implies, existentialism is concerned with our existence here and now, not some abstract future or a nostalgic past. You help clients accept the reality of their present state and their disorder without minimizing its difficulties. You and your clients define their problem accurately. Then, with courage and determination, your clients make use of their freedom to choose the hard work of improvement over hand-wringing, denial, and procrastination. Existentialism may seem to be recommending a kind of tough love, but it is a toughness rooted in a profound respect for the dignity of the individual and a powerful conviction that your clients can find meaning in life by choosing a preferred future and not letting an indifferent universe make the decisions for them.

There is no time like the present, existentialists believe, because there is no time but the present! True, you will not find treatment techniques in the writings of these thinkers. What you will find is a way to put your faith in your clients' power to take charge and charge forward. In his masterwork "Either/Or" Kierkegaard penned this remark: "If I were to wish for anything, I should not wish for wealth and power, but for the passionate sense of the potential, for the eye which, ever young and ardent, sees the possible. Pleasure disappoints, possibility never. And what wine is so sparkling, what so fragrant, what so intoxicating, as possibility!" (Kierkegaard, 1992).

At your best, what you will give to your clients, above any other form of help, is the awesome realization of their own potential, their own power to alter their situation for the better. You will help turn them from observers of life to full participants. Your greatest power is your ability to help them tap the power they themselves possess. Although the esteemed American philosopher and psychologist William James is known as a pragmatist, he often spoke in ways that the existentialists would have found insightful. He once said, "Human beings, by changing the inner attitudes of their minds, can change the outer aspects of their lives." He knew that making free choices may not always bring happiness, but there can be no happiness without making free choices, sometimes courageously and without assurance of success (James, 1899/2007).

Sartre, in his usual bold fashion, provides a brief and excellent summary of the existentialist frame of mind when it comes to creating change in self: "In a word, man must create his own essence: it is in throwing himself into the world, suffering there, struggling there, that he gradually defines himself" (Sartre, 1944).

There are other theories, different counseling methodologies, and various ways of organizing the ones presented here. This overview, however, does provide a good feel for the range of counseling approaches and the theoretic underpinnings of each. Importantly, although every approach has shortcomings, it is also true that each approach noted here has something valuable to offer to the Solution Cycle. This book references a given approach or theory whenever it may contribute to a successful treatment outcome.

Counseling as Central to the Therapy Process

The wall that stands between the activity known as treatment and the activity known as counseling is often not clearly delineated. In the real world of speech and hearing treatment, the clinician may be counseling while doing treatment and may be pursuing a treatment goal while counseling. Sometimes it is difficult to discern, at a given moment, whether a clinician is mainly doing treatment or mainly counseling, and it is usually unimportant to make the distinction if the clinician is achieving satisfactory progress.

You make the distinction between counseling and treatment because you usually need to do both with proficiency if you hope to attain your treatment goals. You make the distinction because counseling and treatment require related but different skills and competencies, and it makes sense to focus on one of these skill sets at a time when you are learning to be an excellent speech-language pathologist or audiologist. Finally, you make the distinction because understanding the relationship of counseling to treatment is critical.

Counseling for Speech-Language Pathologists and Audiologists

The prospect of treatment is what brings you into professional contact with your clients. Your goals may initially be disorder-specific treatment goals. They include objectives like the following:

- Correcting a lisp
- Decoding vocalization with a cochlear implant
- Producing easy onsets
- Constructing two-word utterances

- Following three-step commands
- Using a communication board to indicate wants and needs

If you achieve these treatment goals, you can be said to be successful, even if some desirable counseling outcomes are unmet. To reach ultimate success, defined as your clients' ability to proceed in life without your continued support, you will, however, most likely have to include counseling objectives.

These counseling objectives enable you to consider your clients apart from their disorder, while still considering the effects the disorder has on your clients. For example, counseling may be required to suppress the belief that a particular client's speech disorder is the result of the client's "laziness." Once that client becomes convinced that the disorder is not caused by an aversion to an activity (a counseling goal), the client can make progress toward correcting the disorder (a disorder-specific treatment goal). The distinction between counseling goals and treatment-specific goals are not always clear-cut, but you will be aided in your learning process by establishing the distinction where possible. The example of Ramsey provides an illustration of this scenario.

On rare occasions, you and your clients may correctly decide to achieve counseling goals without directly addressing your treatment-specific goals. When you prepare clients for impending surgery (e.g., laryngectomy, cleft palate repair, cochlear implant), counseling goals are sometimes all that matter. In those cases, the therapy process can still be seen as successful.

The Interviewing and Counseling Environment

The environment in which you interview and counsel clients varies. You could find yourself in an elementary or high school, or an annex to which the student/client comes each week to "see the audiologist (or speech-language pathologist)." You could also be in a university's clinical lab staffed with professors and graduate students learning and conducting treatment or an ENT office with a wing dedicated to speech or hearing treatment.

The venues will differ, but many aspects and challenges of interviewing and counseling remain constant from one setting to another. The quest is always for a process that results in the successful achievement of the goals established by you and your clients.

Interviewing Process and Goals

The initial interview with your clients sets the tone of the experience and the definition of success. Although the interview, as you will see, is a formal interaction and data-gathering process, you and your clients will establish a rapport that will underpin your professional relationship.

Any sound interview has several goals. These include relationship building, determining which tests to administer, gathering data, making a differential diagnosis, recommending a plan of treatment, providing a prognosis, and referring to other professionals (Ivey et al., 2002).

Individual and Group Counseling

Treatment can take place in a one-to-one setting. In this book the one-to-one environment is assumed unless otherwise noted. You may determine—or it may be determined for you—that there will be group sessions. These sessions comprise two or more clients usually, though not always, confronting the same issue or similar issues. The goals of group therapy are not necessarily different from the goals that would be set in a one-to-one framework. The goals are owned by the individual, although well-functioning groups can establish common goals and commitments.

Perhaps the major difference between one-to-one and group sessions comes down to the roles you assume as you adapt to the requirements of each environment. In a one-to-one setting your entire focus is on your individual client. Every technique, every step, every message is directed at that client. In a group session, of course, different clients are subject to different techniques and have separate moments at the center of the process.

Clients in group sessions also interact with each other. Your role sometimes is facilitator or group process leader. In a sense, you never cease being a facilitator; there is always a group present, and that situation is one you must always take into account. When your client is ready, if you have a choice, you may make the choice to engage in a group session because such a session may be the optimal way to achieve generalization of your client's treatment goals. In many school settings, however, group sessions are not always a choice but a requirement because of large caseloads. In these circumstances, you need to make the best of the situation, keeping each client's goals in mind and facilitating those goals among others. Either way, group and individual sessions are both techniques adopted to further the cause of therapy.

Counseling Culturally and Linguistically Diverse Clients

Cultural and linguistic diversity (CLD) in your client demographics is another reality you will encounter, and skilled counseling can be a huge asset in that reality. There is every reason to believe that, throughout your career, CLD will be escalating in most if not every segment of our society and in every age group. Specific knowledge, skills, and alertness to differences among diverse populations make up what is termed *cultural competence*. Cultural competence is in fact a precondition for effective treatment and effective counseling amid CLD. CLD poses specific challenges and those challenges vary according to the makeup of the group.

Cultural diversity includes differences in customs, religious practices and beliefs, social mores, generational attitudes, and the attitudes of one of the groups toward another. Linguistic diversity encompasses those who speak English as a second language (ESL), users of sign language and interpretation, those with regional accents, and people with different educational backgrounds. All these cultural and linguistic variables present opportunities and challenges for you as you engage in treating and counseling individuals with speech, language, swallowing, and hearing disorders. CLD affects every aspect of your work with your clients, because CLD affects every aspect of your clients' relationship with you.

Multicultural counseling and therapy (MCT) is a "metatheoretical approach that recognizes that all helping methods ultimately exist within a cultural context" (Cheatham et al., 2002, p. 291). Clinicians should begin by being aware that there are differences among their clients. Also important is the realization that your clients have family and cultural factors that influence their perceptions of the world (Ivey, Pederson, & Ivey, 2001). These perceptions can affect your clients' interactions with you, their concepts of time and space, and their overall opinions about treatment.

Clinicians should take into account culture related to time, especially if the clinician is used to European American views on time (Ivey et al., 2001). For instance, some individuals in the Native American culture believe one needs to "wait for the right time" (LaFromboise, 1996, p. 5). Speech-language pathologists and audiologists treating these individuals may need to be patient and work within their client's time frame. The idea of "problem" and "solution" is also culturally specific. Developing appropriate and competent interviewing skills and microskills is important in treating and counseling individuals who are culturally and linguistically diverse.

Counseling across the Life Span

Another important aspect of the therapy process is that you will treat individuals across the entire life span, from infants with cleft lip and/or palate who have feeding issues to toddlers with emerging language problems to adolescents with social pragmatic, articulation, or fluency concerns to adults with voice or swallowing issues to elderly adults exhibiting language issues or cognitive decline. Regardless of a client's disorder or stage of life, your role in counseling does not change, nor does counseling below less important.

Your counseling focus will take a familiar trajectory as you engage in therapy at different points in your clients' lives. With clients that range from infancy to early toddlerhood, you will find yourself mainly counseling the parents and caregivers of your clients (Yucel, Derim, & Celik, 2008; Zebrowski & Schum, 1993). As cognitive development increases and your clients become more aware of the affect their environment has on them, as well as their feelings related to their communication disorder, your counseling will shift to focus more on the clients themselves. You will still have moments when you may need to counsel caregivers, parents, and significant others during this stage, but your counseling priority will usually be the clients. As the ages of your clients increase into older adulthood, when you begin to deal with hearing loss, severe receptive or expressive language concerns, or cognitive decline, you will begin again to focus your counseling efforts on the significant others and caregivers of the clients who may now be your clients' children (Holland, 2007).

Review of Key Points

- The two core indicators of a need to integrate counseling into the therapy process are *obstacle dominance*, where a barrier arises between the client and the treatment goal, and *ego impedance*, where the client's self-concept directly hinders the process of therapy.
- The solution-focused approach is effective because it shifts the emphasis from the disorder being treated to the goals the client wants to achieve through treatment. Clinicians help their clients by building on the things they do right, not by focusing on what they do wrong.
- The Solution Cycle is a practical, four-step, nonlinear leadership model that serves as a guide through the counseling and therapy process. Phase One is the learning stage, which involves observation, study, and listening. Phase Two is the development of an alliance base, or Circle of Power. Phase Three is description of a vision of success and associated goals. Phase Four encompasses the achievement of the goals. The Solution Cycle can make use of all the classic counseling models.
- Behaviorism holds that patterns of behavior are impressed upon an organism by environmental influences. The term *operant conditioning* characterizes the way organisms interact with their surroundings to develop their behaviors and habits. Behavior modification, behaviorism's main therapy strategy, uses techniques like positive and negative reinforcement, punishment and extinction, and successive approximation.
- Cognitive therapy distinguishes irrational beliefs from rational or healthy beliefs and works to shift the client's beliefs from the irrational to the rational. People with healthy beliefs experience happiness when they obtain their desires and sadness when they do not. People with irrational beliefs experience bad feelings that actually get in the way of attaining their wants and desires and that cause dysfunctional behavior.
- Rational emotive behavior therapy (REBT) is a well-known form of cognitive therapy in which the clients take three steps to healthy thinking: (1) observe that their irrational beliefs are harmful to them; (2) become capable of thinking differently; and (3) use methods to make progress in changing their thinking in a healthy direction.
- The humanistic approach always puts the client and the client's emotions first. It adopts a favorable view of the client that insists on "unconditional positive regard" for the client, a commitment by the clinician to understand the client on the client's terms.
- For the speech-language pathologist and audiologist, the solution-focused approach begins with the goals jointly set by the client and the clinician, which are always defined as the most desirable outcomes of therapy. Although there are limitations, achievement of your goals is greatly facilitated through the use of counseling skills. They include interpersonal skills, probing, observation,

information gathering, listening, responding, paraphrasing, and summarizing as well as core techniques like planning, decision making, goal setting, alliance building, empathetic interaction, and encouragement.

- Although only the client can be the target, counseling can address the needs not only of the client but also of those around the client. These individuals include client advocates, the client's social and professional networks, and others who can be a factor in the client's improvement.
- The initial interview with the client will set the tone of the experience and the definition of success.
- Treatment can take place in one-to-one settings or in groups.
- Specific knowledge, skills, and alertness to differences among diverse populations make up what is termed *cultural competence*. Cultural competence is a precondition for effective treatment and effective counseling amid cultural and linguistic diversity.
- Multicultural counseling and therapy recognizes that all counseling and therapy approaches must exist within a cultural context.
- You may treat individuals of any age, and counseling takes different forms across the life span.

Practical Exercises

In the chapter, Ramsey's story was used to illustrate the concepts of obstacle dominance and ego impedance. In the space below define obstacle dominance and ego impedance. Then, identify whether the scenarios that follow are depicting a client exhibiting obstacle dominance or ego impedance.

Scenarios

a. Sammy believes that he "cannot do it."

b. Alicia states, "This symptom is getting in the way of achieving my goal. I will never make progress."

c. Louisa says, "With my busy schedule, I can't see how I will ever find the time to practice. I feel like giving up."

d. Carl's previous speech-language pathologist told him that he has a communication disorder and will never improve. She stated that Carl would just have to live with the progress he's made. Carl says to his new clinician, "The conclusions my last clinician made sound right to me. I believe what she said. At this point therapy won't do me any good; I will never improve."

e. Oscar states, "I know I'm the kind of person that never follows through on anything. You told me this is long-term therapy and I know I will give up on it sooner or later. Why bother trying?"

For each of the scenarios, match the speech-language pathologist's response with the correct historical counseling approach (e.g., behaviorism, cognitive behavioral therapy, humanism, existentialism).

Journal Assignment 1: Hard Habit to Break

Your first journal assignment is to choose a habit you have and spend the next 2 weeks changing the habit. You will use a 10-point effort scale (1–10) to rate your overall daily effort in changing the habit (1 = no effort; 10 = high effort). Journal your daily progress at changing your habit using the following guidelines.

Day 1

Choose the habit you will attempt to change.

Rate your perceived effort level at changing the habit on a scale from 1 to 10 (1 being the least amount of effort, 10 being the most amount of effort).

Describe how you plan to change your habit, specifying three or more objectives (goals) and your criterion for each objective.

What are your feelings, thoughts, and attitudes?

How much does this habit affect your quality of life?

How much does this habit affect your peers, family, significant others?

How willing are you to change?

Days 2–12

Rate your overall effort level at changing your habit.

Did you meet your criterion for each of your objectives?

How did your objectives change, or did they?

How did you feel?

What did you think?

What are your attitudes toward changing?

How does this process affect your quality of life?

What impact has this change had on your peers, family, significant others?

How willing are you to change?

Days 13 and 14

Rate your current overall effort level.

Did you meet your objectives?

Reflect on the process of change taking into consideration how change affects your clients, and what strategies you have determined may help your clients deal with that change.

REFERENCES

Andersson, G., Porsaeus, D., Wiklund M., Kaldo, V., & Larsen, H. C. (2005). Treatment of tinnitus in the elderly: A controlled trial of cognitive behavior therapy. *International Journal of Audiology, 44*(11), 671–675.

Barone, O. R., & Tellis, C. M. (2008). *Your voice is your business.* San Diego, CA: Plural Publishing.

Blomgren, M., Roy, N., Callister, T., & Merrill, R. M. (2005). Intensive stuttering modification therapy: A multidimensional assessment of treatment outcomes. *Journal of Speech and Hearing Research, 48*(3), 509–523.

Bothe, A. K., Davidow, J. H., Bramlett, R. E., & Ingham, R. J. (2006). Stuttering treatment research, 1970–2005: I. Systematic review incorporating trial quality assessment of behavioral, cognitive, and related approaches. *American Journal of Speech-Language Pathology, 15*, 321–341.

Camus, A. (1956). *The rebel*. New York, NY: Alfred A. Knopf.

Camus, A. (1961). *Resistance, rebellion and death*. New York, NY: Alfred A. Knopf.

Cheatham et al. (2002). Multicultural counseling and therapy I: Metatheory—taking theory into practice. In A. E. Ivey, M. D. D'Andrea, M. B. Ivey, & L. Simek-Morgan (Eds.), *Theories of counseling and psychotherapy* (pp. 291–328). Boston, MA: Allyn and Bacon.

Conture, E. G. (1990). *Stuttering* (2nd ed.). Englewood Cliffs, NJ: Prentice Hall.

Cook, F. (2012). Solution-focused brief therapy: What is going well? And what else? And what else? Retrieved from http://www.stutteringhelp.org/solution-focused-brief-therapy

Cooper, D. (1990). *Existentialism*. Oxford, England: Basil Blackwell.

Corey, G. (2009). *Theory and practice of counseling and psychotherapy* (8th ed.). Belmont, CA: Thomson Brooks/Cole.

Crowe, T. A. (1997). Counseling: Definition, history, rationale. In T. A. Crowe (Ed.), *Applications of counseling in speech-language pathology and audiology* (pp. 3–29). Baltimore, MD: Williams & Wilkins.

Egan, G. (2006). *The skilled helper: A problem-management and opportunity-development approach to helping* (8th ed.). Stamford, CT: Thomson Brooks Cole.

Ellis, A., & Dryden, W. (2007). *The practice of rational emotive behavior therapy* (2nd ed.). New York, NY: Springer.

Ellis, A., & Knaus, W. (1977). *Overcoming procrastination*. New York, NY: Institute for Rational-Emotive Therapy.

Gable, F. G. (1970). *The third force: The psychology of Abraham Maslow*. New York, NY: Grossman Publishers.

Gustad, J. W. (1953). The definition of counseling. In R. F. Berdie (Ed.), *Roles and relationships in counseling*. Minneapolis: University of Minnesota Press.

Hayes, S. C., Barnes-Holmes, D., & Roche, B. (2001). *Relational frame theory: A post-Skinnerian account of human language and cognition*. New York, NY: Kluwer Academic.

Hernandez, P., & Ikkanda, Z. (2011). Applied behavior analysis: Behavior management of children with autism spectrum disorders in dental environments. *Journal of American Dental Association, 142*(3), 281–287.

Holland, A. (2007). Counseling/coaching in chronic aphasia. *Topics in Language Disorders, 27*(4), 339–350.

Ivey, A. E., D'Andrea, M. D., Ivey, M. B., & Simek-Morgan, L. (2002). *Theories of counseling and psychotherapy*. Boston, MA: Allyn and Bacon.

Ivey, A. E., Pedersen, P. B., & Ivey, M. B. (2001). *Intentional group counseling: A microskills approach*. Belmont, CA: Brooks/Cole.

James, W. (2007). *Principles of psychology*. New York, NY: Cosimo. (Original work published 1899)

Kaderavek, J. N., Laux, J. M., & Mills, N. H. (2004). A counseling training module for students in speech-language pathology training programs. *Contemporary Issues in Communication Science and Disorders, 31*, 153–161.

Kierkegaard, S. (1981). *The concept of anxiety.* Princeton, NJ: Princeton University Press.

Kierkegaard, S. (1992). *Either/or: A fragment of life.* London, England: Penguin Classics.

LaFromboise, T. D., & Jackson, M. (1996). MCT theory and Native-American populations. In D.W. Sue, A.E. Ivey, & P. Pedersen (Eds.), *A theory of multicultural counseling and therapy* (192–203). Pacific Grove, CA: Brooks Cole Publishing.

Manning, W. H. (2000). *Clinical decision-making in fluency disorders* (2nd ed.). Vancouver, Canada: Singular Press.

Maslow, A. H. (1968). *Toward the psychology of being* (2nd ed.). New York, NY: Van Nostrand.

Maslow, A. H. (1999). *Toward a psychology of being* (3rd ed.). Ontario, Canada: John Wiley & Sons.

Menzies, R. G., Onslow, M., Packman, A., & O'Brian, S. (2009). Cognitive behavior therapy for adults who stutter: A tutorial for speech-language pathologists. *Journal of Fluency Disorders, 34*(3), 187–200.

Murphy, J. J. (1997). *Solution-focused counseling in middle and high schools.* Alexandria, VA: American Counseling Association.

Perkins, W. H. (1992). *Stuttering presented.* San Diego, CA: Singular Press.

Phillips, D. T., & Mendel, L. L. (2008). Counseling training in communication disorders: A survey of clinical fellows. *Contemporary Issues in Communication Science and Disorders, 35*, 44–53.

Prins, D., & Ingham, R. J. (2009). Evidenced-based treatment and stuttering—historical perspective. *Journal of Speech, Language, and Hearing Research, 52*, 254–263.

Riley, J. (2002). Counseling: An approach for speech-language pathologists. *Contemporary Issues in Communication Science and Disorders, 29*, 6–16.

Rogers, C. (1995). *On becoming a person: A therapist's view of psychotherapy.* Boston, MA: Mariner Books-Houghton Mifflin.

Rogers, E. M. (1995). *Diffusion of innovations.* New York, NY: The Free Press.

Rosenzweig, S. (1945). The picture association method and its application in a study of reactions to frustration. *Journal of Personality, 14*, 3–23.

Rosenzweig, S. (2002). Rosenzweig picture-frustration (P-F) study. In E. Craighead & C. B. Nemeroff (Eds.), *The Corsini encyclopedia of psychology and behavioral science* (4th ed., 1427–1429). New York, NY: John Wiley & Sons.

Sartre, J. (1944). Characterizations of existentialism. *Action, 29.*

Skinner, B. F. (1953). *Science and human behavior.* New York, NY: MacMillan.

Skinner, B. F. (1959). Teaching machines. *IRE Transactions on Education, 2*(1), 14–22.

Spillers, C. S. (2007). An existential framework for understanding the counseling needs of clients. *American Journal of Speech-Language Pathology, 16*, 191–197.

Twyman, J. S. (2007). A new era of science and practice in behavior analysis. *Association for Behavior Analysis International: Newsletter, 30*(3), 1–4.

Weisbord, M. R. (2004). *Productive workplaces revisited: Dignity, meaning, and community in the 21st century* (2nd ed.). San Francisco, CA: Pfeiffer.

Wolter, J. A., DiLollo, A., & Apel, K. (2006). A narrative therapy approach to counseling: A model for working with adolescents and adults with language-literacy deficits. *Language, Speech, and Hearing Services in the Schools, 37*, 168–177.

Yucel, E., Derim, D., & Celik, D. (2008). The needs of hearing impaired children's parents who attend to auditory verbal therapy-counseling program. *International Journal of Pediatric Otorhinolaryngology, 72*(7), 1097–1110.

Zebrowski, P. M., & Schum, R. L. (1993). Counseling parents of children who stutter. *American Journal of Speech-Language Pathology, 2*, 65–71.

CHAPTER 2

A Framework for Effective Counseling in Communication Science and Disorders

KEY TERMS

- Empathy
- Listening
- Observation

- Preferred future
- Psychologists, counselors, and psychotherapists

- Reflection
- Study

LEARNING OBJECTIVES

After reading this chapter, you will be able to:

- List and describe the benefits of utilizing a solution-focused approach to counseling a client
- List and explain the four phases of the Solution Cycle
- List and explain the Five Intentions of Communication

Solution-Focused Approach to Counseling

Sydney is a bright, attractive, accomplished 26-year-old professional woman. She has a good job, a supportive husband, and a happy family. Sydney also has a fluency disorder. She stutters. She has come to you for help but informs you immediately that she is sure there is nothing you can do for her. She is tense, argumentative, and despondent. Sydney seems defeated before she begins.

You think to yourself, "I didn't become a speech-language pathologist or audiologist to solve people's psychological problems or address their emotional issues. I'm not a trained clinical psychologist or psychotherapist, so what professional right do I have to venture into those arenas?"

You aren't exactly wrong. Yet, clients like Sydney frequently show up pushing a trunk full of obstacles to any progress in the kind of treatment for which you are trained. That large trunk can contain a wide variety of self-inhibiting perceptions, from a straightforward lack of confidence to much more complex psychological issues.

The common element is that the clients must somehow move the baggage out of the way before a path is cleared for you to achieve a measure of success in your clinical endeavors.

You may actually be just the right person to deal with these emotional issues. The American Speech-Language Hearing Association even requires it as one of your professional competencies (American Speech-Language Hearing Association, 2007). Unfortunately, graduate students in speech-language pathology and audiology, as well as clinicians practicing in the field, do not feel well prepared to provide counseling to their clients (Kaderavek, Laux, & Mills, 2004; Phillips & Mendel, 2008). Clinicians also feel a level of discomfort when deciding what counseling to provide their clients, how to counsel clients, and what is within and outside a speech-language pathologist's or audiologist's scope of practice regarding counseling (Phillips & Mendel, 2008).

Scope of Practice

Speech-language pathologists and audiologists should view counseling as more than just giving advice or instruction (Scheuerle, 1992). Counseling requires a specific set of skills and competencies. The counseling you do, however, is certainly no substitute for the dedicated work of a certified psychologist. You are not learning counseling skills to become a professional counselor or psychologist (Phillips & Mendel, 2008). You will not be able to help your clients solve all of their problems, and sometimes you will defer to counseling professionals for assistance. Psychologists, clinical social workers, counselors, and psychotherapists are trained to help clients who have persistent and chronic difficulties adjusting to life issues and changes (Schum, 1986).

For you, counseling is a tool you can employ to help clients achieve their disorder-specific goals or deal with the negative impact the disorder may have on their quality of life. So, yes, as a speech-language pathologist or audiologist, you do counsel your clients although you are not a counselor. The following are guidelines you can use to determine issues that are within and outside your scope of practice.

A counseling approach well suited to do the job is called "solution-focused."

Central Philosophy

The key to a solution-focused approach to counseling is the establishment of clear, short-term goals with a bright spotlight on client strengths and client investment.

Psychologists, clinical social workers, counselors, and psychotherapists: Individuals with advance degrees and certification in the assessment and treatment of those with diseases of the brain, emotional disturbances, and behavior issues.

Within Scope of Practice

- Any issue related to your clients' speech, language, swallowing, or hearing disorder, including bullying, nonclinical depression, resistance, reluctance, grief, avoidance, embarrassment, and similar issues.
- Anything that has a negative impact on your clients' quality of life related to their speech, language, swallowing, or hearing disorder.
- Caregivers', family members', or friends' issues related to your clients' speech, language, swallowing, or hearing disorder.

Outside Scope of Practice (requires referral to a trained counseling professional)

- Diagnosed emotional or psychiatric condition, for example, clinical depression, bipolar disorder, panic or anxiety disorder, as well as others.
- Financial problems not related to the communication disorder.
- Unrelated marital problems.
- Unrelated job issues.
- Drug or alcohol dependency.
- Child custody issues.
- Suicidal tendencies or thoughts.

The following scenario, a faithful rendering of a typical session, demonstrates how the solution-focused approach can work.

Clinician: Your intake form states that you lost your speaking voice about six weeks ago.

Robert: [*Hoarsely*] Five, maybe six, yes.

Clinician: Since that time, has your voice been just like it is now?

Robert: Pretty much. It's worse in the mornings.

Clinician: Is it ever better?

Robert: At times it comes back for a little bit.

Clinician: And then?

Robert: Well, just when I notice that I have a voice, it goes back, back to what you're hearing now.

Clinician: I see. So, it sounds like your voice comes back sometimes when you're not thinking about it.

Robert: Yes.

Clinician: Then, when you think, "hey, I have my voice back," it goes away again.

Robert: I guess that's right.

Clinician: What do you want to accomplish in voice therapy?

Robert: I'd like my voice back permanently, the way it was six weeks ago.

Clinician: Is that our goal, then?

Robert: Yeah, I suppose. Is it possible?

Clinician: I've seen others in your situation achieve it, yes. The question is, do you want to set this as your goal, to get your voice back to where it was six weeks ago?

Robert: Yes.

Clinician: Definitely?

Robert: Yes, definitely.

Clinician: OK, that's our long-term goal. In the short term, we need to make progress toward that goal.

Robert: Right. How do we do that?

Clinician: How about a short-term goal?

Robert: Like what?

Clinician: Well, you say you get your voice back sometimes, even now.

Robert: Yes, but it's temporary.

Clinician: Maybe we can set a goal to find that temporary voice and build on it.

Robert: How do we do that?

Clinician: We'll try a number of things. Do you want to set a short-term goal to find that temporary voice?

Robert: OK, yes.

Clinician: Will you know when you've got it?

Robert: Got what? My voice?

Clinician: Yes, your voice. Will you know when you've got it?

Robert: Sure. I'll hear it.

Clinician: So, you'll tell me when you hear your voice, right?

Robert: Yes. Certainly. But we still don't know what's causing this. My ENT says it's not physical.

Clinician: That's true. We have talked about some possible causes, but we don't know for sure yet.

Robert: But I still think it's important to find out the reason this is happening.

Clinician: I do, too. How about this: along the way, if either of us come upon what we think is a cause of your voice loss, we'll discuss it, OK?

Robert: OK.

Clinician: Something is causing your voice loss, we know that much. Do you believe we can still make progress without knowing the exact cause?

Robert: I don't see why not. What do you think?

Clinician: Yes, I definitely think we can make progress. How about this? Let's try a couple of techniques; you tell me if you hear your voice.

Robert: Sounds good.

The remainder of the session was devoted to a series of brief vocal exercises designed to elicit voice. The scenario presented was very productive from a solution-focused perspective. The clinician and the client set the ultimate goal, for Robert to get his voice back. They established two intermediate goals. The first was to find what Robert called his "temporary voice."

The second intermediate goal was to identify possible causes for Robert's voice loss, for which his ENT had not determined a physical or organic origin. Though the ENT and the clinician may have hypothesized possible causes ranging from an underlying vocal fold paresis (weakness) to something purely functional, there was at this point no urgency to settle the question. Instead, an agreement was made to discuss the matter if a possible cause presented itself. This short-term goal was acceptable and realistic to the client, two essential features of goals in a solution-focused approach to counseling. There are certainly other important aspects of goals (e.g., measurability and doability of the goals) that need to be examined to design well-crafted goals.

Assumptions of a Solution-Focused Approach

There are several assumptions behind the solution-focused approach. The first is that both the clinician and the client are fully invested in the goals and the process (de Shazer & Berg, 1997; de Shazer et al., 2007). Under this assumption, anything less than full commitment by both parties would be deeply flawed. Imagine this sequence, where only the client is asked to invest.

> **Clinician:** Look, Robert, there's no physical problem here. It's up to you to dig down and find out what's going on. I can't do it for you.
>
> **Robert:** I don't know what's causing it. My ENT says it's not physical.
>
> **Clinician:** The ENT can't do it for you either. Surgery won't help you and there are no medications that will get your voice back. It's entirely up to you.

The clinician has given the reins to Robert and told him he is pretty much on his own. Solution-focused clinicians agree that Robert must be committed, but they are just as adamant that the clinician be fully on board, fully invested in Robert's therapy (de Shazer & Berg, 1997; de Shazer et al., 2007). As this scenario shows, the client-only approach may seem to empower Robert by placing responsibility on his shoulders, but that appearance is false. The approach actually undermines him and those who are there to help him. Both the clinician and the ENT are positioned as virtually helpless; these professionals are presented in terms of what they are unable to do. Notice how often the clinician speaks the words *can't* and *not*. Conversely, when only the clinician is required to commit, the situation is not much improved.

> **Clinician:** So, you have lost your voice and the doctor told you there is no physical reason for this to have happened.
>
> **Robert:** That's right. I don't know what to do. It's so frustrating.
>
> **Clinician:** Don't you worry, Robert. I'm here for you. Just put yourself in my hands. Do whatever I ask of you.
>
> **Robert:** Can I do anything?
>
> **Clinician:** All you need to do is trust me. I have helped hundreds of folks just like you, and I'll help you. Don't sweat it. I've got this completely under control.

In this scene, the clinician is clearly overworking the words *I* and *me*. Robert is defined as helpless and passive, practically an observer, while the clinician comes across as something of a magician. This approach seems to be very efficient. Do as I say; ask no questions; follow my directions, and, before you know it, you'll be cured. Actually, this approach is usually time consuming. It gets quickly bogged down as soon as Robert becomes aware that much more will be demanded of him than he was led to believe. He is, after all, the primary agent of his eventual success.

These brief scenarios point to four additional important assumptions you make when you adopt a solution-focused approach. One assumption is that the best approach is a problem-solving approach. Goals are identified as solutions to problems your clients are facing. Remember to include your clients in defining both the problems and the solutions. Another assumption is that the short-term goals must be manageable, doable in a relatively short amount of time. Although it is important for Robert to achieve his ultimate goal, "get back the voice I had six weeks ago," it is critical to establish intermediate or antecedent goals that can be accomplished without excessive stress and frustration.

Overly complex, difficult, or currently inaccessible goals, even significant ones, can be addressed at a later time. Learning the cause of Robert's voice loss is certainly important, but there is not yet a visible path to accomplishing that goal. The clinician simply suggests that "along the way, if either of us come upon what we think is a cause of your voice loss, we'll discuss it." The goal is not discarded or treated lightly, but its enigmatic quality is not allowed to deter Robert and the clinician from making progress elsewhere. The goal being addressed must be achievable with the knowledge and resources currently at hand.

An assumption related to achievability is the premise that you and your clients build on their strengths, on what works rather than on what's wrong. Robert revealed to his clinician that his voice returned at times, although he soon lost it again when he realized it was there. The clinician elicited a commitment to build on that "temporary voice," as stated by Robert. The exercises were couched as efforts to recover the temporary voice, to repeat what Robert had already done. The clinician and Robert saw it as one way to build on a strength.

In addition, by adopting Robert's language, the clinician bought into Robert's perception of his situation and his objectives. The clinician also accepted Robert's description of his goal: "I'd like my voice back permanently, the way it was six weeks ago." The clinician repeated those very words when she clarified the goal to which they were both committing. The fifth and final assumption of solution-focused counseling, therefore, is that the goals must be fully owned by the clients, couched if possible in the clients' own language.

Illustration of the Approach: Miracle Question

Dr. Milton H. Erickson, a psychiatrist, is one of the pioneers in the development of "brief therapy," a common name for solution-focused counseling. His "crystal ball technique" was the forerunner of the "miracle question" (de Shazer, 1990; Sklare,

The Main Assumptions of Solution-Focused Counseling

- Both the clinician and the client are fully invested in the goals and the therapy process.
- Goals are identified as solutions to problems the client faces.
- Although there is always a long-term, ultimate goal, the goals being addressed are achievable with the knowledge and resources currently at hand.
- The clinician and client build on the client's strengths, on what works rather than on what's wrong.
- The goals are fully owned by the client, couched if possible in the client's own language.

Under these assumptions, the clinician emerges as

- Collaborator, not dictator
- Listener and clarifier, not judge and sentencer
- Facilitator, not director

2005). He encouraged patients to look into a crystal ball and imagine a world free of the problems they were facing. When Erickson asked his patients to tell him how they overcame the problem, they revealed a great deal about themselves and what they felt it would take to solve the problem. In 1988 Steve de Shazer wrote about what he called the miracle question (de Shazer, 1988), which he had been using in therapy since the early 1980s.

De Shazer's version of the miracle question consists of asking clients to imagine that they went to bed with the same problem that brought them to therapy. During the night, a miracle happens and the problem is solved by the time the clients awaken the next morning, but the clients do not know there was a miracle. The therapist asks how the clients come to know during the day that a miracle has happened. How would the clients' best friend know the miracle had happened?

Remember Sydney from the beginning of the chapter? Let's see how the miracle question would play out in the following scenario with Sydney and her clinician.

Clinician: All right, Sydney. I want you to use your imagination, OK?

Sydney: OK.

Clinician: You leave this session and go home. You still have the problem that brought you to me. You put your children to bed, watch some TV as usual, and then turn in for the night. During the night a miracle happens while you are asleep. You don't know it has happened, because you are asleep, but because of the miracle your problem is completely solved.

Sydney: The problem? My stuttering?

Clinician: Yes, the problem that brought you to this clinic.

Sydney: So, next morning it is miraculously solved, and I don't know the miracle happened. Is that right?

Clinician: Yes, exactly. Now here's the question. How do you discover that the miracle has happened? Remember, you have no idea there has been a miracle.

Sydney: OK, let me think. [*Pause.*] I don't think I'd know during breakfast, because I hardly talk. I know how to avoid stuttering in front of my kids, so I wouldn't know then.

Clinician: Fine.

Sydney: I'd drive to work. Say hi to everyone; still don't know about the miracle. If I think I might stutter when greeting people, I just wave. I call in my assistant to review the day's appointments. She shuts the door to my office. That's going to be my first indication.

Clinician: What happens?

Sydney: Sheri has been with me for three years. When we're together alone, I usually stutter.

Clinician: Really?

Sydney: Yeah. I am comfortable, so I don't compensate or replace words. I guess I'm unguarded.

Clinician: So, what happens? Imagine it.

Sydney: Sure. I begin to discuss my appointments. I always stutter on the *n* in *nine* when I say "Nine a.m."

Clinician: Always?

Sydney: Yeah. *M*'s and *n*'s are my downfall. Now the miracle has happened, right? I say "nine" perfectly, no hesitation, no seven-second *n* sound.

Clinician: Who notices first, you or Sheri?

Sydney: Sheri. For sure.

Clinician: Sheri?

Sydney: Yes. I won't know right away. I might even think I stuttered. I've actually been told I haven't stuttered when I was sure I had. So, it would be a while before I noticed anything different. Sheri would say something like, "Hey, good 'nine.'"

Clinician: Then?

Sydney: I'd say, "What?" She'd say, "You didn't stutter." When I talked more, she'd comment at some point, maybe after three or four sentences, that I wasn't stuttering. That's when I'd first notice.

Clinician: Interesting.

Sydney: Then I think I'd really begin to realize something had happened. Even with Sheri, when I stutter, it's like a hand grabbing the word from inside my throat, holding it in a tight grip. That hand is so real; I'd notice it wasn't there. At some point I'd notice. Then I'd talk, babble, say anything to check that it was really gone. That hand, that fist, that's my worst enemy. I'd just talk and talk, feeling it gone.

Clinician: Then?

Sydney: When I was convinced it was gone, it would take a long time to be convinced, I'd scream. It would be like getting out of prison when I'm serving a life sentence …

The miracle question exercise revealed a great deal about how Sydney perceives her stuttering and how it affects her life. Sydney disclosed to the clinician how and when she masks her disfluencies. She used powerful metaphors like "a gripping hand in her throat", a "life sentence in prison" to describe her stuttering. Sydney also stated that she is very comfortable with Sheri and does not hide her stuttering from Sheri. Her prediction that Sheri would be the first to make Sydney aware that she did not stutter is a clear indication that Sydney trusts Sheri.

The miracle question can be used with many different clients regardless of age or type of communication disorder. Even a very young client is capable of answering the miracle question. If the client talks about a miracle unrelated to the communication disorder, the clinician is still receiving useful information about the nature of a problem and the impact it has on the client. In this specific example with the young client, the communication disorder may be having a minimal impact on the client's life. If a client, like Sydney, directly addresses the miracle as being related to the communication disorder then the clinician is also provided very valuable information.

De Shazer claimed he used the miracle question during almost every first session with his clients. Speech-language pathologists and audiologists, too, will find that the miracle question is a useful tool to engage clients like Sydney in visualizing her treatment goals and describing the benefits of achieving them. This technique can motivate Sydney to make those goals clear and commit to them. Envisioning her world with the goals achieved can encourage Sydney to proceed with treatment.

Solution-Focused Counseling as a Process

Once Sydney and the clinician agree to carry on, a process has begun. It is a process with four distinct, nonlinear phases comprising what is called the Solution Cycle (**Figure 2-1**). The phases are distinct in that each one has a definition and an identity; specific things happen, and explicit results are achieved in each phase. They are nonlinear in that you may return to or repeat a phase during treatment. Although the phases tend to proceed from one to the next in the order presented in the text, a phase may be revisited or may overlap with another phase during the same session. Phase One, for example, is the learning phase, and it is a phase that never really ends during the process, because learning never ceases. Treatment is rarely neat and tidy. To comprehend a solution-focused approach to counseling, however, a clear and firm grasp of these four phases is extremely helpful for you and your clients.

Overview of the Solution Cycle

As Figure 2-1 indicates, the Solution Cycle begins with the learning phase, where you and your clients discover what you need to know to set and meet your treatment goals. In Phase Two, you and your clients identify individuals who could become allies. These people form an alliance base that can partner with your clients and you in your efforts during treatment and long after. Phase Three encompasses the establishment of your goals and the creation of your clients' vision of the future to which all your work aspires. Finally, in Phase Four, your clients and you perform the tasks required to achieve the vision, to meet the goals you have set.

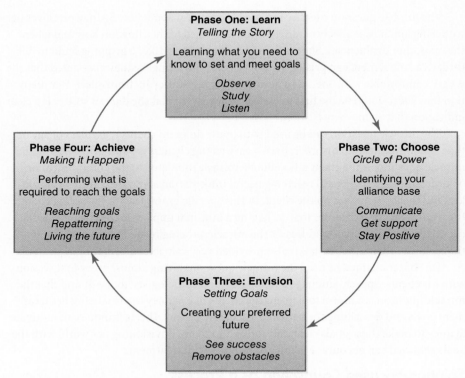

FIGURE 2-1 The Solution Cycle Expanded. There are four nonlinear, distinct phases of the Solution Cycle. Within each phase are objectives that should be targeted and accomplished.

Phase One: Learning: "Telling the Story"

The beauty of the Solution Cycle is the fact that it can be applied to your most comprehensive long-term goal and just as appropriately to a goal you might achieve during a single session. Phase One, learning, is the most elastic of stages. In one sense, it begins long before you see your first client, back in the classroom where a knowledgeable professor introduced you to the disciplines of audiology and speech-language pathology. You call upon and apply that learning throughout treatment.

When actual clients step into your clinic, the learning phase takes on specific meaning and urgency. Information common to all participants is required, and much of these common data are collected on intake forms and during initial interviews. Beyond the developmental, medical, and demographic data, there is information about the clients' issues, attitudes, emotions, motivations, wants, and needs, not all of which will be revealed at once, or easily, or during the earliest sessions. Learning takes place in several important ways.

Observation

As a clinician, you will find observation to be a key learning device. It is something you can do whenever you are in the presence of your clients. In fact, it is something you *should* do when with your clients.

Observation: A process whereby someone focuses attention on another person and looks for signs of attitudes, emotions, thoughts, and beliefs that may be hiding even from the other's own awareness. These signs can reveal themselves in words, facial expressions, involuntary gestures, and even the posture of the body.

The word *observe* has an instructive origin. It derives from the Latin *observare*, "to watch over, look to, attend to, guard, keep safe." In the United States, Memorial Day is "observed" with rituals honoring fallen soldiers in a manner that preserves their memory and ensures they are not forgotten. The word has come to mean "to watch for omens or signs," much in the way magicians caution you to "observe carefully," while they trick you with their sleight of hand. What the magicians are asking is that you watch extra vigilantly to see whether you can catch the hidden maneuver.

When you observe your clients, you too are looking for "omens," signs of attitudes, emotions, thoughts, and beliefs your clients may be hiding even from their own awareness. These omens reveal themselves in facial expressions, involuntary gestures, and even the posture of the body. Much has been written on body language, the messages transmitted, willingly or not, by aspects of the face, hands, and body (Fast, 1970). Eye contact or its lack, a shake of the head or a brief nod, crossing a leg or shrugging the shoulders, any of these observable behaviors can mean something.

When you observe something, you can ignore it or, you can jot it down in your notes for later reference and interpretation. You can also bring it up during the session, as in the following exchange with Sydney, who previously discussed the miracle question with her clinician.

Sydney: Then I think I'd really begin to realize something had happened. Even with Sheri, when I stutter, it's like a hand grabbing the word from inside my throat, holding it in a tight grip. That hand is so real; I'd notice it wasn't there. At some point I'd notice. Then I'd talk, babble, say anything to check that it was really gone. That hand, that fist, that's my worst enemy. I'd just talk and talk, feeling it gone.

Clinician: Then?

Sydney: When I was convinced it was gone, it would take a long time to be convinced, I'd scream. It would be like getting out of prison when I'm serving a life sentence …

Clinician: Sydney, when you just said, "I'd scream," you stopped for a moment and looked toward the window.

Sydney: Did I?

Clinician: Yes. Like this [*clinician demonstrates*].

Sydney: I guess I'm not too surprised. I was thinking of a time when I actually screamed out loud.

Clinician: When you were alone, like in your room?

Sydney: No, I was in the office. I screamed in the office. The senior VP asked me a question and I couldn't get the word out. I just sat there forever. Then I screamed.

Clinician: That was …

Sydney: Incredibly embarrassing. She said, "Let's take a little break." We never mentioned it again.

In this case the astute clinician simply made a reference to a behavior Sydney exhibited: looking away. Although Sydney was not fully aware that she shifted her gaze, its mention triggered an expression of the depth of frustration with her situation. Sydney revealed that her disfluency has had consequences, even in her workplace. These are important insights that shed light on the ways her stuttering has been affecting her life. Observation can be a powerful tool in your efforts to learn what you need to know to counsel your clients effectively.

Study and reflection

Study: A set of learning activities that take place offline, at times other than during sessions.

Observation is immediate and direct study and reflection are learning activities that take place offline, at times other than during sessions. All the classes, projects, labs, and previous client interactions you have had as a student, including your interaction with this book, have built a wealth of knowledge and competence that you bring with you to every counseling encounter.

Reflection: A process of turning one's mind back to an event that happened previously, stopping to think about what occurred. As one reflects on this event, one considers its importance and reaches conclusions that will be of help in planning or determining a course of action.

Study does not end when you become a certified speech-language pathologist or audiologist and begin working with clients. You will study the data supplied during interviews as well as the information gathered from other sources, including relatives, caregivers, school personnel, other healthcare professionals, and acquaintances of your clients. All these sources can play a role in "telling the client's story," providing what you need to know to treat your clients successfully. This is information that you will use to achieve success in therapy.

Reflection is a specific form of study that is important to Phase One of the Solution Cycle. Reflection is literally the act of turning back to something that happened previously and stopping to think about what occurred. When you reflect on a previous session, you turn your mind back to that session. Let's say one day has passed since Sydney disclosed to you that her frustration once caused her to scream aloud in her boss's presence. As you reflect on this revelation, you mull over its importance to your clinical efforts. You reach conclusions that will assist you in planning future treatment sessions and that ensure that you are alert to counseling opportunities and potential obstacles along the way.

Listening

Listening: A two-part process of first understanding and then assessing messages.

Listening is a skill that is essential to the entire learning phase of the Solution Cycle. This skill plays a crucial role in observation, study, and reflection. When you listen you make it possible to understand your clients and their stories; you indicate to your clients that you care about what they think and feel. You make it possible to formulate a response to clients that is based on their own reality. Listening may be one of the most important skills you develop as a clinician. Understanding the listening process and honing your listening competency will improve your counseling efforts in therapy.

Phase Two: Choosing Allies: "Developing the Circle of Power"

The second phase of the Solution Cycle involves identifying and targeting a network of people that will form your clients' "Circle of Power." Members of the circle may be varied, but they have two things in common: (1) they are on the clients' side in their therapy efforts, and (2) each one is in a position to be a positive force in your clients' progress. Failure to recruit a key person into the Circle of Power may inadvertently cause that person to become something other than a supporter, perhaps even a detriment to success.

Development of an alliance base

The Circle of Power, or support network, is really a base of allies enlisted to help clients achieve their goals during therapy and afterward. Potential allies must be sought out and identified. Some are pretty obvious, such as a parent, a spouse, a teacher, or a family physician. Others are less easily identifiable, such as a long-distance friend, a friend on social media, or a grandparent. Who they are and how they are associated with your clients will determine the role they are asked to play in the attainment of your clients' goals.

Membership in the Circle of Power is not fixed and may vary throughout treatment. Different allies may move to the foreground at different times. A friend may be enlisted at the point when your clients begin to practice a technique at school or work. A physician may be needed at a specific time to help mitigate the effects of prescription drugs clients take. Utilizing the Circle of Power effectively over time is a challenge but one with a high potential payoff for you and your clients.

Determining most valued sources of information

Your own professional connections will have access to client information that you need to move effectively through the therapy process. These people include referral sources, other medical personnel, school teachers and assistants, as well as others. You need to decide what you need to know and who is most likely to supply you with that information. These individuals may also help you and your clients discover other people who can be part of the Circle of Power.

Clients

Clients are a major source of information. They are usually the ones who provide baseline knowledge about some of the people or professionals they have seen who can supply additional information, including doctors, other speech-language pathologists or audiologists, as well as additional resources like teachers and allied health professionals. These individuals are integral members of the Circle of Power because they are likely to be valuable informants.

The clinician

As a clinician, you become a major ally of your clients. As primary data gatherer, you are an important source of information. This fact is obvious but can be forgotten during lengthy and sometimes intricate treatment. Whenever you ask a question about your clients and their situation, you need to ask whether you yourself have access to the answer. For example, at a later stage of Sydney's treatment, her speech-language pathologist may wonder whether there is any reason to believe Sydney will have difficulties practicing her new techniques at work. The speech-language pathologist is the one person who knows the embarrassment she felt when she screamed aloud in the presence of the senior VP. In this situation, the ally best equipped to identify a potential difficulty in treatment is none other than the clinician.

The client advocates, social/professional network

The next place to look for helpful information is among the client advocates, all those who may be invested in or affected by your clients' progress in treatment. Parents naturally tend to assume this role, as do spouses, significant others, and siblings. For some, a caregiver will emerge as an advocate. Client advocates have a strong motivation to share certain information, but that information is often biased by the advocates' passionate desire to look out for what they see as the client's best interest. Advocates may actually withhold or distort information if they think they are helping the client by doing so.

The clinician must be aware that client advocates may have their own agenda, and it may be necessary to counsel the advocates themselves to help them play a more constructive role in your clients' efforts toward improvement. Clients may also have reservations about enlisting allies at all. Keep your clients involved in the process of developing their Circle of Power to make sure you are including and excluding the correct people.

Determining the most helpful or influential allies

Informing is only one function of the alliance base. Specific allies can be of assistance in just about every treatment task. Some will help maintain client motivation at critical times. Others will be in a position to provide the feedback that clients often require. Still others can help clients prepare peers and relatives for the changes that treatment will bring about. You must be alert and constantly working to identify and cultivate the allies who will form an effective Circle of Power throughout the process.

When Sydney was imagining the answer to the miracle question, she informed the clinician that her assistant, Sheri, was a special person in her life. What if the clinician decides that Sheri might be a suitable ally at some point in the treatment process? Sydney could explore the possibility with the clinician.

Clinician: You seem to trust Sheri.

Sydney: Yes.

Clinician: A lot?

Sydney: I'd say completely.

Clinician: Do you think Sheri might be willing to help us as we move along?

Sydney: In what way?

Clinician: A number of ways, potentially. One example is real-world practice. If we start working on techniques, you may want to practice them in your day-to-day setting. Sheri might be someone to practice with.

Sydney: Oh, she'd be fine with that.

Clinician: And you?

Sydney: No problem. The office is ready-made for that kind of practice. It's private and comfortable. How else could she help?

Clinician: I might want to get feedback from her on how she views your disfluency.

Sydney: I wouldn't want you to do that too often. She works for me, and imposing on her time like that would make me uncomfortable.

Clinician: But you have no objection if we don't do it too often.

Sydney: No, no other objection. I think her feedback would be dead on.

Clinician: OK. I won't approach her on this without your direct approval each time. That way we'll make sure I'm not imposing on her time. OK?

Sydney: Fine.

The clinician paved the way to enlist Sheri as an ally in the process. The clinician received explicit permission from Sydney to contact Sheri and to seek her in two ways. The clinician showed respect for any reservations Sydney had and made sure her concerns were fully taken into account. A potential ally has now been identified, and her possible roles have been clarified and accepted. The path to success might be just a little smoother.

Phase Three: Envisioning the Preferred Future: "Setting Goals"

Once you have built a substantial base of information and have established your clients' Circle of Power, you are able to collaborate with your clients to discuss the changes your clients will make to establish their ultimate goal. Your clients' long-term goals are considered their preferred future. This is Phase Three of the Solution Cycle. In this stage the solutions or goals are actually framed.

Establishing the mission

The solutions are always viewed in terms of goals. The ultimate goal, the end point that will be the result of the total therapy process, constitutes your clients' and your mission. The accomplishment of that mission is the reason your clients have come to you and are engaged in treatment.

The mission is established by defining the problems that will be solved, enumerating the actions that will be taken to solve the problems, and securing the commitment of the clients and the clinician to make it all happen.

Description of a vision of success

The mission, the ultimate goal, is expressed in terms of a vision of success. This vision is a depiction of the changed circumstances desired, sought, and achieved by the collaborative efforts of you and your clients. It is a description of the clients' world once the mission is accomplished. It is a clear picture of the preferred future.

The preferred future is a future that you and your clients help create. It is distinguished from the passive future, the future you do not help to make, the future that just happens. Solution focus does not mean that solutions occur merely by focusing on them. Solutions occur by working to make them happen. That work is the only difference between the passive future and the preferred future. If Sydney became more fluent, if Robert regained his voice permanently, both would have achieved their preferred future.

> Preferred future: The mission, the ultimate goal of therapy, expressed in terms of a vision of success. This vision is a depiction of the changed circumstances desired, sought, and achieved by the collaborative efforts of clinician and client. It is a description of the client's world once the mission is accomplished.

Overcoming obstacles

Commitment to the preferred future means that nothing is allowed to get in the way of goal attainment. There will be obstacles, but they are not walls forever blocking the road to journey's end. There will be doubts and discouragement, but these are not permitted to drain off the energy and enthusiasm needed to stay the course. Once the commitment is made, the work has begun.

Phase Four: Creating the Preferred Future: "Making It Happen"

You and your clients make a plan. It is a realistic, clear blueprint for change, the specifications for a sturdy bridge from the present, unsatisfactory state to the preferred future. The plan is well thought out. It will remain relevant throughout the process, yet it is flexible enough to adapt to changing circumstances. The plan contains two points of emphasis: (1) the achievement of goals and (2) maintenance and generalization.

Achievement of goals

The first point of emphasis is the achievement of the goals. Every step, every intermediate goal, every action item represents movement toward the ultimate goal or goals. Those long-term goals express the preferred future, the vision, in terms of results, the changes your clients are seeking. Counseling, too, is justified mainly by its ability to propel you and your clients to the long-term goals.

Maintenance and generalization

The second point of emphasis is to make the changes permanent. A change may be the practice of utilizing a hearing aid in the everyday act of communication, or it may be the expansion of expressive vocabulary. Whatever the change, treatment is not complete until the client can maintain the change over time and, where appropriate, generalize the change over a range of communication activities.

Maintenance and generalization are essential to any definition of success in therapy, but such success does not mean that treatment lasts a lifetime. What it means is that the result, the change, the vision of the preferred future, once accomplished, is an enduring reality.

Counseling as Intentional Communication

Counseling is never accidental. You counsel because you choose to counsel, you intend to counsel. Counseling is intentional. Broadcasting your intention to counsel is not

Ways to Become Aware That You Are Counseling

- You stop talking and listen.
- You maintain appropriate eye contact.
- You repeat key words you hear your client say.
- You remove blocks within yourself by maintaining focus and attention on your client.
- You discontinue disorder-specific treatment to attend to your client's emotional response.
- You ask clients how they are doing.

necessary. You need not say to a client, "Just a minute, Sydney, I will now begin a counseling session with you." When you opt to counsel, however, you should be aware that you are doing it.

The following are guidelines to help you become more aware of when you are counseling. Not only should you be aware that you are counseling, you should be aware of the specific intention of your counseling communication. There are five reasons to speak, five intentions you could have when counseling. The five intentions are small talk, information sharing, self-affirmation, persuasion/direction, and feeling (Barone & Tellis, 2008).

Small Talk: Climate, Attitudes, and Motivations

When you discuss matters that seem trivial, you are engaging in small talk. In fact, small talk can be an important and useful form of communication. You might use small talk to get to know your clients, become better acquainted, and develop rapport. Your initial meeting with your clients almost always contains a relationship-building phase, one that comprises mostly small talk.

Small talk can also be used for climate setting. You could open a serious treatment session with small talk to put your clients at ease before moving on. A third use of small talk is relaxation. You might pause midway through a session and chat about nothing vital; you and your clients are just taking a break.

Information: Knowledge Transfer

During the initial interview, you solicit a great deal of data; your main intention is clearly informational. As a clinician, you transmit information regularly to your clients. All the explanations you give, all the instructions, and all the background you supply are informational messages. A message is informational not just because there is information in the message; most messages contain information. A message is informational when your primary intention is to inform.

The most reliable way to check an informational intention is to determine what you want your listener to remember. If it is important that the listener recall what you said, there is a good chance your intention was to inform. If, for example, you give your clients directions to your clinic, you obviously want your clients to remember the directions so the directions can be used to indicate the route to the clinic. The directions are informational.

Affirmation: Self and Stigma, Confidence and Doubt

If you tell your clients that you are working to graduate with your AuD, you are certainly passing along information, but your intention may not be simply to inform. You may intend to affirm yourself, clarify to your clients your status and value. At the beginning of your first session, you provide your clients with facts about yourself. An informational intention is clearly present, though you are also intending to affirm to your clients your ability to stand expertly before them. You are qualified to help them. In this situation, you are unquestionably affirming self.

Self-affirmation is, of course, present in every utterance, though it may not be the primary intention. The moment you begin speaking to someone, you are engaged in a form of self-affirmation. You are asking that another person pay attention; you are in effect stating that what you have to say is important and worth that person's time. There is a degree of self-affirmation in almost everything you say.

Your clients too are affirming self. When self-affirmation is their primary intention, an astute clinician recognizes the fact and recognizes their need to be acknowledged. In the movie *Avatar*, the alien Pandorans greet each other not with a "howdy" or a "what's new." Instead, they say, "I see you." This greeting is an expression of affirmation of the other individual. In a real sense, when your intention is self-affirmation, you are saying to your listener, "Please, see me."

Persuasion/Direction: Behavior and Practices

Often, what you want is for your listeners to make some kind of change, to believe that something is true, or simply to do what you tell them to do. If so, your intention is to persuade, convince, or direct. This intention is common enough in treatment, particularly when you are encouraging your clients to try a technique or to practice during the coming week. At other times, you want your clients to believe that they can improve. This intention, too, is persuasion.

Sydney might believe that she will always stutter on words with the initial /*n*/ phoneme. If your treatment stands a chance of success, you know that she must be at least open to the possibility that she can vocalize /*n*/ more fluently. You may use tools like reasoned argument ("Ninety percent of people in your position show significant improvement"), authority ("I have worked with others who have your disorder, and I have seen them do it. I think you can do it too."), good will ("Why not try?"), or trust ("I haven't led you astray so far, have I?"). You can appeal to the mind and the will. Whatever your specific tactic, if you are attempting to change thinking or to change behavior, your intention is persuasion/direction.

Feeling: Thoughts and Emotions, Willingness and Resistance

Feeling is the last of the five intentions. This intention is not one of thought but one of feeling, affect, or emotion. The clinician's goal in using the feeling intention is to reflect and validate what the client is feeling. Reflecting your clients' emotions or feelings is called empathy. For clients to make a change, they first need to accept that they feel a certain way. Your understanding and acceptance of their feelings is important, too.

Empathy: A process whereby someone feels and reflects another person's emotions or feelings.

In treatment sessions you may want to strengthen an emotion your clients already feel. You might be aware that Sydney feels comfortable with you, as if you are a member of her family or a good friend. Your counseling effort may be designed to make her even more comfortable with you by emphasizing that your values are similar to hers and that you have a sincere regard for Sydney and her improvement. Conversely, you may wish to diminish a feeling Sydney already has, like the fear of making a telephone call. In rational emotive behavior therapy (REBT), exposure is used to reduce a client's feeling about a situation or event.

Although it is certainly a challenge to strengthen your clients' emotional state, it is usually a lot harder to extinguish a negative feeling they may have. The feeling comes from somewhere, possibly a prior bad experience in treatment or an embarrassing moment when speaking in public. The challenge is daunting, because you cannot build confidence until you remove the fear and skepticism that has taken root. Once expunged, fear can be replaced by a feeling of security. If you can counter the negative feelings, you may then be able to build new feelings of confidence or comfort.

These five intentions, small talk, information, affirmation, persuasion/direction, and feeling, all arise at one time or another during therapy. It is important for you to recognize which of them is primary at any given time and to pursue the intention honestly. An understanding of the five intentions will help you shape your counseling methodology and achieve your counseling objectives.

Review of Key Points

- Counseling is no substitute for the work of a certified psychologist, and there will be times when you defer to those professionals. For you, counseling is a tool you can employ to help clients achieve their disorder-specific goals or deal with the negative impact the disorder may have on their quality of life. The counseling approach best suited to do the job is called solution-focused.
- A solution-focused approach to counseling includes goals that highlight client strengths and client investment. Short-term goals should establish progress to the ultimate long-term goal.
- The clinician is a collaborator, not dictator; a listener and clarifier, not judge and sentencer; a facilitator, not a director.
- Techniques like the miracle question get clients into the solution focus frame of reference. The miracle question is a useful tool to engage clients in visualizing their treatment goals and describing the benefits of achieving them.
- The Solution Cycle is a process with four distinct, nonlinear phases: learning, choosing, envisioning, and achieving. This cycle can be applied to your most comprehensive long-term goal and just as appropriately to a goal you might achieve during a single session.
- Learning is the most elastic of the four stages. It begins with your education. With clients, the learning phase includes developmental, medical, and demographic data, information about the client's issues, attitudes, emotions, motivations, wants, and needs. This phase includes observation, reflection, and listening.
- The second phase of the Solution Cycle involves identifying and targeting a network of people that will form the client's Circle of Power. (1) These people are on the client's side in the client's treatment efforts, and (2) each one is in a position to be a positive force in the client's progress.
- Allies consist of the client advocates, all those who may be invested in or affected by the client's progress in treatment, including parents, spouses, significant others, siblings, and caregivers. It may be necessary to counsel the advocates themselves to help them play a more constructive role in the client's efforts at improvement.
- The third stage of the Solution Cycle is to collaborate with your client to depict the changes your client will create, what is called the preferred future. This is the key stage of the Solution Cycle, where the solutions are actually framed.
- The solutions are always viewed in terms of goals. The ultimate goal, the end point that will be the result of the total treatment process, constitutes your client's and your mission. The accomplishment of that mission is the reason your client has come to you and engaged in treatment.
- Maintenance and generalization are essential to any definition of therapy success, but such success does not mean that treatment lasts a lifetime. What it means is that the result, the change, the vision of the preferred future, once accomplished, is an enduring reality.

- Counseling is never accidental. You counsel because you choose to counsel, you are determined to counsel. Counseling is intentional.
- You should be aware of the specific intention of your counseling communication. There are five reasons to speak, the Five Intentions of Communication: small talk, information sharing, self-affirmation, persuasion/direction, and feeling.
- Small talk can be an important and useful form of communication. You use small talk to get to know your client and to develop rapport.
- A message is informational when your primary intention is to inform, to relate something that is to be remembered.
- If you tell your clients you are a fully qualified audiologist, you are passing along information, but your intention may be to affirm yourself, clarify to your clients your status and value. There is a degree of self-affirmation in almost everything you say.
- Your client, too, is affirming self. When self-affirmation is the client's primary intention, an astute clinician recognizes the fact and recognizes the client's need to be acknowledged.
- When you want your listeners to make some kind of change, to believe that something is true, or simply to do what you tell them to do, your intention is to persuade, convince, or direct.
- Feeling is the last of the five intentions. The clinician's goal in using the feeling intention is not to motivate clients to change the way they behave, think, or believe, as in persuasion/direction; rather, it is to encourage change in the way clients feel.
- Although it is a challenge to strengthen a client's emotional state, it is usually a lot harder to extinguish a negative feeling your client may have.

Practical Exercises

List three issues that are within the scope of practice for a speech-language pathologist or audiologist.

List three issues that are outside the scope of practice for a speech-language pathologist or audiologist.

For the following scenarios indicate the client's primary communication intention (i.e., information, small talk, affirmation, persuasion/direction, or feeling).

1. "My new job is demanding a lot from me right now. I think it might be better if we changed therapy from twice a week to once a week for the time being."
2. "Johnny did really well this past week. He seemed focused on practicing his exercises, and I even saw him try to use his strategies when talking to his brother."
3. "You know, I used to be a pretty big deal in this town. I ran my own company … had a lot of people working for me. I made tons of speeches, even wrote articles for the local newspaper."

4. "The traffic was light today on my way into therapy. Maybe more people are on vacation than usual."

5. "Effort? I'm putting so much effort into this therapy. It's all I can do right now to get myself back on my feet. I'm so scared I won't ever be back to where I was before all of this happened. But I'm going to keep trying, keep giving that effort."

Journal Assignment 2: Miracle Question

In this journal assignment you will explore an area or aspect of your life that you may want to change or a challenge you face in your life. Now, answer the following question: "If while you are asleep a miracle happens and the aspect of your life you want to change has changed by the time you wake up the next morning but you don't know a miracle happened, how would you know that a miracle happened as you went about your day? How would the person closest to you know the miracle happened?"

REFERENCES

American Speech-Language-Hearing Association. (2007). *Scope of practice in speech-language pathology* [Scope of practice]. Rockville, MD: Author. Retrieved from http://www.asha.org/policy

Barone, O. R., & Tellis, C. M. (2008). *Your voice is your business.* San Diego, CA: Plural.

de Shazer, S. (1988). *Clues: Investigating solutions in brief therapy.* New York, NY: W. W. Norton.

de Shazer, S. (1990). *How to establish well-formed goals in solution-focused brief therapy* (The Solution-Focused Brief Therapy Audiotape Series). Milwaukee, WI: Brief Family Therapy Center.

de Shazer, S. (n.d.). *The miracle question.* Brief Family Therapy Center. Retrieved from http://www.netzwerk-ost.at/publikationen/pdf/miracle_question.pdf

de Shazer, S., & Berg, I. K. (1997). "What works?" Remarks on research aspects of solution-based therapy. *Journal of Family Therapy, 19,* 121–124.

de Shazer, S., Dolan, Y., Korman, H., Trepper, T., McCollum, E., & Berg, I. K. (2007). *More than miracles: The state of the art of solution-focused brief therapy.* New York, NY: Haworth Press.

Fast, J. (1970). *Body language.* New York, NY: Pocket Books.

Kaderavek, J. N., Laux, J. M., & Mills, N. H. (2004). A counseling training module for students in speech-language pathology training programs. *Contemporary Issues in Communication Science and Disorders, 31,* 153–161.

Phillips, D. T., & Mendel, L. L. (2008). Counseling training in communication disorders: A survey of clinical fellows. *Contemporary Issues in Communication Science and Disorders, 35,* 44–53.

Scheuerle, J. (1992). *Counseling in Speech-Language Pathology and Audiology.* New York, NY: Macmillan.

Schum, R. L. (1986). Counseling in speech and hearing practice. *National Student Speech and Hearing Association, 9,* 1–77.

Sklare, G. B. (2005). *Brief Counseling That Works: A Solution-Focused Approach for School Counselors and Administrators.* Thousand Oaks, CA: Corwin Press.

SECTION II

The Solution Cycle
Phase One: Learning: "Telling the Story"

Section Two focuses on Phase One of the Solution Cycle: Learning. This section includes Chapters 3, 4, and 5. These chapters discuss the use of skilled listening strategies to allow clients to tell their story. Chapter 3 is devoted to responsive listening. In this chapter you learn strategies to assess your client's message and then how to respond effectively. In Chapter 4, you examine the ways you can build positive rapport with your clients and with the important people in your clients' lives. You explore ways to establish a positive attitude and enduring motivation from the first impression through the ongoing relationship to make continual progress in treatment.

Chapter 5 moves from climate setting and attitudinal issues to the crucial task of gathering and transmitting information throughout treatment. From the initial interview, the completion of intake forms and surveys, and your first efforts at probing, questioning, and engaging your clients, you will be provided with guidelines for receiving and giving information that is accurate, complete, timely, and useful to you and to your clients.

CHAPTER 3

Responsive Listening

KEY TERMS

- Attending behaviors
- Blocks to listening
- Challenge
- Hidden messages

- Nonverbals
- Paraverbals
- Probing
- Reflecting emotion

- Responsive listening
- Restatement
- Summarizing
- Verbals

LEARNING OBJECTIVES

After reading this chapter, you will be able to:

- List Carl Rogers's three central components of listening
- List the three key attending behaviors
- Explain the difference between verbals, nonverbals, and paraverbals and their respective contributions to communication
- List and explain the different types of listening blocks
- Explain the two-part process of responsive listening
- Define methods to determine understanding of the speaker's message
- Name and define advanced counseling skills

The humanistic psychologist Carl Rogers expressed the strongest possible commitment to listening in his therapy. His concept of "unconditional positive regard" for the client meant that his chief mission in therapy was to comprehend the client on the client's terms (Kensit, 2000). He was not there to judge the utterances of the client but to listen. He was there to understand not only what his client was saying but also what the client was feeling. Achieving understanding at this level is a difficult and often daunting task, but it is the task of responsive listening.

Rogers wrote a great deal about listening. What he wrote cannot be distilled into a few sound bites. What we will discuss are the three activities central to his take on the listening process (Rogers & Farson, 1957). They encapsulate the challenge of responsive listening for the speech-language pathologist or audiologist engaged in counseling.

First and foremost, Rogers insisted that the listener be prepared to receive and process what he called the "total meaning" of the message being delivered. Rogers asserted that any speaker's message contains this total meaning, which comprises not only the speaker's words but the thoughts and feelings that the speaker embeds in the transmission. There are content and emotion in every transmission. In our terms, all transmissions can have a variety of intentions. Correctly interpreting the speaker's intentions ensures that you get the total meaning.

For Rogers, the second core activity of the responsive listener is to be especially sensitive to the feelings of the speaker. This kind of listening requires a response within you to the emotions that accompany the speaker's message, because these emotions are in fact an integral part of the message itself.

Third, you must pay attention to all the cues that the client is sending your way. That familiar phrase "pay attention" deserves a little scrutiny. Your attention is what is required, and attention involves notice, concentration, awareness, and consideration. Attention is what you pay as a listener, just as money is what you pay as a consumer. In return for money you receive goods or services from a seller. In return for your payment of attention, you receive an accurate message from a speaker. Listening is, at root, the art of making that payment, the art of paying attention.

Attending Behaviors

When you pay money, you exhibit certain behaviors. You may reach into your pocket, retrieve a wallet, and remove cash or a debit card. You may say, "Here you are," or "How much is that?" or provide another cue that you are shelling out some money. You could say you are displaying "money-paying behaviors," although it is hard to imagine why you would put it that way.

When you pay attention, you can be said to be exhibiting "attention-paying behaviors," a term that is usually shortened to "attending behaviors" (Ivey, D'Andrea, Ivey, & Simek-Morgan, 2002). People repeatedly mention a number of attending behaviors as indicators that they are listening to another person (Coakley & Wolvin, 1997). One of the most well recognized of these is eye contact (Riley, 2002).

If you want to indicate to your client that you are listening, you establish steady eye contact with the client. When listening is the clinician's primary activity, the clinician should frequently establish eye contact in conversations with clients. Although different cultures may have different norms, steady eye contact is generally expected of a listener (Bavelas, Coates, & Johnson, 2002). The accompanying facial expression should indicate interest and openness. That expression may vary according to the specific message being delivered, but it is always read as, "Yes, yes, tell me more; I really want to hear this."

Another frequently cited attending behavior is the affirmative head nod. Speakers tend to respond to encouraging nods as an indication to continue without interruption. The head nod may consist of a long, slow motion up and down. If so, the message is, "OK, I'm taking in what you are saying; I'm thinking about it, processing it." A brief nod says something like, "Go on, don't stop." A series of quick nods often indicates enthusiasm about what the listener is hearing. Because you do not wish to imply agreement at this point (you may not agree), you will make sure your face does not signal that you are of the same mind as the speaker, at least not yet. Take care as well that your head nods do not convey impatience or a desire for the speaker to "hurry up."

A third well-recognized attending behavior is, "uh-huh" (Coakley & Wolvin, 1997). What this reveals is that listeners are not expected to sit in total silence. It is natural and appreciated to use verbal cues to signal that you are listening. Aside from, "uh-huh," you can say, "mm-hmm," a quick "yes," or "right," or a simple "mm." You can also use expressions like, "really" or "is that right?" as long as they do not leave the impression that you are skeptical about what the speaker is saying. That would be a judgment, and judgments tend to discourage the speaker or cause the speaker to modify the message.

Your posture when listening also indicates your attitude about the speaker and the message. You want to sit (or stand) in a relatively erect position, perhaps leaning toward the speaker a bit, but not crowding the speaker. Leaning back, crossing arms or legs, sitting on your spine—these closed or slouchy postures will likely be interpreted as indifference or even a measure of hostility.

A lot of people recognize attending behaviors when they think about their "pretending behaviors." These are the behaviors they adopt when they do not actually intend to listen but want to convey that they are really, really interested and really, really listening. Sad, perhaps, but true, most of us have been in the position of having no desire to listen to Bob the Babbler who is determined to share his every opinion with us. Trapped, we fake it. The things we do and utter when faking listening almost always turn out to be the very behaviors we ought to exhibit to indicate that we are interested and that we are listening.

Sydney is a young, professional woman. In the following scenario, Sydney's speech-language pathologist is using a technique called the miracle question to determine factors in Sydney's life that are affected by her stuttering. In that conversation, a great deal of listening takes place. The clinician's attending behaviors are highlighted in brackets as they occur.

> **Clinician:** All right, Sydney. I want you to use your imagination, OK? [*Looks at Sydney; nods slightly.*]
>
> **Sydney:** OK.
>
> **Clinician:** You leave this session and go home. You still have the problem that brought you to me. You put your children to bed, watch some TV as usual, then turn in for the night. During the night a miracle happens while you are asleep. You don't know it has happened, because you are asleep, but because of the miracle your problem is completely solved.
>
> **Sydney:** The problem? My stutter?
>
> **Clinician:** [*Nods.*] Yes, the problem that brought you to this clinic.
>
> **Sydney:** So, next morning it is miraculously solved, and I don't know the miracle happened. Is that right? [*Clinician nods a few times throughout this and smiles slightly.*]

Attending behaviors: Actions, including facial expressions, visible movement, gestures, and sounds, that indicate to a speaker that a person is listening with focus and interest.

Clinician: Yes, exactly. Now here's the question. How do you discover that the miracle has happened? Remember, you have no idea there has been a miracle.

Sydney: OK, let me think. [*Pauses.*] [*During this pause, clinician leans back and relaxes a little to indicate that there is no hurry.*] I don't think I'd know during breakfast, because I hardly talk. I know how to avoid stuttering in front of my kids, so I wouldn't know then.

Clinician: [*Steady eye contact.*] Fine.

Sydney: [*Clinician continues steady eye contact. Inclines toward Sydney to indicate interest.*] I'd drive to work. Say hi to everyone; still don't know about the miracle. If I think I might stutter when greeting people, I just wave. [*Clinician says "mm-hmm."*] I call in my assistant to review the day's appointments. She shuts the door to my office. That's going to be my first indication.

Clinician: [*Questioning look.*] What happens?

Sydney: Sheri has been with me for fifteen years. When we're together alone, I usually stutter.

Clinician: Really? [*Tone is one of interest, not skepticism.*]

Sydney: Yeah. I am comfortable, so I don't compensate or replace words. I guess I'm unguarded.

Clinician: So, what happens? [*Slight shrug*] Imagine it.

Sydney: Sure. I begin to discuss my appointments. I always stutter on the *n* in *nine* when I say, "nine a.m."

Clinician: Always? [*Echo. A question, not a challenge.*]

Sydney: Yeah. *M*'s and *n*'s are my downfall. Now the miracle has happened, right? [*Clinician nods, says "mm-hmm."*] I say, "nine" perfectly, no hesitation, no seven-second *n* sound.

Clinician: Who notices first, you or Sheri? [*Clinician nods, uses palm-up hand gesture to point out Sydney and then an imaginary Sheri.*]

Sydney: Sheri. For sure.

Clinician: Sheri? [*Echo, said with questioning tone, not sarcasm or doubt.*]

Sydney: Yes. I won't know right away. I might even think I stuttered. I've actually been told I haven't stuttered when I was sure I had. So, it would be a while before I noticed anything different. Sheri would say something like, "Hey, good 'nine.'"

Clinician: [*Expectantly.*] Then?

Sydney: I'd say, "What?" She'd say, "You didn't stutter." When I talked more, she'd comment at some point, maybe after three or four sentences, that I wasn't stuttering. That's when I'd first notice.

Clinician: Interesting. [*Couple of brief head nods.*]

Sydney: Then I think I'd really begin to realize something had happened. [*Clinician says, "Yes."*] Even with Sheri, when I stutter, it's like a hand grabbing the word from inside my throat, holding it in a tight grip. [*Clinician says, "mm." Leans forward a bit.*] That hand is so real; I'd notice it wasn't there. At some point I'd notice. Then I'd talk, babble, say anything to check that it was really gone. That hand, that fist, that's my worst enemy. I'd just talk and talk, feeling it gone.

Clinician: [*With great interest in eyes and facial expression.*] Then?

Sydney: When I was convinced it was gone, it would take a long time to be convinced, I'd scream. It would be like getting out of prison when I'm serving a life sentence....

Clinician: [*Steady gaze, voice drops.*] Sydney, when you just said, "I'd scream," you made fists with both hands and sort of shook them.

Sydney: Did I?

Clinician: Yes. Like this. [*Clinician demonstrates.*]

Sydney: I'm not surprised. I have actually screamed out loud. [*Clinician nods empathetically.*]

The attending behaviors add substance and context to the written words in the scenario much as they provide reassurance to Sydney that the clinician is with her and listening.

What we are listening to, the message or transmission, can take the form of verbals, paraverbals, and nonverbals.

Verbals

Verbal comes from the Latin *verbum* and means, simply, "word." Verbals are words, bits of sound (for the hearing) that comprise what grammarians call a "part of speech," a noun, say, or an adjective, adverb, or preposition. You use words to formulate the meanings you wish to transmit to a listener, just as this chapter is using words to get its message across to you.

Your clients will certainly use verbals when speaking to you. A spoken message is made up primarily of words. When you listen successfully, you accurately hear the words spoken to you and you understand those words as the speaker does. How you accomplish this feat is pretty much the crux of the listening process.

Paraverbals and Nonverbals

As you may have noticed while considering attending behaviors, communicators transmit messages by a number of means, not just words. Paraverbals are sounds, sights, touches, and even smells that accompany words (*para-*: beside; *verbals*: the words) and possess or alter intended meaning (Pennycook, 1985).

There is a paraverbal component to every utterance, because words are always spoken with inflection, intonation, or prosody. The inflection conveys meaning or modifies the meaning of the words. Take the sentence, "I didn't say you were wrong."

Verbals: Words, phrases, and sentences used by a speaker.

Paraverbals: Sounds, sights, touches, and even smells that accompany words (*para-*: beside; *verbals*: the words) and possess or alter intended meaning. There is a paraverbal component to every utterance because words are always spoken with inflection, intonation, or prosody. The inflection conveys meaning or modifies the meaning of the words. A vocal sound by itself may be a paraverbal if it is not a word and yet conveys meaning.

If you accent one word, it means one thing. If you accent a different word, the meaning changes. Say the sentence this way: "I didn't say YOU were wrong."

You probably mean something like, "Someone was wrong, but I didn't say it was you." Now change the emphasis: "I didn't say you were WRONG."

That could mean, "I had a strong reaction to what you said, but you weren't necessarily incorrect."

Clearly, even a slight change in inflection can alter the meaning of the sentence, sometimes dramatically. To interpret correctly what your clients are attempting to convey, you must interpret both the words and the "music," the inflection and vocal emphases.

Other oral sounds can be considered paraverbals if they do not have a distinct meaning. For instance, "uh-uh" means "no" and is a verbal, while "mm" is ambiguous and can imply that the speaker is especially interested in what is being transmitted at that moment. The imprecise quality of "mm" makes it a paraverbal.

Other paraverbals are visual, like facial expressions, body language, and hand gestures. Hand gestures as used by people who are deaf constitute verbals, of course; the hearing use gestures mainly as paraverbals. You can get picky here and claim that a wave of the hand to a departing friend means "good-bye" and is a verbal, but such distinctions do not provide much useful guidance to clinicians doing counseling.

Paraverbals can accompany your messages; that is, paraverbals can occur while you are speaking. Paraverbals can also accompany your listening time. In the preceding dialogue with Sydney, you were exposed to attending behaviors, visuals and sounds the clinician produced while Sydney was speaking. The clinician nodded, changed posture, smiled, and uttered sounds like "mm-hmm" to indicate interest and a desire to hear more. It is safe to say that paraverbals are a pretty constant feature of interpersonal interaction, whether you are the speaker or the listener.

Nonverbals also enhance meaning. Like paraverbals, nonverbals are not words. Unlike paraverbals, nonverbals do not necessarily accompany specific words, phrases, or sentences you are uttering at a given moment.

There are many nonverbals, including visuals that accompany your transmission and serve to enhance the communication of a message. Nonverbals can include the position you take with your client—face to face versus catty-corner, say—and whether you are standing or sitting (**Figure 3-1**). For the clinician, positioning may indicate that a specific treatment technique is being adopted; sitting face to face with your client makes it easier to model a speech technique, but be aware that it may signal

> **Nonverbals:**
> Nonverbals enhance the meaning of what someone is expressing. They are not words, and they do not necessarily accompany specific words, phrases, or sentences being uttered at a given moment. There are many nonverbals, including visuals, that accompany a transmission and add meaningful elements to the communication of a message.

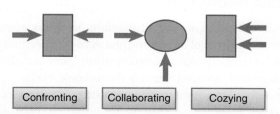

FIGURE 3-1 Positioning. Confronting position is when you sit face to face with a client. Collaborating position is similar to catty-corner. Cozying is often used for mirror work when client and clinician need to see each other for demonstration and observation purposes.

confrontation. Moving slightly to one side in this position may ease the oppositional atmosphere of this position. The collaborating position is similar to sitting catty-corner and can be an effective, comforting seating position. This position is often adopted during therapy sessions, especially when giving a standardized test during an evaluation. The clinician can maintain eye contact with the client and still see the stimulus board during testing.

The cozying position can be used with mirror work when both the clinician and client need to be seen in the mirror for demonstration and observation purposes. Take care when using the cozying position not to position yourself too close to the client. This position can cause discomfort or send the wrong signal if you are positioned too close to the client or are touching the client. You might not sit at all during your sessions. Assuming a position away from the client—in another room, perhaps—during portions of a hearing test is completely acceptable and necessary. Positioning and gestures are considered in more detail as various counseling techniques are explored.

The clothes you wear also send nonverbal messages. You may dress a specific way for therapy sessions. You may dress less formally during some nontherapy interactions with your clients. You might dress up to meet a young client's parents. The point is, what you wear communicates as a nonverbal, and, because your attire is a constant presence throughout an interaction, it can be powerful. The total communication environment, an important set of nonverbals, is discussed later in this section.

To summarize, if you are a hearing individual, you can transmit and listen to (or observe) messages at three levels. You use verbals, words, phrases, and sentences to speak to a listener. Verbals are items that can easily be written down. Accompanying the words are paraverbals. These can be sounds: inflections, intonations, prosody, or expressions like "uh-huh" or "mm-mm" that can convey meaning in a particular context. Paraverbals can also be visual, like facial expressions and hand gestures that augment meaning.

Nonverbals are a third category of transmission. They are not words but can also carry meaning beyond the words and the paraverbals accompanying words.

Verbals, Paraverbals, and Nonverbals

Verbals

- Words, phrases, and sentences you use to speak
- Can be easily written down

Paraverbals

- Accompany verbals
- Sounds, inflection, prosody, intonations, and expression that carry meaning
- Visuals like facial expression or hand gestures

Nonverbals

- Do not directly accompany verbals or paraverbals but also carry meaning
- Background music or silence
- Clothes or accessories you wear
- Seating position you adopt with respect to your client

Nonverbals include sounds like background music or the lack of sound (quiet can also send a message!). Some visuals are nonverbals, like the clothes you wear or the seating position you adopt in respect to the client.

The Communication Environment

The world around you and your clients constitutes a nonverbal and also sends messages. The clinic/therapy room will come to mean something to your clients when they enter it. Perhaps the room will give this signal: "I am about to do therapy; I need to get prepared." You want to secure a pleasant, private, nonthreatening space with comfortable chairs to hold extended sessions and interviews. Your clinic/therapy room and your office provide two different environments that make some forms of communication seem natural and others seem less appropriate. Whatever your choice of location, the environment should promote the purpose of the communication exchange.

You have an implicit (and often explicit) contract with your clients to observe confidentiality. The matters discussed or revealed during treatment must not be discussed or revealed anywhere else, except where clearly permitted by your clients. The space in which your sessions take place must reflect that contract. Doors are closed, and nearby voices cannot be heard. Rules about the use of electronic observation are clarified and observed.

Once you have positioned yourself and your client in a place and in a manner that serves your aims and respects privacy, the task remaining is to communicate, face to face, successfully. Responsive listening is your key to success.

> **Responsive listening:** A communication activity with a specific objective: to comprehend, evaluate, and retain what is being transmitted by a speaker.

The Responsive Listening Process

Listening, as audiologists and speech-language pathologists well know, is an involved physiological process, even when conceived as a purely audiological phenomenon. For our purposes, the physiology reveals a multistep series of activities in which a great deal happens in a very short period of time. From the moment the sounds produced by a speaker reach the ear, a complex task commences, a task requiring significant effort and sustained, intense activity. Listening takes focus and energy and is often anything but easy.

What we call the responsive listening process is a communication activity with a specific objective: to comprehend, evaluate, and retain what is being transmitted by a speaker (**Figure 3-2**). Effective counseling requires an exceptional level of listening competency. It is simply impossible to imagine a good counselor who is not also a good

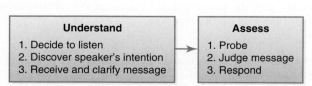

Understand	**Assess**
1. Decide to listen	1. Probe
2. Discover speaker's intention	2. Judge message
3. Receive and clarify message	3. Respond

FIGURE 3-2 The Listening Model. Once a message has been understood and verified by the listener, the message can be assessed and a response formulated.

listener. What "good listener" means is a person with competency at two tasks, achieving understanding of messages and assessing those messages. The Listening Model (Figure 3-2) lays out the steps within each of these two activities.

Achieving Understanding

Listening is a two-part process of first understanding and then assessing messages. That process begins with the decision to listen. As noted earlier, effective listening requires an investment from a listener. The listener must "pay attention," adopt attending behaviors that indicate a determined commitment to get the message being sent. Of course, you need to have a good reason to listen, and there are only two reasons to listen to anyone at any time. The first is self-interest. Some benefit accrues to you, the listener. It could be simply entertainment or important information for continuing therapy.

The second reason is concern for the other person. If you have enough regard for the speaker, that is a sufficient motive to listen. A father listens to his 2-year-old child, not for investment advice but because he loves his child. Listening is not only a way to get information; it is a way to indicate that you care and is, in fact, an act of caring. Once you have established that there is a good reason for you to listen, you must then decide to do so.

In the following scenario, Robert is talking about the experience of losing his voice. Is the clinician primarily listening or transmitting? How can you tell?

Clinician: Your intake form states that you lost your speaking voice about six weeks ago.

Robert: [*Hoarsely*] Five, maybe six, yes.

Clinician: Since that time, has your voice been just like it is now?

Robert: Pretty much. It's worse in the mornings.

Clinician: Is it ever better?

Robert: At times it comes back for a little bit.

Clinician: And then?

Robert: Well, just when I notice that I have a voice, it goes back, back to what you're hearing now.

Clinician: I see. So, it sounds like your voice comes back sometimes when you're not thinking about it.

Robert: Yes.

The Three Indicators That You Have Decided to Listen

- You ask yourself, what does this person want? What is the message?
- You remove all listening blocks and seek to create a quiet, agreeable communication environment.
- You concentrate on the other person's face, tone of voice, and words; you experience a strong desire to figure out what the person is trying to get across; that is, you pay attention.

Clinician: Then, when you think, "Hey, I have my voice back," it goes away again.

Robert: I guess that's right.

Clinician: What would you like to achieve here?

Robert: I'd like my voice back permanently, the way it was six weeks ago.

Clinician: You want the voice you had six weeks ago? Is that our goal, then?

Robert: Yeah, I suppose. Is it possible?

The clinician is doing plenty of talking, to be sure, but there is no doubt the clinician is primarily listening. Listening is not a silent activity. The clinician is doing what good listeners do, seeking understanding. She has decided to listen.

Even before a session, you are "deciding" to listen. As a clinician, you will want to prepare for therapy sessions by first removing possible blocks to listening and creating a suitable space for effective communication.

> **Blocks to listening:** Elements in the environment, in listeners, and in speakers that obstruct a person's willingness or ability to listen effectively.

Blocks to listening

There are three places where blocks to listening can occur: in the environment around the listener, in the speaker, and in the listener (see **Figure 3-3**). The "locations" may overlap, and you may get arguments about just where the block is, but defining the blocks is an important step to removing the blocks.

The first type of block, environmental blocks, consists of sights, sounds, and smells that tend to get in the way of listeners trying to listen. This kind of block is exemplified by the case of a young clinician, Jorge, who was set up for therapy in a preschool. His clients were 4- and 5-year-olds. He was to occupy a small space across a narrow corridor from a classroom. The classroom contained about 20 preschoolers scampering around their inexperienced teacher, a woman new to the profession.

The class emitted the loud sounds of children doing what children do in preschool. The sounds pierced an open lavatory door linking the classroom to the corridor. They traveled through to the room where Jorge was conducting treatment. They were distracting and made listening particularly difficult for Jorge, who was assessing and treating disfluencies, misarticulations, and voice issues among this young population.

Jorge recognized something every speech-language pathologist and audiologist should be aware of: treatment sessions must be carried out in a place that is private, quiet, and without distractions. He attempted to remove the environmental listening block in an exchange with the novice teacher. She was in the midst of a very active class and seemed to have her hands full when Jorge approached her.

Jorge: Hi.

Teacher: [*At the door of the classroom*] Yes?

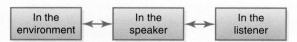

FIGURE 3-3 Blocks to Listening. Listening blocks can occur within the environment, within the speaker, and within the listener. Clinicians should minimize these blocks to the extent that they can.

Jorge: Sorry to bother you, but you know I am conducting therapy across the hall there.

Teacher: Yes. I know.

Jorge: Well, the noise from your classroom travels over to my room, and it's distracting me. [*Pause.*] Maybe you could shut the bathroom door going out into the hall.

Teacher: What?

Jorge: Maybe you could just close that bathroom door; it would muffle the noise. [*Pause.*] Of course, it's not a big deal if you can't. Uh, thanks.

Jorge did not think the conversation went perfectly, but he was a little surprised to learn that the teacher had, soon after that exchange, sought out Jorge's clinical supervisor and told her that Jorge said her classroom was "too noisy." She told the supervisor that she cannot change the way she conducts her class.

Although Jorge's block-removing strategy had drawbacks—a major one being that the classroom sounds did not subside—he did at least devise a strategy to remove the listening block. As a clinician, you may, like Jorge, spend many hours in a room working with clients. You are well advised to be proactive in creating an environment free of blocks like distracting sounds. Jorge's situation provides illustrations of other listening issues later in this chapter, but this section focuses on removing impediments to receiving messages from another person.

Other environmental blocks to effective listening include phone ring tones and text and email beeps. Visuals can also be blocks: an active computer screen, people passing by, lighting that is too dim or too bright, or other sights that may prove distracting. The key is to be aware of the potential blocks that exist in your vicinity and take steps to remove or mitigate them.

Blocks can arise inside you the listener. Hearing loss is an obvious one. More transient physical states can also disrupt listening. Perhaps you are tired because you did not sleep well or it is the end of the workday. Listening is hard work, and fatigue can make it impossible. These impediments have obvious solutions, but that does not mean you will opt for them. If you are tired, you should rest. If you have hearing loss, improve your situation by insisting on a quiet space, positioning yourself closer to the client, and exploring technologies such as amplification and hearing aids.

Your emotional state can also get in the way of listening. The young preschool teacher who met Jorge at the door of her active classroom may have been in an emotional condition that made it difficult for her to get his point. If you just conducted a difficult therapy session and emerged frazzled, take time to calm down before jumping into the next one. If you experience an emotional jolt like an illness in the family, consider rescheduling a clinical session. Even if you are overjoyed because you are about to travel to Maui for a vacation, you may not be in the right frame of mind to listen attentively.

Understanding your physical and emotional states requires a special form of listening. "Listen" to what your body and your feelings are telling you about your ability or willingness to listen. Do not fail to apply the same awareness to your clients as well. Similar physical or emotional listening blocks could be impeding their communication with you.

Listening Blocks

1. Blocks in the environment
   a. Sounds that could distract, such as ambient noises, cell phones, machinery
   b. Visuals, such as computer screens, passing people, windows
   c. Discomforts such as unpleasant odors, harsh temperature, cramped quarters, hard chair
2. Blocks in the listener
   a. Physical conditions such as hearing loss, tiredness
   b. Emotional conditions such as upset, sadness, anger, anticipation
   c. Attitudes, feelings, assumptions about the speaker or the situation
3. Blocks in the speaker
   a. Physical conditions such as an accent, speech disorder, or hyperactivity

Your assumptions and attitudes may be less obvious but very potent blocks to effective listening. A common example involves experienced clinicians who sometimes feel they have "heard it all." This attitude can make them less attentive to the client on the supposition that the client will have nothing new to say. You may make assumptions about young clients—their insights are not to be taken seriously because of their youth. Or you might devalue what an individual with Alzheimer's has to relate.

You can have attitudes about people based on irrelevant attributes like their gender, ethnicity, religion, height, weight, or disability, and these attitudes can create a block to open, effective listening. As a clinician, you learn to remove such blocks by treating every message as a unique opportunity to gain knowledge and appreciation of who that person really is and what that person is trying to get across to you.

To summarize, here is a schema of blocks to listening that you should survey before every important communication exchange. Remove them or ameliorate them; do what you can to reduce their power to get in your way as you communicate.

Once you have resolved to pay attention and have removed all the listening blocks you can, you have taken a major step toward a successful listening exchange. You have entered into the listening process; you have decided to listen.

Determining communication intentions

The next step is to uncover the intention of the speaker. Counseling is "intentional communication" and defined by the Five Intentions of a speaker. As a listener, you are tasked with discovering the intention of the person speaking to you, and it will be one (or more) of those Five Intentions: small talk, information sharing, self-affirmation, persuasion/direction, or feeling.

When you have pinpointed the speaker's most salient intention, you are in a position to understand the message and to know what is expected of you as a listener. If the intention is small talk, you are involved in chitchat, relationship building, climate setting, or just relaxing conversation. If information sharing is the aim, the speaker wants you to remember some things, to increase your knowledge base. When self-affirmation is the intention, the speaker wants you to take notice, recognize the value or status of the speaker. A speaker intending persuasion/direction wants to sway your thinking or get you to act in a certain way. A feeling intention implies a desire to affect your emotions.

When you suspect a particular intention, check it out. Say something similar to the following samples for each intention.

- Small talk: "Oh, you just want to chat about that TV show; OK."
- Information: "So, you are filling me in on what happened last week."
- Self-affirmation: "I can see why you are proud of that skill."
- Persuasion/direction: "I take it you want to try some new techniques in your therapy."
- Feeling: "You'd like me to have more confidence in you."

It is not always necessary to check the intention by referring to it explicitly, but it is important to determine the speaker's intention so that you can get the specific message correctly. Confusion can erupt if you are mistaken about an intention.

Sydney: [*Excitedly*] I met with Sheri in the office yesterday, and guess what? I used the technique you and I practiced, and I hardly stuttered at all! [*Feeling intention: "I want you to be elated about this."*]

Clinician: [*Matter of factly, taking notes*] OK, do you remember the number of times you did stutter during that interaction?

Sydney: Huh?

The clinician probably mistook Sydney's feeling intention for an information exchange. The clinician asked for additional data instead of acknowledging the emotional content of Sydney's disclosure. The session could have gone differently if the clinician had caught the feeling intention.

Sydney: [*Excitedly*] I met with Sheri in the office yesterday, and guess what? I used the technique you and I practiced, and I hardly stuttered at all! [*Feeling intention: "I want you to be elated about this."*]

Clinician: [*Looks right at Sydney, smiles broadly.*] You're kidding! Wow, I'd say you just took a big step forward. Congratulations!

Sydney: Thanks. I can't believe it!

Of course, uncovering the speaker's intention does not mean that the message has been fully transmitted. Sydney's feeling intention may be more complex than the clinician first realizes.

Sydney: [*Excitedly*] I met with Sheri in the office yesterday, and guess what? I used the technique you and I practiced, and I hardly stuttered at all! [*Feeling intention: "I want you to be elated about this."*]

Clinician: [*Looks right at Sydney, smiles broadly.*] You're kidding! Wow, I'd say you just took a big step forward. Congratulations!

Sydney: Thanks. I can't believe it! I bet you're surprised.

Clinician: A little, yes. Pleasantly surprised.

Sydney: I know you weren't sure I'd try out that technique we've been working on. But I did.

Clinician: Yeah, I wasn't sure, but I'm really glad you decided to try it.

At this point, the clinician confirms the strengthening of confidence in Sydney. As a listener, the clinician has received the full feeling message and is prepared to uncover a new intention. That is the way conversations go, from intention to intention. For example, Sydney may now use this expression of confidence (feeling) to propose a more challenging pace of improvement in the future (persuasion/direction). What is clear is that exposing the intention of the speaker is critical to receiving the message accurately and completely.

Once you have ascertained the intention of the speaker, you are in a position to decode the specific message. If you realize the intention is, say, informational, it is time to compile the information the speaker wishes to give out to you. If you become aware that persuasion is intended, you listen for the conclusions the speaker wants you to draw and you listen for the arguments supporting those conclusions. The same holds for the other intentions.

Indicating understanding: Parroting, echoing, restating, reflecting emotion, verifying message

The most critical point of the whole listening process occurs now. Here is where the message is received and clarified. No judgments—positive or negative—about the message are made during this phase. Your task is simply, or not so simply, to reflect to the speaker what you hear. There are several ways to do it. These include parroting, echoing, restating, reflecting emotion and verifying the message.

Parroting is the most straightforward way to reflect the message. It is called the "hearing test" because, like a parrot, you repeat exactly what you hear. This is a way to check that you heard the words correctly.

> **John:** Lisa, you said, "The project will be done by Friday"?
>
> **Lisa:** No, John, I said the project will NOT be done by Friday.
>
> **John:** Oh.

What this example shows is one of the benefits of parroting. You can check that what you thought you heard was exactly what was said. In the example, John obviously failed to hear the word *not* when he repeated what he thought Lisa had said. That little word changed the meaning considerably. Clinicians, like anyone else, are often hopeful of hearing certain thing from clients, and they may "hear" those things even when the clients did not say them.

Parroting is useful also for verifying instructions, directions, and other statements where the precise words are important. During the interview, you collect vital information about your client. Parroting can ensure that you got the client's age right, along with other data.

Clinicians can use parroting to allow the client to hear what the client just said, to allow the client to consider the words the client used.

> **Judy:** When my English teacher calls on me and then tries to rush me, I get so angry I want to walk up to her and slap her.

Clinician: You want to walk up to her and slap her.

Judy: Well, no, I never get physical. I just get this aggressive feeling in my stomach.

Another technique, echoing, is really a version of parroting. You might call it "the clarifying nudge." When you echo you repeat back a word or phrase the speaker uses; you are trying to get the speaker to clarify or say more. It is usually said with a "question mark" on the end, inviting a response.

Robert: I'd really prefer meeting once a week.

Clinician: Once a week? [*Echo*]

Robert: Yes, I think if we meet every two weeks, I'll kind of lose momentum in my improvement program.

The earlier example of Jorge, the young clinician who was bothered by the pre-schoolers in a nearby classroom, illustrates a possible use of echoing. The teacher Jorge confronted was affected by Jorge's use of the word *noise* to describe what was going on in her classroom. If she had echoed the word, it might have prevented a misunderstanding.

Jorge: Sorry to bother you, but you know I am conducting therapy across the hall there.

Teacher: Yes. I know.

Jorge: Well, the noise from your classroom travels over to my room. It's distracting. [*Pause.*] Maybe you could shut the bathroom door going out into the hall.

Teacher: Noise?

Jorge: I'm sorry. That was a really bad choice of words. I meant the sounds. I am finding it a little difficult to hear, since my room is so close to yours.

Whenever you hear a "red flag word," a word that causes you to have a negative reaction, echoing can clear the air by giving the speaker a chance to explain.

Restatement is a type of response that involves repeating what you heard in new words. By using different words from the ones the speaker used, you rephrase what the speaker said; you are interpreting the message and reflecting meaning. Parroting ensures only that you heard correctly; you might parrot a sentence in Chinese perfectly and not have the slightest idea what was meant because you do not understand Mandarin. When you restate the message, you indicate understanding because you are transmitting what you think the speaker meant.

Restatement can take several forms. Paraphrase is a word-by-word restatement that leaves nothing out. In the brief dialogue that follows, the clinician makes an attempt to paraphrase what Rayna is transmitting.

Rayna: I'd like to try a different approach in my therapy.

Clinician: You believe some new directions might give you a better return for the time you spend at the clinic.

Rayna: That's right.

> **Restatement:** Repeating what has been heard in words different from those used by the speaker. Ideally, restatement contains only the meaning transmitted, not implications or assessments of what has been said. Restatement can be a word-by-word paraphrase or a summary.

Watch out! When restating, do not add in your opinion or an inference. Take the example below.

Rayna: I'd like to try a different approach in my therapy.

Clinician: You think I'm on the wrong track in our therapy.

Rayna: No. I'd just like us to consider adding one or two new techniques.

The clinician did not paraphrase but added the inference that Rayna was dissatisfied with the clinician's work. A misstep like this could send the session in the wrong direction, with clinician on the defensive and Rayna trying to explain what she thought was a constructive suggestion. A restatement should be just that, a statement of what the listener thinks the speaker intended to relate. This occurs during the understand phase of the listening process.

A common listening mistake is jumping to conclusions, and that is what happened with the clinician and Rayna. In our language, jumping to conclusions means moving to the assess phase of listening too hastily, without completing the understand phase. You judge the message before you have comprehended it.

There are a lot of reasons you might jump to conclusions. If you tend to become defensive easily, you might, like Rayna's clinician, decode her suggestion as a criticism. If, on the other hand, you are subject to confirmation bias, you have the tendency to view what someone says as corroborating what you already think is true. In that case, you might reach the hasty decision that the speaker is in agreement with you (Oswald & Grosjean, 2004).

The following are statements followed by attempted restatements. All of the restatements have a problem. See whether you can detect what is wrong in each one.

1. John: This price is higher than I expected.
   Restatement: You doubt that you can afford to pay for this.
2. Misty: I was burned once when I agreed to put off my merit increase.
   Restatement: You don't like making sacrifices.
3. Mary: You are asking pretty personal questions.
   Restatement: You think I'm just being a busybody?
4. Sunil: I'm not sure I can afford this level of therapy.
   Restatement: Are you sure you can afford not to engage in this therapy?
5. Cara: I'm not sure I can afford this.
   Restatement: You think the price is too high.
6. Sam: That's the downright ugliest shirt I have ever seen.
   Restatement: You clearly dislike the appearance of my shirt.

In example 1, John says that the price is higher than he expected. Is "You doubt that you can afford to pay for this" a restatement of that sentiment? No, John is saying nothing at all about his ability to pay, just that the price is more than he expected.

In example 2, Misty said she was burned once when she agreed to put off a merit increase. The "restatement" accuses her of not liking to make sacrifices and thus compounds the error of a non-restatement with a personal attack.

Speaking of personal, in example 3, Mary says, "You are asking pretty personal questions." The "restatement" states something Mary never implied, that the speaker is being a busybody. Although it is possible Mary thinks this, it is just as likely that she is a little uncomfortable with the questions but thinks they are entirely appropriate.

In example 4, Sunil says he is not sure he can afford the proposed level of therapy. The response, "Are you sure you can afford not to engage in this therapy?" is not a surprising reaction, but it is not a restatement. In fact, it is a sudden lurch into a persuasive discourse, an indication that listening has actually ended.

In example 5, Cara claims she is not sure she can afford something. "You think the price is too high" is not an accurate restatement. Cara may think the price is entirely reasonable; she just can't afford it.

In the final example, Sam says, "That's the downright ugliest shirt I have ever seen." The response, "You clearly dislike the appearance of my shirt," is for once a pretty good restatement of Sam's sentiment.

Here are the other statements followed by more effective attempts at restatements. You can see whether you can come up with another restatement for each, perhaps a better one.

1. John: This price is higher than I expected.
   Restatement: You didn't anticipate paying so much.
2. Misty: I was burned once when I agreed to put off my merit increase.
   Restatement: In the past, you had a bad experience when you went along with a delay in your merit increase.
3. Mary: You are asking pretty personal questions.
   Restatement: I am asking questions about matters you usually keep to yourself.
4. Sunil: I'm not sure I can afford this level of therapy.
   Restatement: You are uncertain whether you can safely put out the money this therapy is going to cost. (This also works for example 5.)

Reflecting emotion takes you beyond the interpretation of the meaning of what is being said. Reflecting the emotion in a message is a critically important tool to use as you are working to understand the speaker. If a speaker is showing definite emotion in voice or gesture, it is often wise to let the speaker know that you are aware of it and that you want to grasp the emotion fully.

Rayna: [*Raising pitch and intensity, very animated*] I don't want to practice these techniques at school right now.

Clinician: I can see you feel strongly about that.

Rayna: Very.

A change in pitch and intensity can signal a different emotion, even when the same words are used.

Rayna: [*Lowers pitch and intensity, quiver in voice*] I don't want to practice these techniques at school right now.

> **Reflecting emotion:** Using verbals or paraverbals to clarify a feeling that the listener has received from the speaker.

Clinician: The prospect of practicing at school seems to make you a little nervous.

Rayna: Well, yeah. In front of all my friends.

Later sections of this chapter discuss in detail various techniques for reflecting and assessing emotions in the speaker.

Verifying the message is the culmination of the understand phase of listening. After sufficient restatement, verify; that is, check back with the speaker to see that you have received the message accurately and completely. You may use a number of statements or questions to verify understanding of the message.

Once you have verified that your understanding of the message is the same as the speaker's (and not before!), you are in a position to assess what you have heard. Assessment is as much a part of the listening process as understanding. When you assess the message, you take some position on what the speaker has transmitted; you are affected in some way, however small, by this message.

Assessing Messages

Figuring out what you think about what you hear is the act of assessing. There are three steps in assessment of messages: (1) probing to get the speaker's take on the speaker's own message; (2) judging the message to determine what you think about the message and what you are going to do or not do about it; (3) responding to the speaker to transmit your thoughts and feelings about the message.

Probing the speaker occurs right after the understand phase is done, while you are preparing to evaluate what you have heard. At this point you are seeking the speaker's take on what the speaker has said to you. Here are typical probing expressions.

Listener: I see what you're saying. What are your thoughts on this?

Listener: Could you tell me what you think are a few of the pros and cons?

Listener: You've obviously given this a lot of thought. Why do you think it's a good idea?

In many cases, you will refer to the specific points that came out during the understand phase.

Listener: OK, so you want more frequent therapy sessions. What do you see as the benefits and drawbacks of going that route?

Probing should never be rushed, and you do not need to be pushy if the speaker has no more to add. The important thing to remember is to maintain neutrality about

Verifying Statements and Questions

- Is that what you meant?
- I think I've got you now [wait for confirmation].
- Before going on, I want to be clear about what you are telling me.
- Did I miss anything?
- I have a few questions, but, first, do I understand your point correctly?

your own evaluation of the message. Up to this point, throughout the listening process, you have been careful not to reveal whether you approve or disapprove of what the speaker is offering. You are seeking the understanding necessary to determine where you stand. Probing the speaker is the final nonjudgmental interaction before you stop being nonjudgmental.

In fact, after you finish your probing questions, you judge the message. This step may be as simple as, "I agree completely; let's go for it!" or "I am not willing to go along with this." In those instances, you have judged and responded and pretty much completed the listening exchange. Chances are, though, that judging the message will result in the need for you to explain your evaluation, and you may get into a back-and-forth on the validity of your conclusions. At the end of this step, you have determined what you think of the message and are prepared to give your response to the speaker.

Up to this point you have been responding to the speaker throughout the entire exchange. That is why this process is called responsive listening. The exchange ends when you, the listener, give your ultimate response to the message you have heard.

Responding properly at the completion of the process is the listener's responsibility, but a poor response is often worse than no response at all. Here are some characteristics of a poor response.

1. It is based on something other than the speaker's intended message, for example:
   - The "response" was really something the listener wanted to say all along, no matter what the speaker was trying to get across. You can fall into this pattern when you enter a session with an agenda you think is important. You listen to your client with seeming attention, all the way through the listening process. Then, just when the client expects your reaction to what they have said, you shift suddenly and bring up your own agenda item.
   - The "response" is really an implication of the speaker's message or an unrelated thought triggered by the speaker's message. Sydney may be making a point about a difficulty she is having with a particular technique. While making the point, she mentions a colleague, Mike, who seems unreceptive to what she is doing when using the technique. You listen with attention, and then, at the point when your response is expected, you say, "So, is Mike someone you interact with a lot? Do you like him?" If Sydney reacts with confusion or a little frustration, she may be indicating that you have gone off-topic.

Characteristics of a Good Response

- It is based on the intention of the speaker's message.
- It uses the judgments made during the assess phase of listening.
- It is honest and direct.
- It is expressed in terms of future change, what the listener and speaker will do or think differently as a result of the message.
- It states next steps, a later interaction with the speaker.

2. The response fails to use judgments made during the assess phase. Below are two examples.
   - The listener rejects a request despite a seemingly good assessment of its merits. You may think it is a good idea to be agreeable throughout the listening process, but if you end up disagreeing with the speaker, you can cause unnecessary tension when you finally respond. When you do respond, the response should be consistent with the tone of the judgments you made just before. The judge step is just that: your opportunity to evaluate the message you heard. By the time you respond, the speaker should be well prepared to hear exactly what you think of the transmission.
   - The listener seems to be empathetic to the feeling of the speaker but then says that the speaker is reacting too strongly. When you reflect emotion, expressing empathy is usually a positive thing. Once you do so, however, you should not then express surprise at the intensity of the emotion. The whole point of empathy is to indicate that you "get it," that you are fully aware of the emotion of the speaker. Surprise or disapproval is misplaced at that point.
3. It is dishonest or evasive. You undermine all your efforts at listening by not being straightforward with your ultimate response. Do not pretend the speaker's question or issue was not heard. Do not talk around the issue. Evasiveness now is doubly harmful because you have given the strong impression that you favor an open and honest exchange.
4. Vague assurances are given about future change. Avoid phrases like, "Yes, something needs to be done," with no commitment to do anything. The response is the moment to reveal your intended actions, not hide those intentions.
5. It fails to make the next step explicit. Never leave a discussion with a statement like, "We'll have to take this under advisement," and never fail to set a time for a future meeting or interaction. Always use this step to make clear your intended action or lack of action in response to what you have heard.

Responding in the Counseling Setting

For you as a clinician, the response can be a delicate moment in an exchange, particularly when you are counseling. You have listened with care and concern and without bias, and you must now reveal your thinking. This should be done with the same regard for the client, but this is not the time to equivocate or hedge, particularly if you have reached a firm conclusion. If you concur with your client, the conversation will likely go smoothly. The thing is, you will not always concur.

Your client will be disappointed if you end up disagreeing or doing something other than what the client wants, but you will have this going for you: you listened. You heard the client out. You did not dismiss the client's thoughts as out of hand. You have made it clear that you welcome the client's ideas and thoughts; it is just that, on this occasion, you did not see eye to eye. Responding in a way that safeguards the rapport you have built with the client is probably more of an art than a science, but it is an art worth considering and working at.

Points to Remember about the Listening Process

- Listening begins with the decision to listen. You must pay attention, get involved with the speaker, set your concerns aside, focus your "listening energy" on the sender.
- The Understand Phase is a process of discovery—what is this person trying to get across to me?
- No matter what the message, the speaker has always invested at least a little "ego." The speaker has become vulnerable in choosing to transmit, because you can reject.
- There is often, if not always, some emotional content in a message. The very motivation a speaker has to transmit to you implies some emotion.
- The Understand Phase must be separated from the Assess Phase by the listener. That way, you can be sure you have gotten the message before you judge it.
- A response of some kind is almost always expected of a listener.

The next section discusses how to react to feeling messages, but here, first, is a summary of the listening points emphasized so far.

Responding to Emotion

Feeling messages are often the most important messages you receive during clinical sessions. They may come forth during the judge phase of listening, when you respond to something the client has offered, or they may emerge suddenly and unexpectedly, causing you to decide to engage in counseling on the spot.

Discerning Emotional States

It has been mentioned that part of the understand phase of the listening process is to recognize a feeling message and indicate to the speaker that you are aware of it. You may then want to signal that you wish to understand the emotion more fully. When a client like Sydney is exhibiting emotion, there are several possibilities.

1. Sydney may know exactly what the emotion is and why she is feeling it and have no qualms about letting you know all about it.

    Clinician: So, you are angry and frustrated about the fact that you stutter because you are used to having control and you cannot control your stuttering. Also, you believe your stuttering is impeding your career advancement, and that adds to your anger and your frustration.

    Sydney: That's right.

2. Sydney may know the emotion but not the cause.

    Sydney: I get so angry I could scream. Sometimes I do scream. I don't know why, though. I've stuttered my whole life. I'm used to it.

3. She may not know how strongly she feels.

    Clinician: You know you clenched your fists when you said that. What are you feeling?

    Sydney: I did? I clenched my fists? Well, I was a little bit upset maybe, but it's no big deal.

4. She may know more than she is willing to tell you.

> **Sydney:** I know I clenched my fists. I know I have emotions. I just don't want to talk about them.

How important is it for you and Sydney to identify her emotions and clarify why they exist? Emotions can have more or less relevance to what you are trying to accomplish through therapy, but if she has intense and lasting emotions about the issue you are addressing, there is a good chance the emotions will have a significant effect on the process and the outcomes.

Possible Responses to Emotion

How you respond depends in large measure on your beliefs about the role Sydney's emotions are likely to play in her clinical progress. Your choices are varied.

Any direction you take can be problematic. In the best case, you discern the emotions and their causes accurately and use that information to the advantage of the counseling and therapy processes. Discussing feelings always carries some risk, but so does avoiding them.

Responding with Empathy

One way to minimize risk is to respond with empathy. Empathy is the quality of "feeling with," the ability to capture your client's emotion in your own feeling set. When you respond with empathy, you indicate to the client that you understand or may have even had similar feelings to what the client is experiencing. One way to demonstrate empathy is to recount an experience that parallels the client's.

> **Clinician:** I never had a disfluency, but I was once denied a promotion because I never did an audiology internship. That was infuriating because audiology wasn't even required in the position.

> **Sydney:** So, you know what it's like to be passed over for no good reason.

Another way you can show empathy is by describing the client's emotion compellingly.

> **Sydney:** So, do you have any idea what it's like to have this whole speech in your head, and you know you might not be able to get the first two words out because you stutter?

> **Clinician:** It's like that nightmare where you are trying to get to a place and it keeps moving farther and farther away.

> **Sydney:** Exactly. So frustrating.

Some Responses to Emotion

- You can ignore the emotion and move on.
- You can ask about the emotion and discuss it if Sydney wishes to do so.
- You can ask about the emotion and move on if Sydney resists discussing it.
- You can ask about the emotion and, if Sydney resists discussing it, try to convince her that she should discuss it.

An obvious caution is to take care you do not miss the mark. You do not want Sydney to tell you that your example or description is nothing like the feeling she is having. Responding with empathy is not guessing. It can occur when you are actually tuned in to the emotion the client is expressing. Empathy is not pity or compassion, either. It is "feeling with" not "feeling for." Remember, when a client like Sydney gets upset or angry, she may naturally start looking for someone to be angry at—and you are only a couple of feet away. Although clients may sometimes direct their emotion at you, caring and empathetic listening will usually improve the situation.

Advanced Counseling Skills

Dealing with client emotions that are directed at you requires a high level of listening competence. In fact, many advanced listening skills are also advanced counseling skills. They include (1) summarizing and probing; (2) challenging; (3) extracting hidden meaning; and (4) overcoming reluctance and resistance.

Summarizing and Probing

Summarizing is a skill akin to paraphrasing. When you paraphrase, you perform a word-by-word restatement. When you summarize, you select the highlights or create an outline of what the client has said.

Summarizing is called for in several situations. During a lengthy interaction with the client, it can help the communication process to pause, go back, and recap the main points that have been made, either by you or by the client. Good listeners recap to make sure that important items are not lost and to organize the message received from the client. At the end of a session, it is highly recommended that you summarize what happened, creating bullet points that capture the highlights.

> **Summarizing:** Restating the highlights or main points that were expressed by a speaker.

Challenging

Probing has already been identified as integral to the listening process. This skill involves the use of questions and invitations to clients to expand on what they have told you, to disclose more of what is going on in their mind and in their feelings.

You can go beyond probing at times and challenge your clients, reframe their narrative, suggest that there is more to the story than they have thus far revealed. The choice to challenge is made when you are convinced it is worth the risk. Challenges are usually couched as "I-statements," not accusations.

> **Probing:** A listening technique that begins the assessing phase of listening, when the listener makes judgments about what has been heard. Probing seeks the speaker's take or judgment on what the speaker has transmitted.

Clinician: Sydney, I believe that is not all that happened. (I-statement)

Clinician: Sydney, you are wrong. Something else happened, didn't it? (Accusation)

Facts as well as opinions and emotions can be subject to challenge.

Clinician: Sydney, I believe that is not all that happened. (Challenging fact)

Clinician: I am not sure you believe she wanted to cause you harm. (Challenging opinion)

Clinician: Sydney, I get the impression you feel much more strongly about this than you are admitting. (Challenging emotion)

> **Challenge:** An advanced communication technique that asks clients to take a new direction, rethink, or "refeel" what they have just expressed.

Challenging goes beyond probing, beyond a request that Sydney expand on what she has said. When you challenge Sydney, you are asking her to take a new direction, rethink, or "re-feel." It is an advanced technique, and it will prove useful in a variety of contexts.

Extracting the Hidden Message

> **Hidden messages:** An unexpressed notion or thought that is contained in the words that a person chooses to utter, the person's prosody or tone of voice, facial expressions, gestures, or body language.

Hidden messages are often tucked away in the words that are chosen, the prosody or tone of voice, facial expressions, gestures, or body language. Verbals and paraverbals can conceal slivers of communication that, if exposed, may shed light on matters of importance. You extract a hidden message when you are attentive to the verbals and paraverbals and are willing to explore them with your clients. Sydney has already provided an example of extraction of hidden meaning.

Sydney: When I was convinced my stutter was gone, it would take a long time to be convinced, I'd scream. It would be like getting out of prison when I'm serving a life sentence ...

Clinician: Sydney, when you just said, "I'd scream," you stopped for a moment and looked toward the window.

Sydney: Did I?

Clinician: Yes. Like this. [*Clinician demonstrates.*]

Sydney: I'm guess I'm not too surprised. I was thinking of a time when I actually screamed out loud.

Clinician: When you were alone, like in your room?

Sydney: No, I was in the office. I screamed in the office. The senior VP asked me a question and I couldn't get the word out. I just sat there forever. Then I screamed.

Clinician: That was ...

Sydney: Incredibly embarrassing. She said let's take a little break. We never mentioned it again.

The action of Sydney glancing out the window caught the clinician's attention, and the clinician asked about it. A lot was disclosed, embedded in that glance. The technique involves alertness to words or paraverbals that seem out of sync or an addition to what is being explicitly stated. You then ask about what you have observed. You will not always uncover a hidden meaning, but when you do, your client and you just might move closer to a breakthrough. Responsive listening is usually crucial to those positive outcomes.

Listening to Clients with Specific Communication Needs

The term *responsive listening* is especially apt when applied to your clients with specific communication needs. You must respond not only to the messages being sent but also to the unique manner in which those messages are formulated and transmitted by clients with limited access to communication skills. Clients with aphasia, for example, may be unable to retrieve the words that would express their intended meaning. They may resort to paraverbals as their primary mode of communication, or they may require significant amounts of time get across even the simplest messages.

Clients who are deaf or hard of hearing communicate differently, and you work under different assumptions and expectations in any exchange with these clients. Sign language may be your primary communication medium, in which case verbals are visual, and, of course, fluency in sign is your best asset. Clients with cochlear implants present other challenges.

If clients come to you with intellectual or cognitive disorders, the listening process must be adapted to their circumstances and abilities. Although the general principles of effective responsive listening always apply, specific cases will require sometimes significant modifications on your part to receive your clients' intended messages accurately.

Overcoming Reluctance and Resistance

When you practice responsive listening, you will sometimes face the challenge of overcoming your clients' reluctance to tell their full story, their resistance to the fact that there is someone actually listening intently to what they have to say. Resistance can occur with clients who have special needs and those who do not. Resistance can be a feature of clients of almost any age or capacity. Overcoming their reluctance and resistance often requires the cultivation of the kind of openness and respect that can be achieved only by long-term relationship building and a careful, caring willingness to persist in listening.

What your clients choose to reveal to you depends on their comfort level with you, their deep conviction that you are someone they can talk to, someone who not only listens but uses what is learned only in their best interest. Interpersonal communication then becomes a supreme act of mutual trust. Your clients trust you with secrets they may have shared with no one else, with fears that may have kept them from moving forward, and with hopes that may have been inspired by the trust you have placed in them.

Review of Key Points

- Carl Rogers focused on three core listening activities: (1) he insisted that the listener be prepared to receive and process what he called the "total meaning," (2) the responsive listener is to be especially sensitive to the feelings of the speaker, and (3) must pay attention to all the cues that the client is sending.
- Attending behaviors let the speaker know you are listening. These include steady eye contact with the client, the affirmative head nod, and expressions like "uh-huh." Posture and position also can indicate listening.
- What we are listening to can take the form of verbals or words, paraverbals or sights and sounds accompanying the words, and nonverbals.
- Responsive listening is a two-part process of first understanding, and then assessing messages.
- Listening begins with the decision to listen.
- There are only two reasons to listen: self-interest and regard for the other person.
- Blocks to listening can occur in three places: in the environment around the listener, in the speaker, and in the listener. These should be removed before continuing as a listener.
- After deciding to listen, you must uncover the intention of the speaker. The Five Intentions are small talk, information sharing, self-affirmation, persuasion/direction, and feeling.
- After you ascertain the speaker's intention, you decode and receive the specific message, the most critical point of the whole listening process. Key skills include parroting, echoing, restating, and reflecting emotion. Once you have verified that the message has been accurately received, the understand phase is complete. Only now can you move to the assess phase.
- Figuring out what you think about what you hear is the three-step act of assessing: (1) probing to get the speaker's take on the speaker's own message; (2) judging the message to determine what you think about the message and what you are going to do or not do about it; (3) responding to the speaker.
- Feeling messages are often the most important messages you receive during treatment sessions. When a client exhibits emotion, there are several possibilities and you have varied options in responding. You must determine how important it is to your aims for your clients to name their emotions and clarify why they exist.
- Empathy is the quality of "feeling with," the ability to capture your client's emotion in your own feeling set. When you respond with basic empathy, you indicate to the client that you too have had feelings similar to what the client is experiencing.
- Responding with empathy is not guessing. It is not pity or compassion, either. It is "feeling with," not "feeling for."
- Many advanced listening skills are also advanced counseling skills, including (1) summarizing and probing; (2) challenging; (3) extracting hidden meaning; (4) overcoming reluctance and resistance.

- What your clients choose to reveal to you depends on their comfort level with you and their deep conviction that you are someone they can talk to, someone who not only listens but uses what is learned only in their best interest. Interpersonal communication then becomes a supreme act of mutual trust.

Practical Exercises

For each of the following scenarios, identify the client's primary **communication intent** (information, small talk, self-affirmation, persuasion/direction, emotion). Then identify the client's **important experiences**, **paraverbals**, and **feelings or emotions**. Then, practice writing each of **your responses** that indicate understanding.

1. A 16-year-old male is meeting with his speech-language pathologist. He has had therapy for many years for his stuttering and believes that he doesn't need to come for sessions anymore. He says, "I just don't want to come anymore [*strumming his fingers on the table*]. My mom thinks I need to be here, but I think I've learned everything I need to learn. I know my techniques; I just have to do them [*pauses*]. I want to spend my time playing basketball and this therapy just takes up too much of my time [*voice starts to shake a little*]. I'm fine really. I think I just need a break."

2. A father of a child with autism is meeting with the speech-language pathologist for the first time. He says, "We just met with the developmental pediatrician and she told us that our child definitely shows signs of having autism. At first I didn't know what to do or what to say. I was really hoping for a different answer [*wringing his hands*]. Now, I'm ready to face this challenge. That's why we've brought our son to you [*looking straight at the speech-language pathologist*]. I want my son to have all the therapy he can get."

3. A woman is recovering from a car accident and is in a rehabilitation unit. She is a week into a traumatic brain injury rehabilitation program that could go on for several months. She is talking to her speech-language pathologist. "You told me this was going to be hard, and I thought that I had prepared myself for it [*looking down*]. I thought I had the courage it takes, but now I don't think I have it in me [*voice cracks*]. The smallest tasks take so much effort! I just keep breaking down and crying [*holding her hands to her face*]. I don't think I can do it."

REFERENCES

Bavelas, J. B., Coates, L., & Johnson, T. (2002). Listener responses as a collaborative process: The role of eye gaze. *Journal of Communication, 52*(3), 566–580.

Coakley, C., & Wolvin, A. (1997). Listening in the educational environment. In M. Purdy & D. Borisoff (Eds.) *Listening in everyday life: A personal and professional approach* (2nd ed., p. 187). Lanham, MD: University Press of America.

Ivey, A. E., D'Andrea, M. D., Ivey, M. B., & Simek-Morgan, L. (2002). *Theories of counseling and psychotherapy.* Boston, MA: Allyn and Bacon.

Kensit, D. (2000). Rogerian theory: A critique of the effectiveness of pure client-centered therapy. *Counseling Psychology Quarterly, 13*(4), 345–351.

Oswald, M. E., & Grosjean, S. (2004). Confirmation bias. In R. F. Pohl (Ed.), *Cognitive illusions: A handbook on fallacies and biases in thinking, judgment and memory* (pp. 79–96). New York, NY: Psychology Press.

Pennycook, A. (1985). Actions speak louder than words: Paralanguage, communication, and education. *TESOL Quarterly, 19*(2).

Riley, J. (2002). Counseling: An approach for speech-language pathologists. *Contemporary Issues in Communication Science and Disorders, 29*, 6–16.

Rogers, C., & Farson, R. E. (1957). *Active listening*. Chicago, IL: Industrial Relations Center of the University of Chicago.

CHAPTER 4

Small Talk: Climate, Attitudes, and Motivations

KEY TERMS

- Apathy
- Boredom
- Circle of Power
- Cultural awareness
- Cultural literacy
- Dread
- Frustration
- Goals
- Growth
- Long-term goals
- Motivation
- Obsession
- Ownership
- Professionalism
- Purpose
- Rapport
- Reputation
- Short-term goals
- Small talk

LEARNING OBJECTIVES

After reading this chapter, you will be able to:

- Explain the three ways to establish professionalism
- Explain the importance of establishing rapport with a client
- List the key steps to establish a firm handshake
- List and explain the three necessary features in building client motivation

Most experts will tell you that a solution will be effective only if the problem is properly identified and defined. No matter how obvious your clients' issues seem to be—unilateral hearing loss, stuttering, cleft palate—the problem is almost always more complex than it seems at first. This complexity results mainly from the fact that no two clients are identical. No two clients are facing the same exact issues in the same way.

For those reasons, the first phase in understanding problems and reaching solutions is learning, a phase that involves a lot more than retrieving a list of symptoms, disorders, and syndromes (Ivey, Ivey, & Zalaquett, 2010). You need to learn not only the issues challenging your clients but also what sequence of events brought them to you and why. You need to hear their stories. That means your clients must tell you their stories (Egan, 2007; Holland, Neimeyer, & Currier, 2007; Monk, Winslade, Crocket, & Epston, 1997). In a real sense, they must open their lives to you. Learning means getting your clients' stories, getting clients to tell them. Success in the learning phase depends on the quality of the relationship between you and the individual client. This chapter is devoted to achieving progress in the learning phase of the Solution Cycle.

The Clinician–Client Relationship

Throughout the therapy process, you develop some sort of relationship with your clients. With some you will hit it off immediately and encounter few glitches along the way. With others you will experience negativity and frustration. Your relationships with your clients do not remain static; they grow and change, and, if cultivated with care, those changes will be infused with growing trust, responsiveness, and respect. In developing relationships with your clients, you also develop relationships with your clients' advocates and potentially their adversaries. Most of the suggestions made throughout this chapter that refer specifically to clients are applicable to individuals within their Circle of Power, support network, and even those outside that circle.

Professional Standing

Before your clients even meet you, they become aware of your professional standing, and that awareness shapes their view of you and their expectations of you. If you are a student clinician, you cannot anticipate that their regard for you will be the same as it is for the clinical director of your institution or your supervisors, at least at the beginning.

Your professional standing is important because it is, in effect, your reputation, a prized possession that you must safeguard and enhance with each interaction. You may discover that difficulties in counseling can be traced to your clients' initial perceptions about you. Your professional standing is always a significant element of those perceptions. Your reputation is built on your credentials and the things people say about you as a professional. In the following scenario, imagine you are the client and determine what impact this discourse would have on the clinician's professional standing with Kaching, the client.

Clinical Director: Kaching, let me introduce you to your student clinician, Juan. Juan has been with us for—how many years, Juan?

Juan: Three in May.

Clinical Director: Three? Seems like forever. But this is his first semester in clinic. Is Kaching, what, your second client?

Juan: No …well, I …

Clinical Director: Well, never mind. I'm sure he'll be just fine.

This kind of off-the-cuff introduction could cause Kaching to begin having doubts about the services Juan is capable of providing. The clinical director probably meant no harm, but harm could well have resulted from the note of disparagement in her

---

Circle of Power: The people a person depends on or seeks out to enhance that person's effectiveness at whatever task or project the person is doing or contemplating; an alliance base.

Reputation: The regard people have for another because of the other's status, moral standing, expertise, education, wisdom, accomplishments, or any combination of these. One's good name.

introduction of Juan. If Juan is subjected to an introduction like that, he may want to visit with his clinical director and suggest a more positive approach in future meetings with new clients. The following scenario illustrates an improved introduction.

Clinical Director: Kaching, let me introduce you to your student clinician, Juan Fiuza. Juan has been with us for—how many years, Juan?

Clinician: Three in May.

Clinical Director: Yes, I've gotten to know Juan well. He is especially knowledgeable of situations like yours, Kaching.

Juan: Hello, Kaching. Welcome to Steckly Clinic. [*Offers hand.*]

Kaching: Hi. [*Shakes clinician's hand.*]

Clinical Director: OK, I'll leave you. You are in very good hands, Kaching.

The second scenario with the clinical director and Juan is certainly different in both tone and substance from the first. They begin the same way. Juan has been at the clinic 3 years. However, the director's reaction in the first scenario, claiming that "it seems like forever," is ambiguous at best, and the response in the second is unequivocally supportive. The director allows Juan to introduce himself and welcome Kaching; the clinical director concludes with a reinforcing vote of confidence in Juan's abilities.

Juan's professional standing represents the reason Kaching can accept him as her clinician, so it is of great value to Juan. His professional standing is continuously being assessed by Kaching, so he and his colleagues, especially his clinical director, must always behave in a way that enhances it. Once Juan begins interacting with Kaching, it is his responsibility to uphold his professional standing.

Consistency and Reliability

The first requirement is simply to be professional at all times. Juan must look and act as a skilled and confident clinician, and he must do this all session, every session. Studies have shown that a person's trust depends more than anything else on the consistency of the one trusted (Gabarro, 1978; Levin, Whitener, & Cross, 2006). Consistency and reliability can be demonstrated in several ways.

Using Consistency and Reliability to Achieve Trust

- If a session is scheduled, be on time and be prepared.
- Keep commitments and promises. Do what you say you are going to do. Follow through. Finish what you start.
- Show command of your topic and of your process, not arrogantly or conceitedly, but in a straightforward and candid manner.
- Be enthusiastic, but not overly exuberant; do not be enthusiastic about something one minute and unexcited about it the next.
- Stay calm; do not go to extremes. Keep control.

Friendliness and Accessibility

Clients want to know that their clinicians know "their stuff." Clients expect formality at first but want to feel comfortable with the process. Most importantly, clients expect professional behavior (Ivey et al., 2010). Professionalism, however, does not mean a stern face and aloof demeanor. In fact, it is very important to maintain a friendly and open attitude. Eventually, Juan will be counseling Kaching. He will want her to feel comfortable speaking to him about uncomfortable matters. That is part and parcel of what you will need to do as a speech-language pathologist or audiologist. The issues you deal with are personal and affect many aspects of your clients' daily living: how clients communicate with their peers, their children, or their spouses; how their voice is perceived on the phone by their friends; how their swallowing disorder or hearing impairment prevents them from enjoying dinner with their families. Treatment sessions should take place in a nonthreatening, reassuring atmosphere.

> **Professionalism:** Style, manner, and behavior consistent with and demonstrating qualifications in a field of study, career, or expertise.

Unequivocal Boundaries

Professionalism also means that you know your boundaries. Because clinicians deal with issues that are personal to their clients and because clients usually become comfortable with their clinician, you may have difficulty recognizing the line between what is within the realm of speech-language pathology and audiology and what is outside. Anything relating to the communication disorder is within our scope of practice. In the following scenario, see if you can determine whether the clinician stays within the scope of practice or shifts outside of it.

Clinician: So, tell me how things have been with your voice over the past week.

Jaya: I guess okay. When I answered the telephone at work, no one confused me for a man. You know that's been most difficult for me since the surgery. I have all the female characteristics but my voice is still lower, and it bothers me when people think I'm a man on the phone.

Clinician: I think this is the first time you've had a full week where no one has confused you on the phone; that's really great.

Jaya: Yes, but my son is still having difficulty with the switch. He won't talk to me. I really miss the discussions we used to have with each other. It is really upsetting not to have him in my life.

Clinician: Tell me more about how your son's feelings toward the surgery have affected you.

Jaya has undergone male-to-female gender reassignment surgery. The speech-language pathologist has been working on techniques to increase the perception of Jaya's voice as a female voice. The beginning of the discourse is appropriate. The clinician asks for information about how Jaya's voice has been over the week, and the client provides feedback indicating that the week has gone well. Jaya then shifts to providing information about how her transformation has been affecting her relationship with her son. Although Jaya's issues are about how her son and she are not "communicating," the issue is not about how her "new" voice is affecting her communication with her son. The issue is about how her new gender is affecting her communication with her son. The clinician breaches boundaries by asking Jaya to elaborate on this issue. Below is a more appropriate exchange between Jaya and the clinician.

> **Clinician:** I think this is the first time you've had a full week where no one has confused you on the phone; that's really great.
>
> **Jaya:** Yes, but my son is still having difficulty with the switch. He won't talk to me. I really miss the discussions we used to have with each other. It is really upsetting not to have him in my life.
>
> **Clinician:** I can see that this is very difficult for you. Have you talked to your psychologist about this issue with your son?
>
> **Jaya:** No, I haven't seen her for a while.
>
> **Clinician:** I would suggest reconnecting with her to work on the issues you are having between you and your son.

If after this exchange Jaya continues to pursue talking about her son, the clinician needs to be clear that these issues are not within the clinician's scope of practice. If you have developed a positive, supportive, and comfortable relationship with your clients, it can be difficult to redirect clients. If, however, you set your boundaries from the beginning and continue to be clear about them, clients usually understand when you do not engage in discussions outside those boundaries.

Individual Clinician Style and Personality

Clinicians have different styles and personalities. Professionalism does not mean you have to subscribe to one standard model. To be an effective clinician, you need to know and understand your individual style and personality (Riley, 2002). Clients also bring their individuality to the table. Personality and style differences are inevitable, and they need not pose serious problems. Clinicians skilled at responsive listening can adapt their styles and personalities as they process the feedback they receive from their clients.

For example, if you are an animated and garrulous person and one of your clients is quiet and reserved, you may find it beneficial to tone down your interactions with this client. Clients such as this may become overwhelmed by your energetic manner. They may become anxious during treatment if you do not make an adjustment. The same is true if you are a quiet and reserved clinician working with clients who are more outgoing. Increasing your energy and enthusiasm may be integral to keeping your clients' attention and motivation.

That is not to say that you have to try making drastic modifications to your personality and style. Such attempts are not advisable and rarely work out well. You may simply need to change your behavior enough to be more accessible to a particular client. Even then, the change might last only until your relationship with that client is secure. A rule of thumb is to bring your "best" self to every treatment session. You should be attentive, engaged, free from distractions, and responsive. You should also remember the interaction and counseling skills you are learning in this book. Be open to suggestions supervisors and mentors provide you about ways to improve your interaction abilities with clients and client allies.

Rapport

Rapport: A feeling of camaraderie, of having something in common with another person. ("Bad rapport" is the opposite.)

The term rapport implies that there is a positive connection between clinician and client. It means you and your client feel *in sync* or feel alike in important ways. Adjusting your interactions to achieve this "sameness" helps in the initial process of relationship building; you are building "good" rapport. Among the Five Intentions, small talk, information, self-affirmation, persuasion, and emotion, small talk or chit-chat is the intention focused on establishing rapport. Before the initial evaluation you have with clients, and before every treatment session, some of your time will be spent engaging in small talk, which can begin with questions like the ones discussed in the table later in this section.

Small talk: "Chitchat." Discussion of relatively minor matters; used to relax, set a climate, or build a relationship.

When clients enter a clinic, they may feel intimidated and unsure, especially if they harbor preconceptions about seeing a specialist, someone who may make a mysterious diagnosis or cast judgment on them or a loved one. Small talk can work to neutralize those feelings. Small talk can be used to achieve that sameness—we are all human going through the same human situations—whether it's traffic or the weather. The exchange becomes more relaxed with no pressure to come up with the "right answer" or respond to a technical analysis.

Creating the First Impression

Rapport begins with the first impression clients have of you (Barrick, Swider, & Stewart, 2010; Swider, Barrick, Harris, & Stoverink, 2011). Here, the basics of the first impression are addressed. When you meet clients for the first time, it is important to welcome them and introduce yourself. As you noted when clinician Juan met Kaching earlier in this chapter, introductions should not be taken lightly. When you first meet clients, you state your name and what you do, clear up any issues with pronunciation, and determine what you and your clients want to be called. If a client is not alone, you should introduce yourself to everybody present, usually beginning with the client. These are some of the people who will potentially constitute your client's Circle of Power. Eye contact and a firm handshake typically accompany an introduction.

Questions That Initiate Small Talk

- "How was traffic on the way in today?"
- "Is it windy out there?"
- "Did you have any trouble getting here?"
- "Were the directions okay?"

Guidelines for a Firm Handshake

- Stand and step toward the other person.
- Extend your right hand.
- Put the palm of your hand against the palm of your client's hand, past the knuckle.
- Wrap your fingers around your client's hand.
- Establish a firm grip, but not tight enough to hurt the other.
- Shake for no more than 3 seconds and usually a bit less.
- Do not turn your hand so that your hand is above your client's hand. This indicates dominance.
- Do not cover your client's hand with your other hand.
- Maintain eye contact.
- Smile.

In North American culture it is standard to shake hands when meeting someone. In Chinese culture most people bow. In French culture a kiss on both cheeks is customary. In Indian culture a slight forward bow is done simultaneously with hands placed palm-to-palm, fingers upward at the level of the chest. This gesture is called Namaste or Namaskar, meaning, "The spirit in me respects the spirit in you." In the medieval era, two individuals meeting would first at a distance raise their right hand (the hand that usually holds a weapon) to indicate that each person was unarmed. This waving of the right hand became what people customarily do when approaching someone to say "hi" or "hello." When in close range, individuals would then either grasp forearms or hands to greet one another, again to symbolize that each was unarmed. This ritual became the handshake individuals use today to greet one another.

Very few gestures show a lack of confidence and ability more powerfully than a weak handshake (Chaplin, Phillips, Brown, Clanton, & Stein, 2000; Stewart, Dustin, Barrick, & Arnold, 2008). Practice shaking hands with different people. Ask those individuals if you are gripping too hard or not enough. Make sure to pay attention to how those individuals shake your hand (**Figure 4-1**).

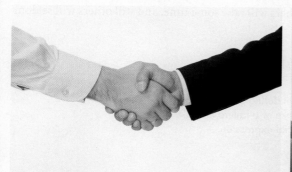
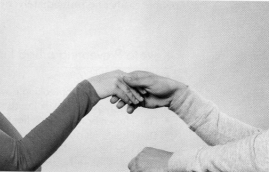

FIGURE 4-1 Handshake. In standard American culture, an effective handshake demonstrates confidence and assuredness. A less effective handshake can indicate decreased confidence or weakness.

Keys to Creating a Good First Impression

- Be punctual.
- Smile.
- Shake hands, and make eye contact.
- Introduce yourself, stating your name and your position.
- Engage in small talk.
- Walk with your client to the therapy room.
- Hold the door open to let your client walk in to the therapy room first.

Your relationship starts with the first impression. How it grows after that depends a lot on how consistent your behavior is with your clients' first impression of you. If you do not make a good first impression, acknowledge the mistake. You will have to continuously work to build up your relationship. If you do make a good first impression, continue reinforcing and enhancing that behavior in every interaction with your clients.

Building the Stable Relationship

Preparation and professional behavior are key aspects of building a stable relationship. Rapport does not end with the initial greeting. The greeting is just the beginning—it sets the stage for what is to come. As you enter into the interviewing and treatment stages, you are continuing to prove yourself to your clients, continuing to build rapport. Your first impressions and continuing relationships with your clients are enhanced by the questions you ask, the way you ask and answer questions, the information you give to clients, how you conduct the testing portion of the evaluation, how you sketch out a plan, and how you implement therapy. Rapport then becomes a gateway to establishing credibility and trust with your clients.

Mutuality of Rapport

Keep in mind that rapport is mutual. You may feel as though you are getting along well with your clients, but you must be adept at determining whether your clients feel the same way about you. Remember, you will make a positive connection with some people easily and immediately; others will take some time, and still others will seldom

Keys to Preventing a Bad First Impression

- Don't be late.
- Avoid shifty eyes or looking down during greeting.
- Don't engage in a weak handshake or a failure to shake hands at all.
- Don't frown or maintain a flat facial expression.
- Don't fail to introduce yourself.
- Don't forget your client's name.
- Don't walk ahead of your client.
- Never ignore your client.
- Don't look unprepared.

see eye to eye with you. When you know you don't enjoy a high comfort level with a client, you may need to work harder to appear at ease. You do not have to be your clients' best friend, but you do have to provide high-quality service, show empathy, and maintain professionalism.

If you get the impression that you and your clients do not have mutual rapport, question clients to understand why they may be uncomfortable, and determine what you might be able to do to help the situation. Clients may not relate well to your style but are okay because they have seen improvements and want to continue working with you. In that case, small talk may be just that, a small matter. When that client is there, you will be all about business. If the lack of mutual rapport is significantly interfering with progress in treatment, and you have done everything you can to remedy the situation, then you may need to refer the client to another clinician.

As you work to develop mutual rapport with clients, especially when difficulties arise, keep in mind the following guidelines.

If you are experiencing difficulties in building rapport with a number of clients, then it would be a good idea to reevaluate your style and approach. Observe yourself on video and analyze your behavior in clinical situations. Take feedback from supervisors or mentors very seriously. Take assertive steps to make the necessary changes in your approach.

Disruptors of Positive Rapport

Aside from your particular style and approach, you may exhibit other attributes that could lead to difficulties in developing rapport with your clients and their advocates. A lack of professionalism—not following through with commitments or promises, continuously being late for treatment sessions, not having a plan in place for sessions, and not maintaining continuity of care—is an example of how you could disrupt building positive rapport with your clients.

Guidelines for Building Rapport

- Do not try to be friends with your clients.
- Do not have an unrealistic expectation that every client will like you. If you get the job done and your clients are satisfied, then your result is positive and appropriate.
- Do not introduce awkwardness into the relationship by trying to be someone other than yourself. If you are funny, be funny. If you do not tell jokes well, don't try to tell jokes.
- Sometimes you will need to adjust your style to appeal to certain clients. If you are outgoing and talkative but your client is shy and reserved, you may need to tone it down a little. The same is true if you are shy and quiet and need to be more dynamic with certain clients. If you both are talkative or both shy and reserved, then someone will have to give a little to make progress in treatment. Usually the responsibility falls on you as the clinician.
- Initiate a discussion with clients concerning any tension or discomfort you are perceiving by saying, for example, "I sensed some resistance toward my last couple of suggestions; tell me if something is bothering you."
- Be patient with the pace of rapport building. As long as the relationship is stable or moving in a positive direction, and not interfering with treatment progress, then there is no need to force the issue.

Alienating someone within your clients' Circle of Power may also affect your ability to develop rapport with your clients. Take Charise, for example. She is a child with an expressive language delay. Her mother likes to come into treatment sessions with Charise; however, during these sessions, she interrupts the clinician by constantly correcting Charise. In the scenario below, determine whether the clinician handles the situation appropriately.

Clinician: [*Holding up figurine of a horse*] Charise, tell me what this is?

Mother: [*Before Charise has a chance to answer, the mother interrupts.*] Charise, you know what that animal is. It's a horse. Remember we saw a horse at the farm yesterday. What does the horse say?

Clinician: [*Sternly*] Mrs. Thomas, you really have to stop interrupting. Charise isn't going to learn to speak if you keep saying things for her.

Versions of this scenario are commonplace in clinical practice. Parents usually think they are being helpful when they interrupt in this way (Egolf, Shames, Johnson, & Kasprisin-Burelli, 1972). The clinician in this case did not handle the mother's interruption in a sensitive and acceptable manner. Even if this is a recurring event with this mother, there is a more appropriate way to handle the mother's interruption than by chastising her in front of her child. The punishment intended for the mother may have a negative effect on how Charise views the clinician as well as how Charise views her mother. A better way to deal with this situation is for the clinician to use this as a "teachable moment," a way to instruct the mother on how to elicit responses from her daughter. Take the following scenario, for example, and determine whether the clinician handled the situation better.

Clinician: [*Holding up figurine of a horse*] Charise, tell me what this is?

Mother: [*Before Charise has a chance to answer, the mother interrupts.*] Charise, you know what that animal is. It's a horse. Remember we saw a horse at the farm yesterday. What does the horse say?

Clinician: Mrs. Thomas, this is a good time to try the technique we talked about last week. Let's give Charise some time to answer—see what she can come up with herself. I'm going to try a different animal [*holding up a cow*]. Charise, tell me what this is? [*Looks at Mrs. Thomas.*] Now we'll wait, keep your eye contact with her [*pauses for 3 seconds*]. Okay, she's not sure. Now, I say to her, "Charise, this animal says, 'moo.' What is it?" We wait again [*pauses for 3 seconds*]. She's still not sure. Now, we help her by leading in to the answer. Charise, what's this animal? It's a c—.

Charise: Cow.

Clinician: That's right, it's a cow. A cow says, "Moo." What does the cow say?

Charise: Moo.

Clinician: Yes, the cow says, "Moo." Now, Mrs. Thomas, you try with this animal [*hands the mother a dog*].

In this example, the clinician works to foster a relationship with the mother. By involving the mother and instructing her on how to extend treatment to the home, the clinician not only reinforces the positive role the mother plays in her daughter's treatment but also helps to ensure that Charise is more likely to generalize her treatment goals. Charise will also be more likely to trust the clinician and see her mother as an advocate to her improvement in treatment.

Positive rapport between you and your clients or between you and one of your clients' advocates is a good thing. Paradoxically, however, rapport can on occasion be a disruption. Mutual rapport can be disruptive to the therapy process if not controlled. Many times clients feel very comfortable with their clinicians. They may be lonely and want someone to talk to, or they may just be talkative and want to use the session time to chit-chat about their lives. If you find yourself constantly focusing your clients back to task, then it is probably a good idea to set some guidelines for the chit-chatting. Let your clients know that you like talking to them and hearing their stories but you have work to do. Over time you will develop multiple strategies to deal with this issue.

For example, you might encourage your clients to tell you stories at the beginning of the session "for a couple of minutes" and then get to work. After you work for a specified amount of time, you might allow your clients to tell you another story. This schedule could turn into a built-in reinforcer for the work you are doing in treatment.

If you find yourself often engaging in discussions outside of treatment-related topics with clients or clients' advocates, and it starts to overlap or interfere with treatment time, then you need to delay those conversations until the end of the treatment session or find another time to have those discussions with your clients or their advocates. Rapport is not an end in itself. A positive relationship paves the way from the first interview with your clients to the implementation of their treatment and ultimately to the successful attainment of their goals. The usual result of good rapport, a positive relationship, and professional respect is a client who is responsive to treatment and well motivated to work toward the goals set.

Client Responsiveness

Clients who are highly motivated to achieve their treatment goals are those who are "connected" to those goals (Barrick, Stewart, & Piotrowski, 2002). This connection between clients and their goals is characterized by three key features: the conviction that they are gaining ownership of the goals, that they are achieving a meaningful purpose in pursuing the goals, and that they are experiencing real growth as they reach these goals. These individuals are called responsive clients. When clients commit to the therapy process, they will likely experience positive long-term results of strong motivation, which is characterized by these three features: ownership, purpose, and growth (**Figure 4-2**).

Achieving Incremental Ownership

Ownership of goals means that the clients feel that the goals are their own, not just yours as the clinician. Ownership of goals does not come all at once. You must counsel

Goals: Intended end points of actions and plans.

Motivation: A connection between a person and an activity that causes the person to be energized and focused when performing that activity.

Ownership: In a motivational context, the sense that one is in control and has options and the resources needed to achieve the desired end.

Purpose: The motivating sense that an activity is worthwhile and meaningful and that there is a good reason to perform the activity.

Growth: In a motivational context, the result of the successful acceptance of a challenge.

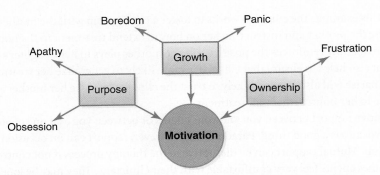

FIGURE 4-2 Motivation Model. A client with decreased motivation may be lacking purpose, growth, or ownership. Assessing the emotions or behaviors exhibited by the client may help to determine which aspect of motivation is deficient or missing.

clients to achieve this feeling of ownership in two respects. First, clients believe the goals are theirs in the sense that the goals are not imposed; they are the clients' by their own choice. The clients chose the goals freely, without coercion or trickery. Second, goals are owned in the same sense as skills are owned: the clients have the firm belief that they possess the knowledge and ability to attain the goals. If a goal is perceived as out of reach, clients cannot be said to have ownership of that goal.

Ownership is usually achieved incrementally, not all at once. The day that clients agree to the goals you set together, their comfort level may not be high. The goals are new; familiarity comes over time. You may need to answer questions like, "Exactly what am I supposed to do here?" Or "What will happen when I achieve this?" Questions like these may surprise you because you thought everything was crystal clear. Be patient. Listen for any sign that clients are feeling alienated from their goals and discuss why this is happening and what you can do to restore their connection to what they are trying to achieve.

Incremental ownership also refers to the fact that long-term goals are attained by way of intermediate or short-term goals. A young client named Ramsey faced several obstacles to improving a lateral emission lisp. His clinician set intermediate goals that addressed his ego impedance and obstacle dominance. Some of the goals addressed skills that Ramsey had to acquire before he could ultimately make this sibilant sound. Other goals dealt with counseling issues. As each of these goals was met, there was a higher probability that Ramsey would experience increased control and greater ownership of the ultimate goal.

As intermediate goals are reached, you should check in with your clients to clarify the progress that was made. You might say, for example, "OK, Ramsey, you can now place your tongue correctly to make an /s/ sound almost without thinking about it. How do you feel about the possibility that you will be able to make that sound whenever you want to do so?" Listen for indications of increased ownership of the ultimate goal and reinforce his sense of ownership with an age-appropriate comment like, "This has been our goal from the beginning. It doesn't seem quite so hard to achieve now, does it?"

Long-term goals: In therapy, the ultimate end points, the desired results, the preferred future.

Short-term goals: An intermediate goal determined to be essential to the accomplishment of longer-term goals. Called MUSTDO goals, an acronym signaling that the short-term goal is measurable, understood, solution focused, time bound, doable, and observable.

Achieving Purpose, Short and Long Term

Along with ownership, your clients must be connected to their goals by purpose (Stajkovic, Locke, & Blair, 2006). They will not be motivated to engage in the treatment process with energy and focus unless they find the goals purposeful. Without purpose they will have no interest. More simply: they must be interested to be motivated, and they will not be interested if they are not achieving a meaningful purpose.

Interest flows from and fuels your clients' sense of purpose, the internal conviction that what they are doing is attractive. *Attractive* is a very helpful word in describing the interest that flows from purpose. The term has two meanings. (1) A thing or person is said to be attractive if it is appealing, beautiful, "nice looking." (2) Something is attractive to you if you are drawn to it, like a magnet draws a piece of metal. (The Latin root *tractus* actually means "dragged" or "drawn." Consider the word *tractor*.) You will set goals like "increase fluency," "effectively communicate wants and needs," or "wear hearing aids in all environments."

Goals like these should be attractive to clients for the reasons mentioned above. There is an aesthetic component to them; that is, they are good, worthwhile, meaningful, even beautiful things to achieve. Clients are certain that time spent pursuing these goals is worthwhile. They believe that once they have achieved the goals, they will be more fully themselves. The path to the goals feels right for them, and they feel strongly that they will be better for having made the journey. It is a journey they are highly invested in taking.

If the goal provides little or no sense of purpose for clients, they are less attracted to it. They will become unmotivated and apathetic. The experience of this extreme state implies that they find the goal uninteresting, uninspiring, trivial, empty, and not worthwhile. As a result, they have difficulty, often great difficulty, generating the internal energy or emotion to engage in the treatment process.

You will find it a challenge to maintain your clients' sense of purpose in both long-term and short-term goals. Practicing short-term goals can be repetitious, tedious, and not easily linked to the long-term goal. Ramsey might find a particular tongue placement activity exhausting; he may be unable to see how this activity relates to the goal of speaking without a lisp. His clinician must help him see that tongue placement is a step in the direction of the goal. The clinician's aim at all times is to maintain clients' interest and avoid the draining specter of apathy, which makes it difficult to muster any effort at all.

You will meet clients who seem to understand the importance of the goals, seem to find the goals purposeful, but who are not engaged in treatment. In these cases, clients seem unwilling to do the work necessary to achieve their desired outcome. The "magnet" of purpose is just not strong enough.

Purpose can also ironically move in the exact opposite direction from apathy, though this occurrence is less frequent. Clients or their caregivers may become more and more consumed with the treatment. The attraction is so strong that it sucks them in and consumes them rather than drawing them in agreeably like a magnet does. The extreme is obsession, exemplified by the client who practices voice techniques until hoarse, the father who corrects his child every time he stutters, the mother who insists her deaf child communicate only through speech and never in sign language. Obsession is an undesirable state sometimes wrongly mistaken for healthy motivation. The end result of obsession, as described here, is often burnout, when clients, exhausted, frustrated, and perhaps resentful, simply give up.

You can easily miss this unhealthy condition if you only see that clients are working hard and taking treatment seriously. You should question your highly engaged clients, their family members, and caregivers about the place of treatment in their lives. For example, you might say to a caregiver, "We agreed you would help your child recognize her disfluency only at specified times. Do you find yourself correcting her more often throughout the day?" Or, "We said you would spend no more than fifteen minutes three times a day on this. Are you exceeding that?" Then discuss the situation; renegotiate the terms to ensure that clients and their advocates are not spending too much time and energy. Obsession is not purpose; it is a problem that must be addressed.

Healthy purpose implies that clients are at the helm, active initiators, fully conscious and very much in control. They are connected to their goals by attraction; interest is high and exhilarating, not chaotic and draining. The goal has its own energy, the ability to draw your clients to it, focus them on its accomplishment, and encourage them to see it through with enthusiasm. Yes, this is an ideal state, but you should always pursue it.

Achieving Growth, Enthusiasm, and Fun

The third way in which you want your clients connected to their goals is through growth. You may be tempted, especially if you are a relatively inexperienced clinician, to try to make the process as easy as possible for clients. Believe it or not, this approach is not recommended. Clients are rarely if ever highly motivated to do something that is very easy. Treatment ought to be challenging to them, but not merely challenging. It should test their skills, take them beyond where they were previously, and bring about growth. At best, you have them operating, in the words of Rosabeth Moss Kanter (1983), at "the edge of their competence" (p. 27). They are growing. That means that they are proving themselves and improving themselves.

Proving themselves

Your clients are demonstrating their resolve, putting their skills and abilities to the test. They are proving themselves. This occurs because of the nature of the treatment work in which they are engaging, the challenge inherent in what they are accomplishing. It has little to do with finding favor in your eyes or simply coming out on top. They are not proving themselves to anyone, except, perhaps, to themselves. Throughout the therapy process, you should be calibrating the degree of difficulty of what you are asking of clients. You should constantly seek that place where the task is not too hard and not too easy.

In the game of horseshoes, competitors lob horseshoes at opposing stakes. The objective is to get the horseshoe in the circle and as close to the stake as possible. A ringer (horseshoe around the stake) wins the most points. If you wanted to teach someone how to play horseshoes, you would need to decide how far that person should initially stand from the stake. The regulation distance for adult females is 30 feet (40 feet for men). If you started a female player 30 feet away from the stake you would not be optimizing her motivation. Placed too far away, she may become overwhelmed, furiously hurling shoe after shoe and missing wildly every time. If you, however, place her too close, she may become bored and lose motivation as she threw ringer after ringer; it was just too easy. Research shows that when learning a new task, individuals should start at a place where they can obtain a 50% success rate (Whalen & Schreibman, 2003). In horseshoes, you would choose a distance where the player would manage to get about 50% of her tosses inside the circle (near the stake). As she improves, you will place her farther and farther from the stake.

Video game designers are also well aware of the growth aspect of motivation. They keep players at the controller hour after hour by starting them at a "level" where they achieve about a 50% success rate. As soon as they might get bored, say at about 80% success, the game moves them to a higher "level," and they are soon back at 50% ready to prove themselves at this level. The process continues from level to level. What the horseshoe player and the gamer are doing is not only proving themselves but also improving themselves.

Improving themselves

Personal growth is achieved as the client improves. Clients become better, improve, and grow by their acceptance of a challenge (Egan, 2007). The challenge extends their skill, makes them more than they were before. Self-improvement, real growth, is essential to the kind of challenge that connects them motivationally with their goals. As with the horseshoe player and the gamer, you will keep your clients highly motivated, challenged, and growing during treatment if you continuously monitor the level of difficulty so you can avoid two extremes: too easy and too hard.

As the process becomes too easy, it becomes less and less a source of growth. Clients find it increasingly difficult to generate the energy to complete the task. This difficulty may ultimately lead to boredom. When this happens, there is no test, no excitement, no challenge or growth. With some clients, of course, you will lower the level of difficulty of a task with the intention of empowering clients with a feeling of success. After that, you build on success by increasing the level of difficulty.

As the process gets too hard, either it becomes more than their skill level can take or it becomes overwhelming because there is too much to do in a short period of time. They then move toward a scattered focus, possibly panic or extreme anxiety. Some clients eventually just give up.

As a clinician you should distinguish growth from purpose. Your clients may find a goal purposeful, but your exercise regimen may be too hard or too easy. They could, for example, be bored, but not apathetic. Balanced growth requires that the task be reasonably difficult. The task should extend your clients' skills, improve them. To achieve growth, clients should be encouraged to give their very best as they work toward a goal they find meaningful and desirable. That means that when they have made the great effort and reached the goal, they are better! They have grown.

Avoiding Obsession and Dread, Apathy and Boredom

As you counsel your clients, keep them connected to their goals and activities in a healthy way. Monitor, discuss, and question continuously. Be prepared to alter your clients' goals and activities to maintain their conviction that throughout treatment, they have ownership, purpose, and growth. They are truly connected. Make sure that they are not demotivated by any sense of frustration, obsession, apathy, dread, or boredom. In this way, you evoke client responsiveness from one session to the next until, together, you reach a successful outcome.

The Limits of the Best Relationship

All relationships have limits. The time will come when your clients either meet all their goals and are dismissed from treatment or reach their potential and need only maintenance sessions with you. In most circumstances, the ultimate goal of your treatment is to make clients their own clinician. The present chapter began with instruction on the Learning Phase of the Solution Cycle—getting to know your clients, getting to know your clients' story. To be able to learn about your clients, you discovered that you have to develop rapport with them, get "in sync" with them, be on their wavelength. You learned that building a relationship with your clients and your clients' advocates is integral to the therapy process. You looked at various approaches and counseling techniques that can help in the relationship-building process.

If you effectively foster a strong and productive relationship, you can greatly increase the probability of successful treatment. Still, the relationship will not erase the limitations inherent in a degenerative disorder such as dementia or a chronic mental incapacity. Once you have built the best possible relationship with a client, your professional competence, along with the potential of the individual client to make progress, will finally determine the treatment outcomes that will be achieved.

The Primacy of Professional Competence

We have observed that maintaining professionalism and demonstrating professional competence start with the first impression you give to your clients and their advocates. Your clinical supervisors, colleagues, and mentors can help or hinder your first impression. For a student, how they introduce you to clients, how they treat you in front of clients, and what they say about you to clients either fosters trust and credibility between you and your clients or creates an awkward and sometimes irremediable situation between you and clients. Ultimately, however, the responsibility is on you

---

Frustration: The feeling that one is not in control, is without options, is being forced against one's will.

Obsession: In a motivational context, interest that has become extreme to the point of excluding other possible interests. Characterized by high energy and narrow focus.

Apathy: A lack of interest and enthusiasm caused by a sense that an activity has little or no purpose. Apathy leads to a loss of energy and poor motivation.

Dread: An emotion that can arise when one engages in or contemplates situations with which one is seriously ill prepared to cope. Dread can come about when an activity is seen as far too difficult or dangerous.

Boredom: A lack of desire to perform an activity because it is not challenging, is perceived as too easy.

to create a good first impression and follow through with consistent, predictable, and professional behavior.

The Willingness to Be Helped

The clinician–client relationship is a two-way street. Despite your best efforts, if clients do not want to be helped, success in treatment is improbable, perhaps unattainable. In these cases, you have to be willing to part ways until the clients are ready to put forth the effort to make changes. As long as you made every attempt and possible accommodation to provide a path for your clients' journey, you should not take offense at their unwillingness to accept the help you have given. Keep tabs on those clients by sending reminder letters inviting them back to treatment. You might even call them once in a while to check in on them.

Some Ethical Guidelines

Not only are there limits to the best relationship but there are also boundaries to the best relationship. If you find yourself in a situation where mutual rapport goes beyond a general liking of either your client or a client's advocate, remember to maintain professional behavior and boundaries. If a client is underage, then in no way should you pursue a nonprofessional relationship with that client. If the client is of legal age, then it is professionally appropriate for you to refer the client to another clinician before engaging in a romantic relationship with the client. The same guidelines hold if you and a client's advocate are interested in developing a deeper relationship. Referral to another clinician helps so that professional boundaries are maintained.

Client confidentiality is also an important ethical consideration for you to keep in mind at all times. The Health Insurance Portability and Accountability Act (HIPPA, 1996) mandates that you not disclose any client information to anyone other than those your clients have specified. This disclosure includes the information you are allowed to leave on a voicemail, how your clients prefer to be contacted, as well as those to whom you may give information over the telephone. Be careful not to talk about clients or provide any identifying information about your clients in public forums, including professional conferences, social networks, emails, or when talking on a cell phone in public.

> **Cultural awareness:** Sensitivity to differing norms for greeting and interacting, based not on stereotypes or assumptions but on actual differences that exist among various cultures.

Some Cultural Guidelines

Cultural awareness and linguistic awareness are very important. When your clients include people from other cultures, you may need to be sensitive to different norms for greeting and interacting and to practice cultural literacy (Ivey et al., 2010). Do not stereotype clients or make assumptions based on things you have heard about their culture. Rather, when you assess or treat clients with different cultural and linguistic backgrounds, you should be aware that the norms and behaviors with which you are familiar may vary or be unacceptable. Areas where these issues could arise include the following.

> **Cultural literacy:** Knowledge and understanding of specific cultural norms and practices. This knowledge enables a person to navigate comfortably within that culture.

Areas Requiring Cultural Awareness or Cultural Literacy

- Initial greeting and handshake. For example, in some cultures women do not shake hands with men.
- Eye contact. Whereas mainstream North American culture favors fairly steady eye contact during face-to-face interactions, people of other cultures may show respect by looking down or away.
- Role of authority. You may anticipate questions and feedback when you propose a treatment option, but in some cultures, your words may be taken as the final authority and not questioned.
- Role of family and community. In some cultures, an elder in the family or local community could veto a plan apparently agreed upon by you and your client. Extended family members may be very involved in decisions about the client's care, or not involved at all.
- Time. Some cultures place a high value on punctuality; others interpret appointment times more loosely. You may need to inform your clients of the consequences of arriving late. In both cases, no offense should be taken.
- Keep in mind that different cultures have different views and stigmas associated with certain disorders.

When working with clients from other cultural backgrounds, you should keep the above "awareness areas" in mind. Observe clients' behavior for clues to what is appropriate. Do not hesitate to ask clients whether a particular arrangement is "comfortable." Make appropriate changes. Discuss any concerns with your supervisor.

Review of Key Points

- The first phase in reaching a solution through the Solution Cycle is learning, a phase that involves getting clients to open their lives to you, getting their story.
- Be professional at all times. Your professional standing is really your reputation, a significant element of the perception your clients have of you, the reason clients can accept you as their clinician.
- Professionalism means that you know your boundaries. Do not confuse the line between what is within the realm of speech-language pathology and audiology and what is outside.
- Rapport is the feeling that you are in sync with your clients. Good rapport begins with the first impression clients have of you and helps in the initial process of relationship building. Small talk is the intention focused on establishing rapport. Before every therapy session, some of your time will be spent engaging in small talk.
- Follow the guidelines for a good, firm handshake. Nothing shows a lack of confidence and ability more than a bad handshake.
- It is important that rapport is mutual. If the lack of mutual rapport is significantly interfering with progress in therapy, and you have done everything you can to remedy the situation, then you may need to refer the client to another clinician.
- If you are experiencing difficulties in building rapport with a number of clients, then it would be a good idea to reevaluate your style and approach. Take assertive steps to make the necessary changes in your approach.
- Clients highly motivated to achieve their treatment goals are "connected" to those goals by three key features, ownership of the goals, purpose in pursuing their goals, and growth as they reach the goals. These individuals are called responsive clients.
- Ownership of goals is incremental and means that the clients feel that the goals are their own, not just yours as the clinician.
- Clients will not be motivated to engage in the therapy process with energy and focus unless they find the goals purposeful. Without purpose they will have no interest.
- Therapy ought to be challenging and bring about growth. Clients are proving themselves and improving themselves.
- All relationships have limits. The ultimate goal of your therapy is to make clients their own clinicians, able to leave therapy with long-term improvements.
- The clinician–client relationship is a two-way street. Despite your best efforts, if clients do not want to be helped, success in therapy is improbable, perhaps unattainable. In these cases, you have to be willing to part ways at least temporarily.
- If a client is underage, then in no way should you pursue a nonprofessional relationship with that client. If the client is of legal age, then it is professionally appropriate for you to refer the client to another clinician before engaging in a romantic relationship.

- Client confidentiality is also an important ethical consideration for you always to keep in mind. The Health Insurance Portability and Accountability Act (HIPAA) provides excellent guidelines in this area.
- Cultural awareness and linguistic awareness are very important, not to stereotype but to be aware that the norms and behaviors with which you are familiar may vary or be unacceptable in other cultures.

Practical Exercises

For each of the following scenarios, indicate whether the client's issue is something that is within your scope of practice as a speech-language pathologist or audiologist or is outside your scope of practice and warrants a referral to a licensed psychologist, social worker, or psychiatrist. Briefly explain your answer.

1. Sharon, a 65-year-old, states, "I have had so much trouble communicating with my husband since his stroke."
2. Caden, a 12-year-old, states, "My parents want me to get a cochlear implant, but I don't want one. They say it will improve my life, but I don't agree with them. I'm happy the way I am."
3. Maribel, a 25-year-old, says, "I'm so upset that I haven't made more progress since I left the rehab center. My speech-language pathologist said I would keep improving. But I don't see it. This all wouldn't have happened if I didn't try to drive home after that party. Since the car accident, I swore I wouldn't drink again. But it's so hard. I was out with my friends the other night and I did have a drink. It was only one, but I wanted to have more. If I don't start to see more improvement, I'm scared I'll really start drinking again."
4. Ignacio, a 33-year-old, says, "At my last job I didn't have to talk much. My stuttering really didn't bother me at all. But now that this new job requires me to be on the phone more … and those monthly budget reports to my division, I'm freaking out. I thought this would be a step up, a good career move. What if I can't do it?"
5. Zoey, a 42-year-old, says, "This therapy will not make me better. I stay the same week after week. This disorder has changed me; I'm nothing now. My life is not worth living."
6. Noah, a 52-year-old son of your client, says, "I haven't seen my dad in years. I don't know why he made me his power of attorney. He didn't even call to tell me he was sick. I just received this call from his lawyer saying that I needed to come and make these decisions for him. How can I make a decision about life support when I don't even know what he would want to do?"
7. Sataya, a 28-year-old, states, "A hearing loss? He's only eight months old. I don't want him to wear those hearing aids, but my friend said that then I would have to teach him sign language. I want him to be able to talk. She said he won't talk if I teach him sign language. Then what? Where will he go to school? Will he be able to get a job, get married?"

Journal Activity 3: Make a Good First Impression

Introduce yourself to five new communication partners. These individuals could be people within your community, at work, or at school. In your journal, reflect on the following questions: How did you introduce yourself? What first impression did you make? How did the individuals react to you (take note of each person's paraverbals)? How did you develop positive rapport? What small talk did you engage in? What would you do differently if you were to rewind and make the introduction all over again?

REFERENCES

Barrick, M. R., Stewart, G. L., & Piotrowski, M. (2002). Personality and job performance: Test of the mediating effects of motivation among sales representatives. *Journal of Applied Psychology, 87*(1), 43–51.

Barrick, M. R., Swider, B. W., & Stewart, G. L. (2010). Initial evaluations in the interview: Relationships with subsequent interviewer evaluations and employment offers. *Journal of Applied Psychology, 95*(6), 1163–1172.

Chaplin, W. F., Phillips, J. B., Brown, J. D., Clanton, N. R., & Stein, J. L. (2000). Handshaking, gender, personality, and first impressions. *Journal of Personality and Social Psychology, 79*(1), 110–117.

Egan, G. (2007). *The skilled helper* (8th ed.). Belmont, CA: Thomson Brooks/Cole.

Egolf, D. B., Shames, G. H., Johnson, P. R., & Kasprisin-Burrelli, A. (1972). The use of parent–child interaction patterns in therapy for young stutterers. *Journal of Speech and Hearing Disorders, 37*, 222–232.

Gabarro, J. (1978). The development of trust, influence, and expectations. In A. G. Athos & J. J. Gabarro (Eds.), *Interpersonal behavior* (pp. 290–303). Englewood Cliffs, NJ: Prentice Hall.

Health Insurance Portability and Accountability Act of 1996, 42 U.S.C. § 1320d-9 (2010).

Holland, J. M., Neimeyer, R. A., & Currier, J. M. (2007). The efficacy of personal construct therapy: A comprehensive review. *Journal of Clinical Psychology, 63*, 93–107.

Ivey, A. E, Ivey, M. B., & Zalaquett, C. P. (2010). *Intentional interviewing and counseling: Facilitating client development in a multicultural society* (7th ed.). Belmont, CA: Brooks/Cole, Cengage Learning.

Kanter, R. M. (1983). *The change masters: Innovation and entrepreneurship in the American corporation*. New York, NY: Simon & Schuster.

Levin, D. Z., Whitener, E. M., & Cross, R. (2006). Perceived trustworthiness of knowledge sources: The moderating impact of relationship length. *Journal of Applied Psychology, 91*(5), 1163–1171.

Monk, G., Winslade, J., Crocket, K., & Epston, D. (1997). *Narrative theory in practice: The archeology of hope*. San Francisco, CA: Jossey-Bass.

Riley, J. (2002). Counseling: An approach for speech-language pathologists. *Contemporary Issues in Communication Science and Disorders, 29*, 6–16.

Stajkovic, A. D., Locke, E. A., & Blair, E. S. (2006). A first examination of the relationships between primed subconscious goals, assigned conscious goals, and task performance. *Journal of Applied Psychology, 91*(5), 1172–1180.

Stewart, G. L., Dustin, S. L., Barrick, M. R., & Arnold, T. C. (2008). Exploring the handshake in employment. *Journal of Applied Psychology, 93*(5), 1139–1146.

Swider, B. W., Barrick, M. R., Harris, T. B., & Stoverink, A. C. (2011). Managing and creating an image in the interview: The role of interviewee initial impressions. *Journal of Applied Psychology. 96*(6), 1275–1288.

Whalen, C., & Schreibman, L. (2003). Joint attention training for children with autism using behavior modification procedures. *Journal of Child Psychology and Psychiatry and Allied Disciplines, 44*(3), 456–468.

CHAPTER 5

Information: Knowledge Transfer in the Counseling Process

KEY TERMS

- Adversary
- Advocates
- Case history
- Chief complaint
- Information
- Intake form
- Interviewing

LEARNING OBJECTIVES

After reading this chapter, you will be able to:

- Define information as a communication intention related to the interview process
- Explain the key components of the interview process
- List and explain the fundamentals of an informed client
- List and explain the needs of an informed clinician
- Define the three types of knowledge that will be important for your clients
- Explain why it is important to keep clients and client advocates informed throughout the therapy process

Of the Five Intentions of Communication, information is what comes to mind most often when people think of communication (Barone & Tellis, 2008). Many people believe that information sharing is the heart of communication. Although important, information sharing is not the primary intention of every communication exchange, even as it is an intention that you cannot do without. Information is knowledge, and knowledge is power.

As a clinician, you will find that the possession of certain information is crucial to your success in treating and counseling your clients. Your client's case history, the primary language spoken in the client's home, your client's diagnosis, and your recommendations for treatment can all be considered items of information. Clients too must secure a base of information as they proceed through treatment. Caregivers and other allies will likewise benefit from receiving relevant and timely information.

> **Information:** In therapy, the factual, practical, technical, and developmental knowledge needed to proceed and achieve success.

This chapter focuses on what clinicians, clients, and allies ought to know to be appropriately informed. You will learn the essentials of the interview process as well as skills required to conduct a successful interview. Interviewing is vitally important when you are seeking knowledge about your clients as well as acquiring information about influential people in your clients' lives (Ivey, Ivey, & Zalaquett, 2010).

The Fundamentals of an Informed Clinician

You will want to take time to inform yourself about each and every client you see. How will you know when you are informed? You will know when you become convinced that you are equipped with the knowledge needed to collaborate with your clients in setting appropriate treatment goals and taking the steps necessary to achieve those goals. If treatment is unsuccessful because of something you did not know, conventional wisdom says you are not accountable. Perhaps not, but if the information is something you could have discovered earlier, if it is data you should have inquired about, then your lack of knowledge created an obstacle that could have been avoided.

Guidelines for an Informed Clinician

The guidelines listed below help you identify and categorize the items you need to discover and retain about your clients. Most of these items should be collected during the interview process, which is discussed in detail later in this chapter (see **Figure 5-1**).

1. The clients' intake forms constitute the starting point of information gathering. Filling out the forms begins the process of developing the clients' case histories. The case histories comprise information about your clients' speech-language or hearing record, including issues, disorders, and treatment history. The case histories also contain background data on family, education, and occupation histories, along with medical, social, developmental, and related information.

Case history: The client's case history is the starting point of information gathering; it covers information on the client's speech-language or audiological record, including issues, disorders, and past treatment, as well as background data on family, education, and occupation, medical, social, and related information.

Interviewing: The interview process is an informational give-and-take between therapist and client, client advocates, and adversaries. It is designed to capture relevant client information in a structured manner. During the interview, clients tell their stories, and the clinician provides necessary information to the clients.

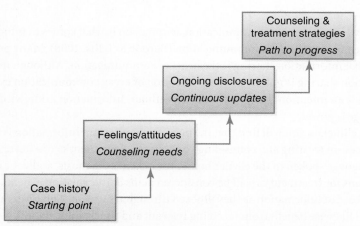

FIGURE 5-1 Client Information Guidelines. Information clinicians need to know about their clients throughout the therapy process.

2. Once compiled, the case histories offer cues to help you explore your clients' attitudes and feelings. A careful and professional examination of the items in a case history provides insight into matters that may become significant as you proceed. Discuss each item with your clients. You might discover, for instance, that a client's apparent apprehension is due to an earlier unsuccessful attempt at therapy or that a family member's negative opinion about therapy is influencing a client's decision about wearing hearing aids. Conversations like these can reveal some of your clients' hopes and fears as you and they enter into the therapy process. The conversations also can give clues about your clients' potential counseling needs.

3. Information gathering continues throughout your association with your clients. As a clinician you never stop listening, questioning, and observing to acquire helpful information about your clients. You will continually augment, sift, and refine that information as you achieve a better understanding of their case histories and current situation, attitudes, and feelings. Incomplete information is brought up-to-date, and incorrect information is amended. With richer and more accurate knowledge about your clients, you are better able to fine-tune your treatment goals and techniques. You also can identify areas where counseling may be needed.

Basic Facts About Your Clients and Clients' Peer Relationships and Social Connections

The interview process should be designed to capture relevant client information in a structured manner. Most of the crucial facts you require are elicited in an intake form, which may well be completed before you first meet your clients. You gather the remaining information during face-to-face discussions.

Your clients' advocates are usually an integral part of their life, and those advocates play a sometimes pivotal role in how your clients progress in treatment (Beatson, 2006). Many clinicians are familiar with such terms as *caregiver*, *loved ones*, and *family and friends* when indicating the people in a client's support network. We use the terms *ally* or *advocate* as a way to speak generally about all of the people in your clients' lives who have a positive influence or who are supportive of the therapy process. The term adversary is used to categorize individuals who have a negative influence or who are not supportive of your clients' efforts in the therapy process. You want individuals who play a positive role in your clients' therapy; you want allies, not adversaries. In the early stages, the question is, what do you need to discover about your clients' advocates to help you build an alliance with them?

You will want to know how influential an advocate is in an individual client's life and thinking. The advocate's influence is the result of a number of factors: relationship to the client, longevity of the relationship, feelings the client has about the advocate, importance of the advocate in the client's life, as well as the overall amount of time the client and the advocate spend together or in communication. When your clients mention names of potential allies, it is a good idea to write down the names along with any

> **Client advocates:** People influential in a client's life. They tend to be assertive in their commitment to what they see as beneficial to the client. They can be helpful in the therapy process, but they may, under certain circumstances, become adversarial.

> **Adversary:** An individual who has a negative influence or who is not supportive of a client's efforts in the therapy process.

other significant details about their relationship to the particular client. Much of this information can be gleaned in discussions with your clients. You may not want to delve into this individual's story right away, especially if it would be a digression from the discussion you and your client are conducting.

At some point you will want to probe more deeply to get a better picture of the kind of role a particular acquaintance might play. Then, of course, make a note of your findings and reflections. Review these findings frequently, and you will be more prepared when an ally is needed. Possible adversaries, too, should be noted.

Basic Knowledge of Clients' Specific Communication Issues

Intake form: The clients' intake forms constitute the starting point of information gathering. Filling out the forms begins the process of developing the clients' case history. The forms ask for the information associated with the case history.

During the interview process, beginning with the intake form, the clients answer questions about the specific communication issues that led them to seek your services. These questions appear in written form, and you augment these data when you discuss your clients' answers. Although you may use a standard intake form, the information you obtain will differ depending on the clients' age and disorder. Still, the cautions listed below can alert you to factors you should consider as you interpret clients' written responses.

These are a sampling of the factors that warn you to proceed with care as you conduct the interview. If you suspect your clients are misinterpreting a question, be sure to seek clarification until you are certain they have given a full and accurate answer. The information you receive from intake forms is usually basic and needs further probing throughout the interview.

Continuous Listening and Observing

Your most dependable means of gathering sound information is your ability to listen responsively to your clients and observe them attentively throughout the interview and related interactions. Double-check any written or oral response you suspect may be erroneous or off the mark in some way.

What you are doing during this early stage is introductory. You are introducing yourself to your clients while they are being introduced to you. You are using your questioning and interpretive skills to gather critical information about your clients and their communication issues. The questions you ask and the answers you receive should enhance your credibility with them and allow you to establish the appropriate tone for treatment as well as the appropriate goals of treatment (Ivey et al., 2010). The relevance and efficacy of those goals depend on the quality of data you collect during this phase.

Reasons for Caution When Reading Client Information Forms

- Clients may not have an accurate understanding of an item.
- Linguistic or cultural diversity may be a factor, leading the clients to misinterpret the intent of an item or have difficulty answering it.
- The age and ability of clients can greatly affect both the written responses and later discussion.
- Client attitudes, positive or negative, can also influence responses.

Basic Knowledge of the Treatment Options

If the interview and discussions go reasonably well, there will be no crucial gaps in the information you have collected, and your perception of your clients' attitudes and motivations will be clear and accurate. You can then diagnose needs and determine the most appropriate treatment directions to take, the ones most likely to yield significant progress in resolving speech-language or hearing issues.

Frequently, treatment options suggest themselves early in the interview process. Consider these three examples. A 19-year-old client who stutters reveals to you that she will do anything to become fluent. A 3-year-old client who is profoundly deaf has cochlear implants and an obvious inability to decode rudimentary speech. An 83-year-old client arrives with his daughter, who immediately informs you of her father's recent stroke and ongoing dementia.

Cases with features similar to these will likely point you toward specific treatment paths to the exclusion of others. In fact, as you grow professionally, you will get better and better at determining appropriate treatment strategies early on. In situations like those presented above, you may see value in not launching immediately into a particular treatment strategy. You might instead begin with traditional counseling practices focusing on feelings and attitudes. You may well uncover an issue that must be addressed before a given treatment can be effective.

That client with new cochlear implants might need to deal with the dread that can accompany a world where unfamiliar auditory stimuli are creating a strange and frightening environment (Blume, 1999). The important task is to find the right balance between your tendency to focus rapidly on promising courses of action and the requirement to keep an open mind and avoid jumping to conclusions too hastily.

As a clinician, you use the initial client interviews and discussions to gather information useful to your collaboration with your clients. This information includes basic facts about your clients and basic facts about their advocates, peer relationships, and social networks. You acquire a solid knowledge of their specific speech-language or hearing issues through interviewing and discussion coupled with continuous listening and observing.

These efforts culminate in a professionally structured hypothesis of the problem and render basic knowledge of the how to proceed with the evaluation, treatment, and counseling options most likely to generate positive results.

The Interview Process

During the interview, you gather the bulk of information about your clients (Ivey et al., 2010). That is because much of the interview involves informational give-and-take between you, your clients, and their advocates and adversaries. During the interview, you help your clients tell their stories, and you provide necessary information to your clients. Before you begin the interview, you must build rapport with your clients (Barrick, Swider, & Stewart, 2010). Small talk is an important intention in this relationship-building stage. During the interview, you continue to develop your relationship with your clients, but your primary intention quickly moves from small talk to information.

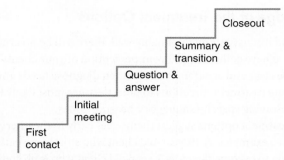

FIGURE 5-2 Interview Process. The interview process has distinct stages.

The credibility you have with your clients is essential to the successful exchange of information throughout the interview. If clients do not believe in you, they will be less likely to share information with you, especially sensitive and relevant information (Hubble, Duncan, & Miller, 1999; Ivey et al., 2010). Much of what builds credibility happens before you even meet your clients. Your clients may be influenced by the things people say about you, by your credentials and degrees, and by the testimony of others who have achieved successful results with you.

Credibility continues to build during your first contact with your clients and your initial meeting, often involving small talk. How you relate to your clients is important. As you move through the interview, you also reveal yourself. Your clients begin to trust you (Levin, Whitener, & Cross, 2006). Your line of questioning shows your knowledge. Your interpretation of events and experiences proves your reasoning ability. As you and your clients interact, your credibility is being firmly established. The next section guides you through the process of the interview to achieve the most success in this crucial form of information exchange (see **Figure 5-2**).

First Contact

Clients often make the first contact with clinicians. They are the ones seeking help. This contact usually occurs over the telephone or through email. The first contact becomes the first impression your client has of you. If you are not timely in your response, if your voicemail message is too informal or curt, if your receptionist is not friendly and helpful, clients may be turned off from treatment before they have met you. Here are some guidelines to follow to ensure the first contact a client has with you is positive:

1. Respond within 24 hours to clients' requests for appointments.
2. Instruct receptionists to answer the telephone with a proper greeting, for example, "This is the Speech-Language and Hearing Center; Steve speaking. How may I help you?" Receptionists should also know the protocols for providing information about your facility, setting up appointments, confirming appointments, obtaining pertinent information about clients, and directing clients to appropriate resources when they have questions.

3. If you do not have a receptionist, set up your voicemail with detailed information for your clients. A sample script is, "You have reached Sanaya Patel at the Speech-Language and Hearing Center. Please leave a detailed message with your full name spelled, the date you are calling, your reason for calling, and your preferred way to be contacted. I will return your call within twenty-four hours. If this is an emergency, please dial nine-one-one or proceed to your local hospital's emergency room."

4. If you have an email account only for clients, you may want to set an automatic reply stating, "Thank you for your request. I will respond by email within 24 hours."

When returning clients' calls, you need to keep in mind the Health Insurance Portability and Accountability Act (HIPAA) of 1996 and not disclose any personal health information to anyone but the client. You should ask for clients by name. If the person answering the telephone is your client or is the parent of a client younger than 18 years who made the initial call, you can identify yourself by full name, title, and affiliation. If the person answering the telephone is not your client, you should state who you are, by full name, and indicate that you are returning the client's call.

When leaving a voicemail message for clients, you should also state your full name and indicate that you are returning the client's call. Be careful not to breach confidentiality by providing too many details in the message. Remember to include a return telephone number and to restate your name and number at the end of the message. For example, "This is Sanaya Patel and I am returning Sophia's call. She can return my call at 555-5555. Again this is Sanaya Patel and my number is 555-5555." Speak slowly and articulate your words carefully.

Once clients come to your office, you should have them sign a HIPAA form indicating how they would prefer to be contacted (telephone, cell phone, email), who they authorize that you can provide information to, and whether or not you can leave information on a voicemail (detailed or not).

Initial Meeting

Sometimes the initial meeting is the first contact you have with your clients. In a hospital, inpatient rehabilitation center, nursing home, or school setting, clients may not directly contact you. You will probably meet them for the first time when you enter their hospital room to conduct your evaluation or when you remove them from a classroom for testing. If the initial meeting is your first contact, then there is extra pressure to make a good first impression.

You will want to master specific skills to create a good first impression. When meeting your clients, make eye contact, introduce yourself, and extend your hand to provide a firm handshake. State your full name and then how you would like clients to refer to you. This becomes important especially if your ID or badge states your full name. For example, if your name is Katharine and you prefer to be called Kate, indicate that preference to clients during the introduction. It is appropriate to introduce yourself to all individuals present (client, parents, caregivers, spouse, or others).

Making a good first impression also includes walking beside your clients as you go to the room where treatment takes place, asking "get-to-know-you" questions, debriefing clients about the facility (especially if clients have been referred to your facility by an outside professional), and, if all else fails, talking about the weather.

Question and Answer

A situation novice clinicians often find nerve-racking is transitioning from the small talk phase to actually beginning the interview. One way to prepare yourself is to summarize how the evaluation will proceed. Consider a statement, such as the one below, to transition from small talk to the start of the interview.

Clinician: Let me tell you what we'll do today. First, I'll ask you some questions. Then we'll move on to testing. I'm going to run you through a couple of tests. Some things may be difficult for you to do, but I just want you to try your best. After we are done testing, I'll go over the results with you and discuss your options. So, let's begin. Tell me why you are here today.

Many new clinicians prepare a list of questions and have a difficult time straying from the list, wanting to ask only the questions on the list and in the order they are written on the paper. Preparation is good, but remember to be flexible. Your role in the first interview is to guide your clients through the story-telling process. Begin with an open-ended statement such as, "From your intake form, I see that you have been referred by Dr. Hernandez. Tell me a little about what's going on." Or simply, as stated above, say, "Tell me why you are here today." Once you have the general picture, you can begin asking more pointed or yes/no questions about certain events to get a clearer understanding of your clients' story. Remember, you are gathering specific information, as discussed earlier in this chapter.

Clients and client advocates may be good historians. These individuals are able to accurately recount the chronology of events leading to their visit with you. They need little guidance as they recall and state events from the onset of the problem to the present situation. With good historians, make sure to clarify important dates and summarize events periodically to double-check that you are receiving the message accurately. Consider the following scenario with the mother of Hosannah, a new client.

Clinician: Tell me a little about what's going on.

Parent: My pediatrician told me to come. She said that my daughter, Hosannah, is not where she should be in her speech development. I was wondering about this before our last visit to the pediatrician. I can understand Hosannah pretty well, but people who don't know her have a very hard time understanding her. Even my husband has trouble sometimes. Certain sounds are not as good as others, and when she talks in sentences, I guess I can see how she's more difficult to understand.

Clinician: When did you first notice a problem with Hosannah's speech?

Parent: I guess when she started preschool three months ago. The teachers told me at our first parent–teacher meeting last month that they have a hard time understanding Hosannah. After that meeting, I started to pay attention to how she sounds and also how people react to her when she speaks.

Clinician: Can you tell me about Hosannah's development? When did she start crawling and walking? When did she sit up? When did she start talking?

Parent: She reached all of those milestones at the right time. I think she sat up for the first time at close to four months and a couple of months later she could sit on her own. I remember when she crawled for the first time. We had a big snowstorm at the end of November right around Thanksgiving so she was eight months old. She started saying words at around a year old; she was babbling before that though. She even said *mama*, *dada* earlier than a year, maybe nine or ten months old.

In this scenario Hosannah's mother is aware of what is going on with her daughter. She has begun to realize there is a problem and is able to answer questions with details and interpretation. The mother can also recount specifics about when Hosannah reached her developmental milestones. This parent is an excellent historian.

Unlike Hosannah's mother, there are clients and client advocates who are not such good historians. These clients need more help in telling their story. Take the following situation between a clinician and a client's mother. This mother needs more guidance throughout the interview.

Clinician: Tell me why you are here today.

Mother: My pediatrician told me to come.

Clinician: Why did your pediatrician think you should bring your daughter here?

Mother: I think she thinks there is something wrong with her speech.

Clinician: Are you concerned with your child's speech?

Mother: Not really. I understand her pretty well, but other people have a hard time.

Clinician: When did you first notice that people have trouble understanding her?

Mother: I guess when she started preschool. Her teachers said something to me.

At this point the clinician needs to start probing more to get details from the client's mother.

Clinician: When did she start preschool and what did the teachers say?

Mother: She started school three months ago. The teachers told me at our first meeting that she is difficult to understand. I started listening a little more closely to her and watching how others react when she talks. I guess I have noticed that people don't understand her as well as I do. Now that I think about it, my husband has trouble sometimes, too.

Clinician: Can you tell me about her development? When did she start crawling and walking? When did she sit up? When did she start talking?

Client: Oh, I don't remember.

Clinician: I know it can be hard to remember all of those dates. Let's start with sitting up. Can you remember anything about the time of year when it happened?

Client: Yes, actually, it was the Fourth of July. We met our friends for a picnic and she sat up, she was leaning against my legs a little but that was the first time. She was born in March, so she must have been four months old.

In this scenario, the clinician has to ask a lot of questions to get information from the client's mother. The clinician even uses a strategy to help the client's mother recall when her daughter reached certain milestones by associating the event to the time of year when it happened. Depending on the situation and the memory of the person being interviewed, you may need to use strategies like these to get more information from the person. Asking questions about the chronology of events is also a helpful strategy when interviewing. Questions like, "So, what happened first?" "When did you first notice an issue?" and "What happened next?" are ways to facilitate clients' recall of events during the interview.

When clarifying concepts throughout the interview, take care not to ask leading questions. A leading question assumes a message clients do not necessarily intend but is what the clinician desires to evoke. For example, a clinician may ask a client, "You avoid speaking situations because you do not like the sound of your voice, don't you?" This question suggests that the sound of the client's voice prevents the client from entering speaking situations. The phrasing of this question, especially ending with "don't you," also implies a challenge to the client at a stage in the treatment process when a challenge may not be warranted. The clinician should have asked the question in a nonleading form, for example, "Why do you avoid certain speaking situations?" Clients now have the opportunity to answer the question based on how they feel without anything implied from the clinician.

Summary and Transition

Once the body of the interview is complete, you should summarize your clients' story to make sure you have the time line correct and important information identified. Take a moment to clarify any concepts and ask clients whether they have any other information to add. For example, you may say, "Let me summarize what you just told me. Please let me know if what I have isn't correct or if I'm missing any key points." Then you would proceed by recapping the interview.

At this point you should be able to identify your client's chief complaint. A chief complaint can be characterized in a number of ways. It is the primary motive, the reason your client has come to you for an evaluation. It is what is bothering your client the most. It is, importantly, what your client wants to begin working on first in treatment.

Chief complaint: The chief complaint can be characterized in a number of ways. It is the primary motive, the reason a client comes to a clinician for an evaluation. It is what is bothering the client the most. It is, importantly, what the client wants to begin working on first in treatment.

Client Interview Guidelines

- Provide a summary of the evaluation.
- Transition into questioning by asking a general open-ended question.
- Guide clients through the story-telling process.
- Use the chronology of events to help guide clients (e.g., "What happened first, second, etc.?").
- Intersperse open- and close-ended questions as needed.
- Restate important dates and concepts to ensure accurate transmission of information.
- Do not ask leading questions.

At this point you should state what you believe is the client's chief complaint and clarify whether you are accurate in your assessment of what is most troubling to your client. If you are unsure, then you should question the client further before moving forward. In the scenario below, Annabelle is a 6-year-old child with a unilateral hearing loss who just began wearing a hearing aid.

Clinician: So, Annabelle, your mom and I have spent a lot of time talking about you and what's going on with your hearing aid. I want to ask you a few questions now. Is that okay? [*Annabelle nods.*] The first thing I want to know is how you feel about wearing your hearing aid.

Annabelle: It's okay. I hear my teachers and my friends better. I usually don't even know it's there. The tube itches my ear a little and that bothers me, but it's getting better.

Clinician: Yeah, it takes some time for your ear to get used to the plastic, but I'm glad it's getting better. Is there anything else that bothers you about using the hearing aid?

Annabelle: [*Pauses.*] There is one boy in class who keeps making fun of me. He doesn't always say something, but when my hair is in a ponytail he can see the hearing aid; then he laughs and teases me.

Clinician: How does it make you feel when he teases you?

Annabelle: I get embarrassed, and it makes me want to take off the hearing aid.

Clinician: It sounds like this boy's teasing is really bothering you. Is there anything else that is bothering you about your hearing aid?

Annabelle: No, the plastic tube and that boy at school are what bother me most.

After only a few questions, the clinician in the above scenario can identify the client's chief complaints. One is the discomfort the client feels with the tubing in her ear and the other is the boy teasing her at school. Once you have summarized your client's story and clarified your client's chief complaint, you should transition to the next phase of the evaluation. In Annabelle's case, a potential issue, teasing, has surfaced. It may become an ongoing concern, and the clinician would be wise to note it and check its effect at intervals in the future.

Closeout

At the end of the evaluation you must always take time to provide information to clients on how they performed during the evaluation. You will summarize results, provide recommendations, make referrals, and clarify the next phase of the process. During evaluations, novice clinicians often find the closeout to be a difficult task. It is the pinnacle of information exchange where you, as the professional, provide clients with your professional judgment and opinion. This judgment is based on the analysis of all the information you acquired throughout the evaluation, beginning with your initial meeting, proceeding through the interview, and culminating in the results compiled from your testing.

Guidelines for Administering a Closeout for an Evaluation

- Acknowledge and thank the client for participating in the process.
- Restate key concepts from the interview.
- Briefly review the purpose of each of the tests you administered.
- Concisely and directly state your assessment, diagnosis, recommendations, and referrals.
- Provide your prognosis for recovery based on your client's motivation, client's support system, client's willingness to participate in evaluation, client's current health status, and client's performance in stimulability testing or trial therapy.
- Ask whether your client has any questions, and answer questions appropriately.
- Clarify your client's goals.
- Provide your client with brochures, pamphlets, web site links, or information he or she can read at home.

During the closeout, you may have to give diagnoses that are unexpected or unwelcome. Definitely acknowledge that this type of information might be difficult to receive, and state that you understand that clients will have many questions as the information starts to sink in. At this moment be sure to let your clients know that you are on their side, will answer questions to the best of your ability, and will provide direction and support to the highest standard of care.

At the end of every treatment session, you should also take time to summarize and, in essence, close out with your clients. You should recap what you accomplished during the session. Indicate progress your clients have made toward goals. Clarify with clients that the goals you are working on are still important. Review homework assignments and provide information about what will be addressed in the next session. If you are treating a young child, you should end sessions a little early so you can speak with the parent or guardian about the child's progress, goals, and future treatment.

The Fundamentals of an Informed Client

During the interview process, you have a responsibility to gather the information you need to begin treatment, but your responsibility does not cease there. You must also make sure that your clients receive and appropriately process the information they require to proceed in a productive fashion. Clients must absorb a considerable amount of information and possess a strong motivation to succeed in addressing targeted communication issues.

Basic Knowledge for All Clients

All clients need to obtain a common cache of basic knowledge. This knowledge may be (1) practical, (2) technical, or (3) developmental (Jarvis, 1992; Khatib & Nikouee, 2012; Masciotra, Morel, & Ruiz, 2012) (see **Figure 5-3**).

1. Practical knowledge encompasses the information your clients need to attend sessions and perform the tasks and projects associated with the clinical process. The physical location of sessions, the date and time of sessions, and the means of transportation to and from sessions are examples of practical matters.

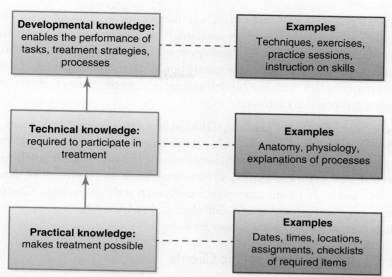

FIGURE 5-3 Types of Knowledge. Clients need to have information and knowledge that help them through the different stages of the therapy process.

An individualized checklist of items that clients need for sessions is another bit of practical knowledge. The list can be wide-ranging and might include items like a note-taking device, specific literature, bottled water, hearing aids, and homework due each session. With such a checklist each session can run more smoothly with less worry over needed items that might otherwise be forgotten.

2. Technical knowledge is what clients need to know to participate effectively in treatment. This type of knowledge can include anatomical data that helps explain more precisely what clients are doing or not doing when speaking or listening, what parts of the anatomy are functioning adequately or inadequately and why, as well as specific physiological changes that may be necessary for improvement.

Technical knowledge can likewise describe instruments and devices you intend to employ with particular clients, how these devices are used, and how they help collect information. Clients should be informed about the purpose of any piece of equipment you may use with them.

The appropriate level of technical knowledge for particular clients depends on clients' age and mental capacity, the amount of knowledge they require to obtain the optimal benefit from the technology being employed, and the explanations necessary to satisfy their curiosity or need to understand.

3. Developmental knowledge, the third type of basic knowledge, is information given to assist clients in performing the tasks, techniques, and strategies established to generate desired improvements. Clients need to know how to do all the things you ask of them during treatment and between sessions.

Developmental knowledge can include instructions on techniques that will be practiced and skills that will be acquired. It can also encompass the thinking behind a particular treatment strategy or series of steps that clients will take to achieve their goals. Developmental knowledge describes what a particular accomplishment "feels like" as well as what is happening when that accomplishment is successfully achieved.

Every client will acquire practical, technical, and developmental knowledge throughout the clinical process. The value of this knowledge is obvious: it enables clients to make progress. As you counsel clients, you use this information to help increase comfort with new stages and techniques for improvement. You will find that these descriptions and explanations can enhance motivation and collaboration. Clients tend to experience greater ownership and control when they know what is going on, what they are being asked to do, and why they are doing it.

Basic Knowledge for Specific Clients

Practical, technical, and developmental knowledge is common to all clients, but it is always tailored to the unique speech, language, swallowing, or hearing disorder for which a particular client is being treated. You must be selective, not overly generic or overly detailed, in the information you transmit to a given client. Follow these guidelines when you are framing your discussion of basic knowledge with your clients.

Basic Knowledge of the Treatment Process

Knowledge of the treatment process itself is valuable. When clients know what to expect during treatment, they have a context that helps them understand how their current activity will lead to the desired outcomes. Clients can mark progress in the journey and be assured that the destination is getting ever closer.

To be sure, information about the treatment *process* can be overwhelming, especially if the process is complex and expected to take significant time. Revealing the process in smaller steps might be advisable. Often you can simplify your explanation, omitting details that might confuse your clients.

The most important aspect of information about the treatment process is its link to the goal. However you choose to describe the process to your clients, you must make very clear that the process will lead to the accomplishment of the goal. There may be

Guidelines for Providing Basic Knowledge to Clients

- The information relates specifically to this client's issues. The relevance of what is transmitted is self-evident.
- The information does not overwhelm but is given in manageable "doses."
- Information is passed on when it is needed. That usually means that you give the information to the client at the point at which the client will be making use of it.
- Information is reinforced by repetition, by use of audiovisual aids, and by delivering it in written format, especially if you expect the client to make use of it.

times when you ask clients to "take it on faith" that the steps will be productive. In these cases, explanation of the process may only confuse clients or distract them from completing the activity you are facilitating. Eventually, when you take the initiative to explain a process, you then connect that process to the intended result.

The Dangers of Insufficient Information

Whereas too much or overly complicated information can be daunting and confusing, insufficient information thwarts the whole point of giving information. Clients end up with an inadequate description or an inadequate explanation. This can leave them frustrated or just misinformed. If clients act on insufficient information, they may not act in the way you intend.

Give thought to what it is you are explaining or describing and make sure you have painted a full and complete picture, even if you are simplifying that picture. Always allow for questions. These questions will help you bridge any gaps in your clients' understanding.

Transferring Information Throughout the Counseling Process

Maintaining the flow of information with your clients throughout treatment is important. Listen and observe to keep updated and accurate information about all you need to know to keep your clients engaged and to counsel appropriately. Give required information in a timely fashion so your clients remain knowledgeable along the way.

Knowledge Progression for All Clients

All clients must be updated regularly on their progress and on what is expected of them. You can use the first few minutes and last few minutes of each session to recap and give a status report detailing the matters that clients should be aware of. There is a progression of knowledge as your clients move through the treatment process. It is your responsibility to see that your clients accumulate the information as it is needed, see how that information builds on what went before, and achieve a confident understanding of each new layer of knowledge.

Knowledge Progression for Specific Speech-Language, Swallowing, and Hearing Issues

What, then, do clients need to know about their own issue or disorder? The key to answering this question is the phrase *need to know*. This principle is a useful one for determining what and how much information to transmit to clients as well as when to transmit it. Ask, "What does this client need to know to achieve the goals established at this particular point in treatment?" Such knowledge includes the particular steps in a technique or process, the details of the practice regimen that you are proposing, and ways to monitor progress. Those items constitute the minimum knowledge required and fit the "need to know" standard.

Counseling indicates what further information ought to flow to your clients. Some lose motivation if they do not understand the reasons you chose a particular technique. Some feel uninformed if they have no solid grasp of the theory behind a process. Many need assurances from you that they can actually do what you are proposing before their next session. Asking clients whether they "feel informed" is crucial to ensuring that clients are informed, as the following scenario illustrates.

Clinician: OK, Mahin, you know what you need to practice during the next two weeks.

Mahin: Yes.

Clinician: If you forget, all the steps are written down on the sheet I gave you, right?

Mahin: Yes, they are clear. Since we practiced them here, I know how it goes.

[*Clinician has made sure that Mahin truly does know the steps well enough to perform them on her own.*]

Clinician: Great. What other information could you use at this point? [*Clinician is asking, open-endedly, whether Mahin feels fully informed.*]

Mahin: Well, I'm not really sure why I'm doing this; I mean, I know how to do it, but what's the point?

Clinician: You're not sure how this will help you?

Mahin: I can see that it might help me overcome my shyness, since I have to practice with people I don't know, but what else will it do for me?

Clinician: You mean how does it relate to the goals we set …

Mahin: Yeah.

Clinician: OK, you know one of our intermediate goals is to participate more in discussions with your family and friends.

Mahin: Yes, but I don't see how this exercise helps that goal.

Clinician: Let me explain how it works. You are still getting used to your new hearing aids, and you are beginning to realize how often you missed out on the conversations going on around you. Asking a question to a person you don't know and listening throughout the response will help you to learn to keep focus throughout an interaction with another person.

Mahin: I get it. You don't want me to drop out of conversations as much as I used to.

Clinician: Yes, that's right.

Mahin: Thanks. That really helps.

In the scenario the clinician showed patience, responsive listening, and a willingness to give Mahin all the information she felt she needed. If she would benefit from knowing statistics related to the success of a particular technique, the clinician should feel free to supply those data. In fact, Mahin did ask about the purpose of the exercise. In this situation the clinician decided correctly to go beyond the "need to know" standard. By making this decision, the clinician was able to increase Mahin's understanding of the reason for the exercise. Information can generate confidence and motivation. It can help create a positive attitude and diminish anxiety. Yes, too much information can overwhelm or confuse, but you often have to give more than the minimum information. Many times you have to go beyond the "need to know basis" if you desire a highly successful outcome. Careful listening and questioning reveal the level of information your clients really need.

Knowledge Stages of the Therapy Process

Throughout treatment, clients must be kept informed of their progress in the most specific terms. Later stages of treatment may require a more sophisticated comprehension of the concepts involved in the process to gain a more advanced grasp of the steps through which the clients are advancing. Failure to keep clients abreast of this relevant information can cause frustration, confusion, and sometimes serious missteps. A common consequence of not being fully informed is regression or plateauing. Intelligent attention to your clients' needs for information is as critical to your counseling efforts as any other focus.

Informing Advocates and Allies

Information should also flow to client advocates. The nature of this information, its frequency, and its timing are all matters of judgment, but there are guidelines to use when determining what to tell client advocates and when to tell them.

Knowledge Progression as the Process Advances: Why Keep Them Informed?

The journey through therapy frequently builds toward ultimate success, the achievement of the long-term goals. The information you give at the beginning may be rudimentary, enough to get started. As the process continues, you may be called upon to impart more sophisticated data. Without those data, clients may flounder or be unable to comprehend what you are asking of them. Keeping them informed requires patience and an ability to couch sometimes-technical matters in terms your clients can grasp. This task is especially difficult with a person who is young or has receptive language problems. All along the way, however, your job is to render the information your clients need to continue progressing and to do so with confidence and enthusiasm.

Guidelines on Giving Timely Information to Clients and Advocates

- Client advocates should know enough to be able to return information to the clinician in a usable form and render assistance to clients as the clinician deems helpful.
- Advocates should receive clear instructions on how they can assist the clients on specific occasions when they are enlisted to help.
- Without explicit client permission, clinicians may not give advocates access to confidential information about clients' progress, disorder, or personal information.

Knowledge Required by Advocates and Allies for Specific Issues

Different advocates need different kinds and levels of knowledge about the issues you and your clients are dealing with. A high school athletic coach may need simple information, like where to position a client who is hard of hearing, whereas the parents of a third grader need much fuller information on symptoms, techniques, rationales, and ways to help. Each advocate must be assessed and given the right information at the right time in the most effective manner.

Remember, advocates may come and go during treatment. One may be called into service repeatedly or continuously. Another may be solicited only once and for a short period of time. The content and timing of the information you give the advocates depend on their roles in helping your clients. Careful planning and attention to the needs of your clients enable you to use this Circle of Power to the full benefit of your clients.

Knowledge Required by Advocates and Allies throughout Therapy

If an advocate is called upon once or infrequently, the advocate usually requires only the information needed at the moment you call upon that person. Ask yourself how exactly the advocate is to assist you and what exactly the advocate needs to know to render that assistance. Advocates and other allies play an integral role in your clients' journey through therapy, and they need to be informed throughout the process.

Review of Key Points

- Information sharing is what most often comes to mind when people think of communication. You and your clients need specific information to be successful in treatment.
- An informed clinician is a clinician equipped with the knowledge needed to collaborate with a client in setting appropriate therapy goals and taking the steps necessary to achieve those goals.
- The client's case history, the starting point of information gathering, covers information on the client's speech-language or audiological record, including issues, disorders, and treatment history, as well as background data on family, education, and occupation, medical, social, and related information.
- An informed client possesses the information required to proceed in a productive fashion, including (1) practical, (2) technical, and (3) developmental knowledge.
- Practical, technical, and developmental knowledge is always tailored to a particular client's unique speech, swallowing, or hearing disorders. Knowledge of the therapy process itself can be valuable as long as it is linked to the goal.
- If the client acts on insufficient information, the client may not act in the way you intend.
- The interview process involves information exchange between you, the client, and the client's caregiver, spouse, family, or friends. The credibility you have with your client is essential to the successful exchange of information in the interview.
- The first contact, often made by the client, becomes the first impression your client has of you.
- Never disclose any personal health information to anyone but the client. Once the client comes to your office, you should have the client sign a HIPAA form indicating how the client would prefer to be contacted, who you can give information to, and whether you can leave information on a voicemail.
- When clarifying concepts throughout the interview do not ask leading questions. Follow the guideline for interviewing clients.
- Closeout occurs at the end of every session and at the end of an evaluation; you take time to provide information to clients on how they performed during the evaluation or treatment, summarize results, indicate progress toward goals (for treatment), provide recommendations, make referrals, and clarify the next phase of the process.
- There is a progression of knowledge that must be transmitted as the client moves through the therapy process. It includes "need to know" data about their own issue or disorder.
- Counseling indicates what further information ought to flow to your clients to keep them motivated and feeling informed.

- Information should also flow to client advocates and associates of clients. The nature, frequency, and timing of this information are all matters of judgment, but there are guidelines.
- Different advocates need different kinds and levels of knowledge about the issues you and your clients are dealing with.

Practical Exercises

Preparing and Helping Clients Tell Their Story

To help with the following activity, take some time to answer the questions below.

One of the biggest issues I face in my life is _____

I find it difficult when I have to _____

I get anxious when I have to _____

A recurring issue I face in my life is _____

The thing that scares me the most is _____

The thing that gives me the most trouble is _____

The person I have most difficulty with is _____

The main issue with my relationship with that person is _____

My life would be better if _____

I wish I _____

Analyze the answers to the questions above. Try to identify a recurrent theme or issue. State the issue or problem explicitly.

Now, answer the questions below.

I have had this problem since _____

This problem started when _____

This problem started because _____

The things that make this problem worse are _____

The things that make this problem better are _____

To make this problem better, I would _____

In-Class Activity 1: Developing Interviewing Skills

Put yourselves in groups of three.

- Assign one person to be the client, one person to be the clinician, and one person to be the evaluator.
- The clinician begins by introducing her- or himself and providing a firm handshake. Then the clinician states the following, "*Based on your answers to the previous statements, tell me about the issues you are currently experiencing.*"

- The clinician should then guide the client through a 5-minute exercise to help the client tell his or her story. Keep in mind listening skills, responses to indicate understanding, and attending behaviors (from Chapter 3). Also focus responses to guide the client through his or her story (funneling technique). Clinicians should not assess the message or create a response at this stage.
- The evaluator should keep track of time. At the end of 5 minutes, the evaluator stops the discussion. The evaluator takes 3 minutes to provide feedback to the clinician. The goal of the feedback is to help clinicians to identify positive qualities about themselves as interviewers and to help clinicians become better interviewers. Feedback should be constructive, specific, positive, and helpful.
- The client should then provide feedback to the clinician about the interviewing process. Did the clinician help in the story-telling process? Did the clinician seem attentive? Were follow-up questions logical and helpful to the process?
- Continue the activity until all three members of the group have had a chance to play all three roles (client, clinician, evaluator).
- Reflect on the experience with in-class discussion.

REFERENCES

Barone, O. R., & Tellis, C. M. (2008). *Your voice is your business.* San Diego, CA: Plural Publishing.

Barrick, M. R., Swider, B. W., & Stewart, G. L. (2010). Initial evaluations in the interview: Relationships with subsequent interviewer evaluations and employment offer. *Journal of Applied Psychology, 95*(6), 1163–1172.

Beatson, J. E. (2006). Preparing speech-language pathologists as family-centered practitioners in assessment and program planning for children with autism spectrum disorder. *Seminars in Speech-Language Pathology, 27*(1), 1–9.

Blume, S. S. (1999). Histories of cochlear implantation. *Social Sciences & Medicine, 49*(9), 1257–1268.

Hubble, M. A., Duncan, B. L., & Miller, S. D. (1999). *The heart and soul of change: What works in therapy.* Washington, DC: American Psychological Association.

Ivey, A. E, Ivey, M. B., & Zalaquett, C. P. (2010). *Intentional interviewing and counseling: Facilitating client development in a multicultural society* (7th ed.). Belmont, CA: Brooks/Cole, Cengage Learning.

Jarvis, P. (1992). Learning practical knowledge. *New Directions for Adult Continuing Education, 55,* 89–95.

Khatib, M., & Nikouee, M. (2012). Planned focus on form: Automatization of procedural knowledge. *RELC Journal: A Journal of Language Teaching and Research, 43*(2), 187–201.

Levin, D. Z., Whitener, E. M., & Cross, R. (2006). Perceived trustworthiness of knowledge sources: The moderating impact of relationship length. *Journal of Applied Psychology, 91*(5), 1163–1171.

Masciotra, D., & Morel, D., & Ruiz, J. (2012). Transmitting technical knowledge or developing action: An enactive approach and the ASKAR method in TPE. *Therapeutic Patient Education, 4*(1), 1–10.

SECTION III

The Solution Cycle
Phase Two: Choosing Allies: "Developing the Circle of Power"

Chapter 6
Affirmation: Self and Stigma, Doubt and Confidence

Chapter 7
Alliances: Getting Support

Section Three focuses on Phase Two of the Solution Cycle: Choosing Allies. In Phase One, Section Two, you learned how important it is to make a good first impression, build rapport with your clients, and continue fostering that relationship throughout the therapy process. Small talk was a highlighted intention in Phase One. Section Two also pointed out that information exchange is an important intention especially as you learn about your clients' story. Information is transferred between the clinician and clients mainly during the interview. You continue sharing information with your clients during therapy, but you determine how much information clients and their advocates need to be most successful. Chapter 6 considers another one of the Five Intentions of Communication, self-affirmation. Chapter 7 discusses the Circle of Power or alliance base that you and your clients build throughout your relationship.

Affirmation: Self and Stigma, Doubt and Confidence

KEY TERMS

- Activity limitations
- Disability
- Ideal self
- Impairments
- Participation restriction
- Self-affirmation
- Self-concept
- Self-esteem
- Self-image
- Shame
- Stigma

LEARNING OBJECTIVES

After reading this chapter, you will be able to:

- Define and clarify the relationship among terms related to self-esteem: self-affirmation, self-concept, self-image, self-esteem, ideal self
- Identify major causes and counseling approaches to increasing congruence between self-image and the ideal self
- Identify effective counseling strategies to counter the effects of stigma and shame
- List the techniques for restoring self-esteem and a can do attitude in clients

Client Self-Concept

Self-affirmation is one of the Five Intentions of a speaker. Whenever clients start a sentence with the word *I*, they are affirming themselves or something about themselves. They are making a direct or indirect assertion about the way they think and feel about themselves. It is present in many utterances and can point the way to powerful counseling opportunities. In this chapter, you will learn how your clients' self-image affects the progression of therapy.

Self-affirmation depends on self-image. Once self-image is defined, you can explore the ways self-image affects the clinical process. Clients display different behaviors at different times depending on how they see themselves, and these behaviors can vary throughout therapy. In one session a client could be strong, ready to

> **Self-affirmation:** One of the Five Intentions of a speaker. A direct or indirect assertion by a speaker about the way the speaker thinks and feels about himself or herself.

Self-image: How people see themselves, their current state—beautiful or ugly, smart or dumb, good or bad, fat or thin, or something in between. Self-image does not always reflect reality. In effect, self-image depicts how far people think they really are from their ideal self.

Self-concept: According to Carl Rogers, "The organized, consistent set of perceptions and beliefs about oneself." Self-concept has three features: self-esteem or self-worth, ideal self, and self-image.

Self-esteem: Self-esteem is the value one places on oneself, acceptance or approval of self. Self-esteem is a sense of self-worth. Largely formed during childhood, self-esteem is thought to be learned through experience, and not something that can be taught.

Ideal self: The person one would like to be, the fulfillment of one's supreme wishes and ambitions, one's desired state.

conquer the world; in the next session that same person could feel defeated and unsure of how therapy will help.

Self-image may deter progress in therapy when clients become ashamed or feel stigmatized by the presence of a communication disorder. You will examine the effects of shame and stigma and the consequent need for counseling, and you will learn to be sensitive to the impact-related factors such as culture and societal perceptions can have on the therapy process.

As your clients face their insecurities and doubts, their feelings of helplessness and frustration, you will examine the ways counseling can empower them to persevere and finally achieve their therapy goals.

When you counsel, you are often, if not always, addressing your client's self-image. You must develop a clear understanding of the meaning of self-image, its role in effective counseling and therapy, and the ways self-image evolves under the impact of important events in the lives of your clients.

What Self-Image Is

For our purposes, self-image can be defined as Carl Rogers understood it (Rogers, 1951). He began with the broader term, self-concept, which he said was "the organized, consistent set of perceptions and beliefs about oneself" (Rogers, 1959, p. 481). Self-concept has three features: self-esteem or self-worth, ideal self, and self-image (**Figure 6-1**).

Self-esteem is the value you place on yourself, your acceptance or approval of yourself. Self-esteem is a sense of self-worth. Largely formed during childhood, self-esteem is thought to be learned through experience and is not something that can be taught (Blascovich & Tomaka, 1993).

Individuals with high self-esteem are confident in their abilities and do not worry about what others think of them. They are self-accepting and generally optimistic. The two main benefits of a high self-esteem are feelings of happiness or pleasantness and the inclination to take initiative (Baumeister, Campbell, Krueger, & Vohs, 2003). In therapy, clients who have high self-esteem are usually more willing to attempt new strategies and techniques even if the techniques are seen as awkward or embarrassing. These clients are more likely to generalize concepts learned in therapy to other social and professional environments much sooner than clients with low self-esteem.

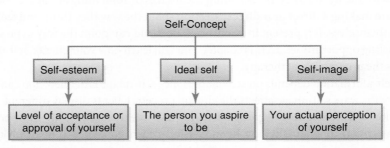

FIGURE 6-1 Self-Concept. The three features of self-concept are self-esteem, ideal self, and self-image.

Individuals with low self-esteem view themselves more negatively. They tend not to exhibit confidence in their abilities, are inclined to worry about or care what others think of them, show a desire to be or act like others, and are generally pessimistic (Rogers, 1959). Clients with low self-esteem have more difficulty believing that they can make improvements with therapy. They may exhibit apprehension about learning new techniques or strategies and may express doubt about their abilities to acquire new skills.

Counseling should focus on reducing barriers constructed by low self-esteem. Such counseling is crucial to building confidence and optimism about the outcomes of therapy. Using positive reinforcement as a reward for specific client behaviors that reflect high self-esteem and show a desire for self-improvement have been shown to be more effective than haphazard praise in hopes of boosting self-esteem (Baumeister et al., 2003).

Self-esteem can be measured in a variety of ways. The most widely used method of measuring self-esteem is the Rosenberg Self-Esteem Scale (Rosenberg, 1999). This 10-item scale is designed to measure individuals' degree of agreement regarding statements about themselves. For example, "On the whole, I am satisfied with myself" and "I feel that I'm a person of worth, or at least on an equal plane with others." The revised Janis-Field Feelings of Inadequacy Scale (JFS) is a multidimensional scale of self-worth and can be used with adults (Fleming & Courtney, 1984). The School Short-Form Coopersmith Self-Esteem Inventory is an appropriate tool to use with middle school students ages 13 to 15 years (Hills, Francis, & Jennings, 2011).

The ideal self is the person you would like to be, the fulfillment of your supreme wishes and ambitions, your desired state. The fictional wizard Harry Potter once came upon the Mirror of Erised, which is said to reflect the "deepest and most desperate desire of our hearts." (*Erised* is *desire* spelled backward.) In that mirror Harry Potter saw what Rogers would have called Harry's ideal self.

Self-image is just how you see yourself, your current state—beautiful or ugly, smart or dumb, good or bad, fat or thin, or something in between. Self-image does not always reflect reality. In effect, self-image depicts how far we think we really are from our ideal self. A person who stutters may believe his occasional disfluencies are clearly obvious to his colleagues, though, in reality, his colleagues may not notice them at all. In contrast to the previous example, an adolescent client may think she pronounces her /r/ phoneme correctly all of the time but cringes when she hears an audio recording of her mispronunciation of the phoneme during speech. A grandfather may believe he hears all aspects of conversation, though he is confused when he does not recollect key components of a story because he never heard them in the first place.

Harry Potter's headmaster told him, "The happiest person in the whole world would look in the Mirror of Erised and see a reflection of exactly the way he or she is." In Rogers's terminology, the happiest person in the world is the one whose self-image and ideal self are exactly the same, or as close to congruent as they can be (**Figure 6-2**). Individuals whose self-image is congruent with their ideal self are likely to have high self-esteem. Those whose self-image is far from their ideal self are likely to have trouble with self-esteem.

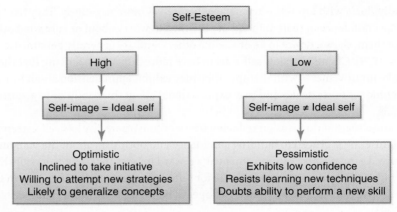

FIGURE 6-2 Self-Esteem. An individual whose self-image and ideal self are congruent often exhibits higher self-esteem than an individual whose self-image and ideal self are incongruent.

The Role of Self-Concept in Success and Failure of the Clinical Process

When determining whether speech-language-hearing therapy is an appropriate treatment option for clients, clinicians must be aware of not only the impairment the client faces but also the impact the impairment has on the client's ability to perform activities of daily living and fully participate in social and occupational settings. The World Health Organization's (WHO, 2015a) International Classification of Functioning, Disability, and Health (ICF) uses disability as a term that encompasses impairments (negative changes to the body's anatomy and physiology), activity limitations (problems in performing particular tasks or functions as a result of the impairment), and participation restriction (difficulty with or decreased involvement in social and occupational situations) (World Health Organization, 2015b).

The severity of the disability dictates the necessity for a particular treatment. Hearing loss is an impairment—a change in the structure and function of the hearing mechanism. Activity limitation is the individual's inability to detect sounds at those frequencies affected by the impairment. Participation restriction, then, is the individual's decreased involvement in conversations because of the hearing loss. Not all individuals experience impairments the same way. Two people with the same hearing loss can be given the same recommendation for hearing aids, but one may choose to purchase the aids while the other does not. The decision these individuals make is based on their perception of how much the hearing loss affects their quality of life.

Evaluating the severity of the disability is multifactorial. The ICF Checklist is a practical tool that can be used to assess individuals' perceptions of their functioning and disability (World Health Organization, 2015b). An astute clinician uses this checklist to assess how clients' current (self-image) and desired (ideal self) states affect their perception of themselves related to their communication impairment as well as their views on therapy. Remember that congruence between clients' current self and ideal self leads to a happy self. Clients who do not view their impairment as having a

Disability: A term that encompasses impairments (negative changes to the body's anatomy and physiology), activity limitations (problems in performing particular tasks or functions as a result of the impairment), and participation restriction (difficulty with or decreased involvement in social and occupational situations).

Impairments: A negative change to the body's anatomy and physiology.

Activity limitation: A problem in performing particular tasks or functions as a result of an impairment.

Participation restriction: Difficulty with or decreased involvement in social and occupational situations.

negative impact on their ability to participate in life situations may not be candidates for therapy.

The cases presented in the following paragraphs depict four individuals with different perceptions about the congruence between their current self and their ideal self and how these perceptions can affect both counseling and the clinical process. Olivia, a successful mortgage broker, is a person who stutters. The actual stuttering disfluencies she exhibits in her speech (e.g., blocks, prolongations, and part-word repetitions) are considered her impairment. Her inability to produce fluent speech is her activity limitation. If evaluated on the percentage and duration of stuttering moments as well as the number of concomitant secondary behaviors she has in a 2-minute sample of her speech, Olivia would be classified as having a moderate stuttering disorder.

Olivia's stuttering, however, does not reduce the professional impact she has in meetings with clients and colleagues. She has a large group of friends and is outgoing and amiable in social situations. She notices the stuttering moments in her speech, but they do not bother her in the least. Her participation restriction is completely unaffected by her impairment. Olivia's current self (at least related to her stuttering) is congruent with her ideal self. Her level of functioning regardless of her impairment classifies her as "not having a disorder"; her disability is mild. Therapy is not warranted in her case.

Clark, a colleague of Olivia's, is also a person who stutters. He rarely has stuttering moments in his speech, but when he does his whole life seems to fall apart. The thought of those moments embarrasses him so thoroughly that he avoids speaking situations completely. He would rather text or email his clients than call them on the phone. Leading meetings at work is one of his most feared situations. He enjoys going out with friends but often sits listening and rarely adds his own comments.

In this case, Clark's impairment and activity limitation are considered fairly mild, though the impact they have on his life is pretty severe. Because his current self is incongruent with his ideal self, he is a candidate for therapy. Counseling would also be a necessary component to his treatment to help him deal with the social and occupational barriers present in his life related to his stuttering. Clark has a stuttering disorder, and his disability is significantly qualified by his avoidance of life situations.

Clark's and Olivia's cases, though different, are fairly easy to assess. Sometimes, though, it is more difficult to delineate the best course of action on the basis of clients' responses. Len, for example, is a 58-year-old teacher who has an undiagnosed hearing loss. He has been a teacher for 30 years and prides himself on his attentiveness and devotion to student learning. The students praise him as their "best teacher." When asked by his physician at a routine appointment whether he is having trouble hearing, Len adamantly states that his hearing is fine. Len's family and his students disagree. His wife complains that the television volume is so high that it hurts her ears. Len's students wonder why he talks so loud during lectures and are confused when he does not always respond to their questions in class. In Len's case, his current self is congruent with his ideal self, though his current self is far from congruent with reality as perceived by everyone with whom he communicates.

Counseling becomes a priority with clients like Len. If he can be persuaded to have a hearing test, sometimes the hard facts of the audiogram will shed light on the reality of his impairment. A course of trial therapy may be offered. Len could be given a temporary hearing aid to use for a couple of weeks. Discussing the potential barriers Len faces related to his self-concept is important to understanding why Len may be opposed to admitting that he does have difficulty hearing in certain environments.

Argyle (2008) proposes four factors that can affect your self-esteem and consequently your self-concept: others' reactions to you, your comparison of others to yourself, your roles in society, and your identity. In the right circumstances, any of these factors can promote a positive self-image. With Len, however, all four could constitute potential barriers to a positive self-concept and may influence his denial of the hearing impairment and subsequent social and occupational ramifications. Effective counseling could remove these barriers by making Len aware that his misperceptions may be due to cultural or public stigma as well as his own biases.

Whereas Len's error is the misperception of his current self, some clients make a different mistake. They have an unattainable view of their ideal self. These are the clients who strive for an ideal self that is beyond their capacity. Caregivers can also fall prey to this overly optimistic perception.

Marilyn's 19-year-old son, George, was diagnosed with autism, low cognitive abilities, and low IQ as a young child. George has had speech-language services with several different speech-language pathologists since his diagnosis. Every time the speech-language pathologist indicated that George's goals were met, Marilyn switched clinicians for a new perspective and evaluation. She hears the same assessment from each clinician: "George is functioning at his cognitive and intellectual capacity. No other speech-language services are warranted at this time." Even so, Marilyn demands to have George in therapy. She is willing to pay out of pocket for the expense. No one can begrudge Marilyn for her dedication and devotion to her child, but the ideal self she desires for George is beyond his cognitive and intellectual capacity.

Counseling Marilyn on the reality of the situation is imperative. Marilyn needs to state her goals for George. The clinician and Marilyn then can sort the goals into attainable and unattainable based on George's documented level of functioning. This process is not an easy task. Many times, caregivers and clients have to grieve the loss of the unattainable goals, the shattered dreams. They need to work on aligning their own or their loved one's current self with an attainable ideal self.

Society often insists that you should "never give up," that "quitters never win," and that "anything is possible." Recognizing limits, however, is not giving up; it is part of a process of setting new goals that are in line with the reality of the situation. Spending time, energy, and focus on goals that are possible is much more productive than constantly reaching for the impossible.

In George's case maintenance and generalization of the client's current self are the priority. Recommending that George attend group therapy or a day program setting to maintain his current social skills and communication abilities may be excellent options. The clinician could also teach Marilyn communication strategies to work on at home with George to help him generalize his learned skills.

Clinicians who adopt a solution-focused approach to therapy address clients' desired goals and construct a detailed picture of what their clients' lives will look like once clients' goals have been met and their problem has been resolved or dealt with acceptably. With Olivia, Clark, Len, and Marilyn, clinicians should look to these individuals' past experiences to determine times when aspects of their goals were already being expressed or successfully addressed to some degree in their lives. These moments will form the building blocks for the construction of appropriate and effective solutions. To some extent, these past experiences provide an example of a time when the clients' self-image was more congruent with their ideal self.

How self-image changes

Amado, a young man from the Philippines, came to a speech-language pathologist to work on modifying his accent for job interviews. He and his clinician had the following exchange in an early session.

Clinician: What do you notice about the way other people react to you, Amado?

Amado: Whenever people hear the way I talk, they know that I'm not from around here.

Clinician: Does that present a problem for you?

Amado: Before, no. Some people like my accent, but it's hard to find a job with my accent.

Clinician: How do you know your accent is causing difficulties for you in looking for a job?

Amado: It's not hard to figure out. Some places have turned me down because they say I'm not what they are looking for. I know what they are looking for. Someone who doesn't sound like me.

Clinician: Do you think you sound bad in some way?

Amado: I did like the way I talk, but now I just want to talk like I'm from around here so I can fit in! Every time I talk now, it is like I am saying, "Look at the stupid man."

Clinician: You feel that having an accent tells some people you are stupid?

Amado: It tells me I am stupid.

The clinician has been alerted that Amado's self-image is suffering because of his perception that some other people devalue him because he speaks with an accent. In his "Mirror of Erised," he sees a version of himself that speaks with no accent. Interestingly, he has had an accent as long as he has spoken English, but he has not had a self-image problem about his accent until lately. Amado's clinician needs to determine the impact of his self-image on his motivation to modify his accent. On the surface, he would seem to be motivated by his affected self-image, but it is possible that he has come to believe himself too "stupid" to be able to speak the way he wants to speak.

In addition, Amado might have a tendency to set his goal unrealistically high. Accent modification is not accent removal. Given his possible feelings that any accent, even the vestige of an accent, might be an impediment, he could object to anything short of complete accent removal. For most clients, that is an unrealistic therapy goal. A useful counseling goal might be to help Amado see that significant accent modification will likely accomplish what he wants in his job search. He may also need help in restoring a positive self-image independent of his progress in modifying his accent.

You saw in the scenario that Amado's self-image underwent a change for the worse when he began seeking a job and noting people's apparent reaction to his accent. Self-image is dynamic. It changes continuously as events unfold and the perception of events evolves. Amado went from liking the way he spoke to believing his accent signaled that he was stupid. Accent modification will probably have an effect on his self-image, but how big an effect and what kind of effect remain to be seen.

With effective counseling, you can monitor a client's self-image and work to improve it. In Amado's case, his self-image is entwined with the progress he makes in modifying his accent. Counseling will be an important component throughout this process. It is difficult to imagine significant progress without it.

Cautious counseling: Understanding the limits

You should be aware of the limits to what even highly creative and competent counseling can achieve. As always, you must avoid the mistake of counseling independent of your therapy goals. You are a speech-language pathologist or audiologist attending to defined communication issues with your clients. You counsel to support and promote progress toward the improvement of those issues. No matter how tempted you may be, you are not justified in launching off on a separate mission to enhance your clients' self-image.

You are also well advised not to make the error of believing that reaching a counseling goal will magically address your therapy goals. Psychotherapists have been accused of falling into this trap: all they need to do is get the patient to see that her phobia is due to a traumatic childhood event and—*poof!*—the fear melts away and the patient is fine forever after. Likewise, as in Amado's case, you are mistaken if you believe that all you have to do to address Amado's accent issue is counsel him so successfully that he no longer is bothered by any accent he may have.

Obviously, a laudable result of counseling is a marked improvement in Amado's self-image; however, he came to you for help in modifying his accent, and, as long as this remains a goal defined by you and your client, your work is not complete until you reach the goal. You may also encounter situations where progress is slowed because the self-image of your clients is gravely affected by the communication disorder. In these situations the difficulties can become so overwhelming that the best course of action is to refer your clients to a licensed psychologist or counselor. After assessing the circumstances you can decide whether it is a good idea to continue your therapy or delay therapy until your clients are ready to resume.

The Variety of Roles Clients Play

Impact roles can have on clients

The roles clients play in society can have an impact on their self-image and their self-concept. This possibility was discussed in the scenario with Len, the teacher in denial about his hearing loss. Being a respected teacher is important to Len, as is his role as a devoted husband. Just acknowledging that he has trouble hearing could shake his confidence—make him feel like he is getting old or incapable of performing his job-related tasks. Actually wearing a hearing aid may drive him completely over the edge.

Amado also assumes many roles in daily life, each with its own features and challenges. He distinguished at least one of the roles he plays, that of job seeker.

Clinician: Amado, you told me how you feel about your accent during a job interview.

Amado: Yes, I feel lousy.

Clinician: You speak English with others, right?

Amado: My American friends, sure.

Clinician: How do you feel about your accent with them?

Amado: I don't know. I was always comfortable with them; they never made me feel like I was different.

Clinician: Has that changed?

Amado: Yes, some. After looking for jobs, I got sensitive about my accent. Even with my friends now I wonder sometimes; maybe they are nice to my face, but once my back is turned, what do they say?

Clinician: Do you think you are right to be suspicious?

Amado: Not really. They don't act any different. But I can't help it. This is really bothering me.

Clinician: How about at home? With family?

Amado: Yeah, when I don't have to speak English, it's all good. I feel like myself, maybe relieved, you know?

Amado needs to understand that he plays different roles in different situations and that these roles can alter his self-image.

Clarifying the different roles

As a clinician, you should explore the roles your clients play in society and determine what they require from your clients. One activity you can work on with your clients is the development of a "Spider Chart." This chart is used to assess the roles your clients play at different times in their lives (see **Figure 6-3**).

Have clients place their name in a circle in the middle of a piece of paper and then draw spokes out from the circle and identify the different roles they play in their life on each spoke (e.g., job seeker, son, husband, daughter, teacher, mother, friend). For each of these roles, have your clients identify one or two issues they face related to their communication disorder.

Obviously, the issues associated with Amado's accent or Len's hearing loss change as their roles change. Amado feels much more comfortable speaking with his family than he does in his role as a job seeker or friend. Len may be more likely to trial hearing aids at home than he would at school. This is true of all clients and applies to virtually all speech-language, swallowing, hearing, and voice disorders. Counseling and therapy must take into account various roles and their impact on the individual. You are not only

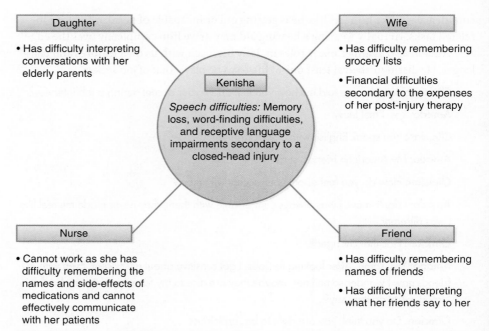

FIGURE 6-3 The Spider Chart. Using a Spider Chart allows clients to identify the prominent roles in their lives as well as the various difficulties they experience as a result of their communication disorders.

improving your clients' ability to correct or mitigate a disorder, you are helping your clients function better in their real world, in the great assortment of roles that they play.

In the 2010 movie *The King's Speech*, George VI is an individual who stutters. The movie makes many remarkable points about stuttering. Among them are the clearly different effects of the king's stuttering on the various roles he plays—that of parent, friend, husband, and, of course, the monarch who rallies his people with wartime radio broadcasts. His speech-language pathologist, Lionel Logue, counsels him to recognize these roles and treat his stuttering differently for different occasions.

In addition, Logue has to make George VI aware that his stuttering behaves differently when he is playing different roles. The stress of the broadcasts intensifies the severity of the disfluencies, and as a result he must employ a multitude of techniques to deliver a speech effectively. As a father speaking to his two daughters, he requires far fewer strategies to communicate. When you counsel, you will assist your clients in navigating the various roles they play and determining what is likely to be required to function acceptably in each of those roles.

Stigma and Shame

When Communication Disorders Stigmatize

The roles clients play in society are dynamic and not limited to a single word or definition. Len is not just a teacher. Len is the students' "best teacher." His role at the school and in his community carries prestige; it defines a portion of Len's character, his personality, and his identity. Because others view him in a positive light, Len's self-esteem is likely enhanced by his role as a teacher.

Relatives, friends, and colleagues of your clients are usually well meaning; however, they can be clueless about the impact their words and looks may have on your clients. When Len's friend alerts him that there is something in his ear, the friend may not be aware of Len's embarrassment at the sudden realization that the clear tube leading from Len's hearing aid to his ear canal is more visible than he previously thought. Sometimes, sadly, people are just plain malicious or mean. The effects of their behavior on clients can range from irritating to devastating. An impairment becomes stigmatized when it is labeled not only as a disorder but as a socially undesirable disorder. Len may be stigmatized by his hearing loss because of his belief that hearing loss signifies a change in his identity—"elderly, old, retirement age." When a prospective employer of Amado is impatient with Amado's accent, the employer is being insensitive; when that same employer indicates that individuals with accents are not suitable to work in this organization, the employer is stigmatizing. Unlike mere insensitivity, which is certainly painful enough, stigma carries the implication that Amado is unwelcome, a detriment to the institution and its people, a potential embarrassment, a blemish on its reputation.

An added challenge occurs when Amado experiences the force of stigma; then he is likely to feel many emotions—anger, sadness, shock—but perhaps the worst emotion is shame, the abject feeling that he is a disgrace, unworthy to be in the company of the stigmatizers. His self-image takes a direct hit; in the judgment of others he is found guilty, subject to shunning, name calling, and worse. The counseling challenge is to enable Amado to regain his sense of self-worth and his ability to thrive in his social environment.

Self Stigma and Public Stigma

There are two forms of stigma: self-stigma and public stigma (Corrigan, Larson, & Rüsch, 2009). Public stigma relates to how people in general understand and react to individuals with communication disorders. This type of stigma can be defined by stereotypes, prejudices, and discrimination. Stereotypes are beliefs adopted by individuals within one group about individuals from another group: "All individuals who wear hearing aids are old." When stereotypes are agreed upon and endorsed by one group about another group, they become prejudices. Often prejudices evoke negative emotional reactions about a group: "Individuals who wear hearing aids are old and cannot perform their job functions because of their hearing loss." The behavioral reaction to a prejudice is called discrimination and can manifest in one of three ways: opportunity loss, coercion, and segregation (Crocker, Major, & Steele, 1998).

Your culture comprises people with a common set of beliefs, values, and practices. Culture exalts what it considers consistent with those customs and can also disparage and belittle what is inconsistent. The culture itself may stigmatize what it considers an affront to its common beliefs, values, and practices. In mainstream U.S. culture an individual who stutters might be deemed a person with an impairment, certainly not someone subject to public stigma.

Shame: The abject feeling that a person is a disgrace, unworthy to be in the company of those who stigmatize. Self-image takes a direct hit; in the judgment of others the shamed one is found guilty, subject to shunning, name-calling, and worse.

Stigma: An impairment labeled not only as a disorder but as a socially undesirable disorder. Unlike mere insensitivity, stigma carries the implication that a person is unwelcome, a detriment to an institution and its people, a potential embarrassment, a blemish on its reputation.

Most if not all communication disorders have been or are subject to public stigma, some more than others. In practice, individuals who stutter can be stigmatized when their stuttering is associated with characteristics inconsistent with their culture's values. The individual who stutters may be perceived as lacking confidence, as nervous or timid. Once these associations are made, the individual who stutters may indeed be subject to the shame of a public stigma.

When individuals are aware of stereotypes, agree with stereotypes, and then apply them to themselves, public stigma is defined as self-stigma (Corrigan, Watson, & Barr, 2006; Watson, Corrigan, Larson, & Sells, 2007). Self-stigma negatively affects self-esteem. The research is quite clear that stigma can affect the attainment of goals and the positive outcome of therapy (Corrigan et al., 2009).

When clients experience stigma and shame, you should immediately begin counseling to determine the extent and effects of what is stigmatizing. Then you should counter the resultant impact on self-image, confidence, optimism, and motivation. The following guidelines should be considered when dealing with clients experiencing stigma.

Facing Doubt, Erasing Doubt

When, for whatever reason, self-image begins to suffer, when clients start to lower their opinion of themselves and their abilities, then the gap between their self-image and ideal self starts to looks unbridgeable. Their own Mirror of Erised shows them an image increasingly out of reach. Doubt replaces confidence. Success in therapy is threatened to its very foundations.

Inability and Frustration

"I just can't do it." As a clinician, this is a line you never want to hear. And, yet, it is a line you are almost certain to hear with your clients at one moment or another. Clients

Counseling Clients Experiencing Stigma

- Encourage the client to tell stories about what is stigmatizing and how it makes the client feel. Create an integrated narrative that gives a good sense of the client's beliefs and experiences.
- Set goals and construct a plan to counteract the effects of stigma and ensure that it does not obstruct the therapy process. The goal is not to remove stigma but to empower clients to continue the pursuit of their goals and participate in therapy in the face of stigma. A solution-focused approach centered on what can be done rather than on what cannot be done is effective in managing stigma.
- Use clients' relatives, friends, and associates to enlist an alliance base to confront the stigma. Peers, support groups, and mentoring services are helpful in managing stigma (Corrigan et al., 2009).
- Set aside time during every session to address and update the state of affairs in regard to the stigma and efforts to mitigate its effects. Be aware of any changes, particularly an intensification of the negative impact on your client.
- Monitor progress in challenging the stigma.

sometimes feel frustration, the sense that no matter how hard they try they don't progress. The "can't do" attitude is accompanied by the loss of ownership or control and can have a number of causes, including the impact of the kind of stigmatizing discussed earlier. Causes like those are related to an issue of self-image, and counseling is indicated when that is the case.

Of course, a possible cause of the feeling of inability is actual inability. Clients sometimes accurately assess that they are not—or are not yet—able to perform what is being asked in therapy. They may need training, practice, or deeper knowledge of the activity or task. A new intermediate goal or set of goals must be defined to get clients back on track. This procedure is not unusual; a great deal of therapy proceeds from insight gained from one session to the next. Sometimes you discover that you are trying to move too quickly or without sufficient preparation. The remedy, of course, is to adjust the goals and recalibrate the assigned activities.

Frustration springing from a lowered self-image is a different matter. Clients are in fact able to perform the defined task, but the self-image issue is holding them back. Your responsibility at that point is to address self-image and get the therapy process back on course. The effort is always linked to therapy goals, to move the clients from "can't do" to "can do."

The following are counseling strategies you can employ to help clients identify and develop positive goals related to what they will do rather than what they will not do to achieve success.

1. *Scaling questions.* This strategy is used to help clients develop a perception of their issues along a continuum. You can ask clients to rate their satisfaction, confidence, and effort related to their communication issue. You should use some predetermined scale to keep track of clients' perceptions. For example, when asking clients, "On a scale from one to ten, one being the most dissatisfied you have been with your issue and ten being the most satisfied you have been, how would you rate yourself today?" If clients rate themselves at a 2, you would follow up by asking them to explain why they rated themselves at a 2 today and what they think would need to happen or what they could do to improve their satisfaction. You and your clients would then work on assessing current goals or generating new ones.

2. *Exception-seeking questions.* You should use these questions to assess the times when the clients' issue was not as severe or was nonexistent in the their lives. You can ask clients, "Was there a time in the past when the issue did not affect you as much? What strategies did you use at those times? What factors influenced you at that time?" The goal of these questions is to probe clients to generate reasons for why the issue had a less severe impact on them during those previous times and then to repeat the strategies that worked in the past to lessen the current effects of the issue.

3. *Coping questions.* This line of questioning is designed to help clients see that even in the most hopeless of situations, there is still something they are doing to manage the issue. You may say something like, "I can see how difficult this issue has been for you, but you still figure out a way to get yourself to our sessions

every week. How do you do that?" By validating their feelings and then providing them with an example of something they are doing to cope successfully with the situation, clients challenge their problem-focused narrative with solution-focused talk.

4. *Problem-free talk.* You can use other aspects of your clients' lives (e.g., environments where they feel confident or relaxed, roles that empower them) to uncover resources clients can use to deal with situations that do not evoke the same confidence or comfort (Jones, 2008). If clients get nervous speaking in front of colleagues, you may talk about speaking situations that do not make them nervous, such as talking with family and friends. The problem-free discussions should appear to clients like small talk, chit-chat, or topics seemingly irrelevant to therapy. Look for clients' personal resources elicited during such conversations that you could use as strategies to help your clients in their more difficult situations.

The Quit Option

A particularly undesirable outcome of deep frustration is the increasing attractiveness of quitting, stopping therapy and reverting to life as it was. Frustrated clients feel helpless, without options, painted into a corner. The new patterns of behavior you are targeting have always been to some extent daunting. They involve untried skills and unrehearsed techniques. They are unfamiliar, uncomfortable, perhaps a little embarrassing. The new pattern must be worth all the trouble it takes to abandon the familiar and form brand new habits.

When you add doubt and frustration to the already difficult task of adopting a new pattern, the impulse to quit becomes that much more tempting. It is not only important but urgent to counsel clients effectively to forestall the temptation to abandon therapy for the comfort and familiarity of the old ways.

Power and Perseverance

The key in these dangerous moments is to reestablish your clients' sense of personal power and their willingness to persevere. You must restore the clients' energy, in a word, their commitment to the goals of therapy.

Commitment requires not only energy but focused energy, energy directed toward a goal, a target. This goal-centeredness or sense of direction is focus. Focus refers to your clients' perception of their goals and their attitude toward the goals. Strong, energetic focus has a number of elements that you must assert during your counseling encounters.

Your clients' individual conviction of command and possession of their goals yields the personal power that makes perseverance possible. A decisive surge of strength flows from inside your clients. It is constant, constructive, and liberating. This personal power is always rooted in the conviction that they can accomplish their goals and bring the therapy process to a successful conclusion. Personal power derives in part from the sense of control and resourcefulness.

The Focus of a Committed Client

- Clients have a robust conception of where they are going, what they are out to accomplish. Reinforce: clarify and redefine goals as often as needed to keep goals from becoming murky or indistinct.
- Clients see the therapy goals as meaningful and worthwhile. Reinforce: keep highlighting the impetus of their therapy, the value of the targeted improvements to their quality of life.
- No matter what step they are taking, clients do not lose sight of their goals. Reinforce: keep the goals front and center; review them every session.
- Clients have a powerful conviction that obstacles can be overcome. Reinforce: a great danger when clients face doubt and frustration is obstacle dominance; do not let these obstacles obstruct their vision of the goals they are out to achieve.
- Clients tend to see their goals, no matter how complex, as one goal, not many. Reinforce: goals themselves become obstacles when they are too numerous or complex; keep them simple and clear.
- Clients have a remarkable optimism that they will successfully reach the goal, yet they are utterly realistic about what it will take to do so. Reinforce: you are addressing self-image to support optimism, the exhilarating conviction that success is within their grasp.

Control or ownership implies options, alternatives as your clients engage in their therapy efforts. They do not feel backed into a corner, unable to make a move. Instead, they feel free to choose from among a variety of possible ways to go. In your counseling, you must clarify the range of options available to clients, insist that multiple choices are available.

Conviction and Commitment

Committed clients possess the means to achieve their goals. Resources are available to them. They are literally "resourceful," full of the resources they need to succeed. They are secure in the knowledge that the tools required are at their command. There is an honest optimism, an irresistible strength, a movement from can't do to can do. Your clients' ideal self, their own Mirror of Erised, becomes an image of themselves that they deeply want to realize. Not only do they want to become that self but also they believe unequivocally that they can do so. And not only do they believe they can become that self but also they are convinced that the therapy journey on which you and they have embarked will, because of their firm commitment, enable them one day to look in the Mirror of Erised and see a reflection of themselves exactly the way they are.

Review of Key Points

- Self-affirmation is one of the Five Intentions of a speaker. Whenever clients start a sentence with the word *I*, they are affirming themselves or something about themselves. Self-affirmation depends on self-image. When you counsel, you are often addressing your client's self-image.
- Self-concept is made up of self-esteem, ideal self, and self-image.
- Self-esteem is a sense of self-worth. Clients with high self-esteem are generally optimistic and are typically more willing to attempt new strategies in therapy. Clients with low self-esteem do not typically exhibit confidence in their abilities.
- An individual's ideal self is the person that he or she would like to be.
- Self-image is just how we see ourselves and may not always reflect reality. Clients whose self-image is congruent with their ideal self are likely to have high self-esteem; clients whose self-image is further from their ideal self are likely to have lower self-esteem.
- The WHO classifies *disability* as a term that encompasses impairments, activity limitations, and participation restrictions.
- Impairments are negative changes to the body's anatomy and physiology.
- Activity limitations are problems in performing particular tasks or functions as a result of the impairment.
- Participation restriction is difficulty with or decreased involvement in social and occupational situations.
- When clients' participation in life activities is reduced, they may be more appropriate candidates for therapy.
- The four factors that can affect your self-esteem are others' reactions to you, your comparison of others to yourself, your roles in society, and your identity.
- There are limits to what counseling can achieve. At one end, you must avoid the mistake of uncoupling counseling from your therapy goals. At the other end, you should not think that reaching a counseling goal will fully address your therapy goals.
- No matter how successful counseling is, your work is not complete until you reach the goal.
- Clients assume many roles in daily life, each with its own features and challenges. The Spider Chart activity is one you can do with your clients to assess the roles they play in their lives. As a counselor, you will assist your clients in navigating the myriad roles they play and determining what is likely to be required to function acceptably in each of those roles.
- A speech-language, swallowing, hearing, or voice disorder stigmatizes when it is labeled not only as a disorder but also as a socially undesirable disorder. Unlike mere insensitivity, stigma carries the implication that clients are unwelcome, a detriment, or a potential embarrassment.
- One of the worst emotions clients experience along with stigma is shame. Self-image takes a direct hit; clients are subject to shunning, name calling, and

worse. A counselor's challenge is to enable clients to regain their sense of self-worth and ability to thrive in their social environment.

- Your culture comprises people with a common set of beliefs, values, and practices. Culture itself may stigmatize what it considers an affront to these beliefs, values, and practices. In some cultures individuals with a speech-language pathology or hearing disorder can be stigmatized.
- When clients present with stigma and shame, you should immediately begin counseling to determine the extent and effects of the stigmatizing and to counter the resultant impact on self-image, confidence, optimism, and motivation. Set goals, construct a plan to counteract the effects of stigma, and ensure that it does not obstruct progress in therapy.
- When self-image begins to suffer, the gap between clients' self-image and ideal self starts to looks unbridgeable, and doubt replaces confidence. Clients are able to perform the defined task, but the self-image issue is holding them back. You must address self-image and get the therapy back on course.
- A particularly undesirable outcome of deep frustration is the increasing attractiveness of quitting therapy and reverting to life as it was. When you add doubt and frustration to the already difficult task of adopting a new pattern, the quit option becomes that much more tempting. It is then urgent to counsel clients effectively to forestall the temptation to abandon therapy.
- Commitment to therapy requires not only energy but focused energy, energy directed toward a goal, a target. Clients have a robust conception of where they are going, and no matter what step they are taking, clients do not lose sight of their goal. They believe that obstacles can be overcome, and they have a remarkable optimism that they will successfully reach the goal.
- Control implies options and resourcefulness, because clients feel free to choose from among a variety of possible ways to go and are secure in the knowledge that the tools required are at their command.

Practical Exercises

For this assignment, you will create your own Spider Chart. This chart will help you to identify the different roles you play within your life. Begin by writing your name in the box within the circle. Then, think about all the roles you play within your life (e.g., sister/brother, daughter/son, mother/father, spouse, graduate student). Write one of those roles in the box after the first spoke. Continue adding spokes and boxes for each of the other roles you play in your life.

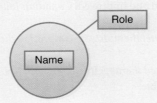

Now, repeat the process for a client you have, a family member, significant other, or a friend. Complete the wheel to the best of your knowledge.

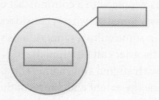

For this assignment, identify the potential impairment, activity limitations, and participant restrictions for each client.

1. 53-year-old male who recently underwent a total laryngectomy
2. 67-year-old female who is recovering from a left-hemisphere stroke and who has been diagnosed with Broca's aphasia

REFERENCES

Argyle, M. (2008). *Social encounters: Contributions to social interaction.* Piscataway, NJ: Aldine Transaction.

Baumeister, R. F., Campbell, J. D., Krueger, J. I., & Vohs, K. D. (2003). Does high self-esteem cause better performance, interpersonal success, happiness, or healthier life-styles? *Psychological Science in the Public Interest, 4*(1), 1–44.

Blascovich, J., & Tomaka, J. (1993). Measures of self-esteem. In J. P. Robinson, P. R. Shaver & L. S. Wrightsman (Eds.), *Measures of personality and social psychology attitudes* (3rd ed., pp. 115–160). Ann Arbor, MI: Institute for Social Research.

Corrigan, P. W., Larson, J. E., & Rüsch, N. (2009). Self-stigma and the "why try" effect: Impact on life goals and evidenced-based practice. *World Psychiatry, 8*(2), 75–81.

Corrigan, P. W., Watson, A. C., & Barr, L. (2006). The self-stigma of mental illness: Implications for self-esteem and self-efficacy. *Journal of Social and Clinical Psychology, 25*(8), 875–884.

Crocker, J., Major, B., & Steele, C. (1998). Social stigma. In D. T. Gilbert & S. T. Fiske (Eds.), *The handbook of social psychology* (Vol. 2, *4th ed.*, pp. 504–553). New York, NY: McGraw-Hill.

Fleming, J. S., & Courtney, B. E. (1984). The dimensionality of self-esteem: II. Hierarchical facet model for revised measurement scales. *Journal of Personality and Social Psychology, 46*(2), 404–421.

Hills, P. R., Francis, L. J., Jennings, P. (2011). The School Short-Form Coopersmith Self-Esteem Inventory: Revised and improved. *Canadian Journal of School Psychology, 26*(1), 62–71.

Jones, D. (2008). *Becoming a brief therapist: Special edition the complete works.* Lulu Enterprises: UK Ltd.

Rogers, C. (1951). *Client-centered therapy: Its current practice, implications and theory.* London, England: Constable.

Rogers, C. (1959). A theory of therapy, personality and interpersonal relationships as developed in the client-centered framework. In S. Koch (Ed.), *Psychology: A study of a science. Vol. 3: Formulations of the person and the social context.* New York, NY: McGraw-Hill.

Rosenberg, M. (1999). *Society and the adolescent self-image* (4th ed.). Darby, PA: Diane Publishing Company.

Watson, A. C., Corrigan, P., Larson, J. E., & Sells, M. (2007). Self-stigma in people with mental illness. *Schizophrenia Bulletin, 33*(6), 1312–1318.

World Health Organization. (2015a). Classifications. Retrieved from http://www.who.int /classifications/icf/icf_more/en/

World Health Organization. (2015b). Disabilities. Retrieved from http://www.who.int /topics/disabilities/en/

CHAPTER 7

Alliances: Getting Support

KEY TERMS

- Adversary
- Ally
- Circle of Power
- Interaction Process Model
- Reciprocity

LEARNING OBJECTIVES

After reading this chapter, you will be able to:

- Describe the Circle of Power as an alliance base of acquaintances able to assist in the achievement of therapy goals
- Clarify how the Circle of Power can supply allies and adversaries as a clinician and client seek to achieve their goals
- Practice ways to enlist the help of a potential ally
- Use the Interaction Process Model to plan and conduct a successful meeting to enlist the help of a potential ally
- Apply the lessons learned about the Circle of Power to clients in a group therapy process or support group process

Most of us have been a part of one kind of circle or another. If you like to make bed covers, you might join a quilting circle comprising people literally sitting in a circle stitching away at intricately patterned coverlets. To get ready for the big final, you may find yourself in a study circle. To ask the Almighty for a favor, you could be part of a prayer circle. You have a circle of friends and a circle of intimates. This chapter looks at another one of your circles, the Circle of Power.

This is a circle of people "around" you. They are the people you depend on or seek out to enhance your effectiveness at whatever task or project you are doing or contemplating. Managers have a Circle of Power at work. That circle may include subordinates, peers, superiors, or people outside the organization. Without these associates, the manager's job cannot get done, and the manager will likely fail. Your clients too have a Circle of Power, people who can help your clients achieve the goals they set

> Circle of power: The people a person depends on or seeks out to enhance that person's effectiveness at whatever task or project the person is doing or contemplating; an alliance base.

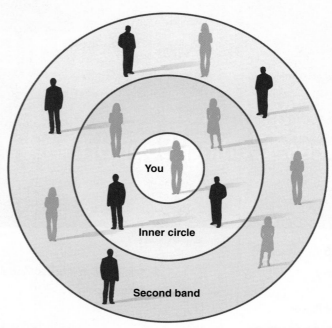

FIGURE 7-1 The Circle of Power. The circle includes clients as well as the influential people in their lives. Those closest to the clients are located in their inner circle, and other allies are located in the second band of the circle.

in therapy. That circle includes you, of course, and it widens to include all who might serve as allies promoting and abetting the improvements sought by your clients (**Figure 7-1**).

Those closest to your client, the most intimate, the ones with the greatest influence, the ones held in the highest regard, occupy the inner circle. These can include a parent or close relative, a beloved coach or teacher, a best friend. Rarely are more than four or five people within the inner circle. The second band of the Circle of Power contains people associated with your client, influential, but not to the degree of those in the inner circle. Although you have no definitive way to place a person in the inner circle or in the second band, these categories remind you to consider the degree of influence a potential ally has on your client.

Identifying Allies

You have a number of ways to identify this alliance base, this Circle of Power. Often, potential allies emerge during discussions about other things. A clinician was working with Sydney, an individual who stutters. The clinician decided to use the technique known as the "miracle question." The "miracle" was this: Sydney's stuttering disappeared while she slept one night. The clinician asked Sydney the miracle question. How would she come to realize that her disfluency had been miraculously resolved during the night? When asking Sydney to answer the miracle question, the clinician noticed what seemed to be a special relationship Sydney had with her assistant. The scenario picks up on the morning after the miracle happened.

Sydney: I'd drive to work. Say hi to everyone; still don't know about the miracle. If I think I might stutter when greeting people, I just wave. I call in my assistant to review the day's appointments. She shuts the door to my office. That's going to be my first indication.

Clinician: What happens?

Sydney: Sheri has been with me for three years. When we're together alone, I usually stutter.

Clinician: Really?

Sydney: Yeah. I am comfortable, so I don't compensate or replace words. I guess I'm unguarded.... *M*'s and *n*'s are my downfall. Now the miracle has happened, right? I say, "nine," perfectly, no hesitation, no seven-second *n* sound.

Clinician: Who notices first, you or Sheri?

Sydney: Sheri. For sure.

Clinician: Sheri?

Sydney: Yes. I won't know right away. I might even think I stuttered. I've actually been told I haven't stuttered when I was sure I had. So, it would be a while before I noticed anything different. Sheri would say something like, "Hey, good 'nine.'"

Clinician: Then?

Sydney: I'd say, "What?" She'd say, "You didn't stutter." When I talked more, she'd comment at some point, maybe after three or four sentences, that I wasn't stuttering. That's when I'd first notice.

Clinician: Interesting.

In the scenario, the clinician quite rightly pursues the implications of the "miracle." Your knowledge of the Circle of Power, however, might cause you to change the direction of the dialogue. Imagine the clinician cycling back to gather more information on Sheri, a potential member of Sydney's Circle of Power.

Clinician: I think this imaginary miracle brought out some useful information. Right now, I'd like to hear more about your assistant.

Sydney: Sheri?

Clinician: Yes, Sheri. You've known her for how long?

Sydney: Five years. She was in another department when I met her. We clicked right away, and three years ago I got a chance to hire her away. I guess I talk to her as much as anybody I know.

Clinician: You are close.

Sydney: Very. I mean she's very professional, knows I'm her boss, which is never a problem because no one works harder than she does. I guess I just trust her.

Clinician: How did this trust develop?

Sydney: I think it began quite a while ago. I'd talk to her and she'd listen.

Clinician: Don't people listen to you?

Sydney: Sheri's different. Most people, when they hear me stutter, they get nervous, you know? Their eyes dart around like they want to be somewhere else. Sometimes they finish my sentences or just huff and puff like they're impatient with me.

Clinician: But Sheri's different.

Sydney: Yes. Nothing about her changes when I stutter. The conversation goes along like there was no stuttering at all. That's what I meant when I said I sometimes don't even know if I stuttered or not—with her.

Clinician: Does she know you've started therapy?

Sydney: Sure. She recommended it.

Clinician: Really?

Sydney: Yes. A few weeks ago I told her I had tried therapy for my stuttering twice as a kid and once before as an adult. She said why not try again. She said techniques might have changed or I might find a speech therapist who suits me better. She helped me decide to come to your clinic.

Clinician: Sheri seems to be on your side in all this.

Sydney: That's why I trust her; she's really in my corner, you know?

Ally (also called, advocates): In therapy, someone who may be invested in or affected by progress in treatment; perceived as someone who actively supports the client's efforts to achieve therapy goals. An ally is usually a member of the client's Circle of Power.

A conversation like this one provides useful information on Sydney's close associate, Sheri. She is clearly one of Sydney's client advocates, one of those who may be invested in or affected by Sydney's progress in treatment. As a client advocate, Sheri is perceived by both Sydney and Sheri herself as someone who actively supports Sydney's efforts to become more fluent. Sheri is precisely the kind of person you might at some point enlist to work with your client in practicing a new technique or getting over a barrier to therapy that arises. Sheri then becomes an ally, a member of Sydney's Circle of Power. Peers and friends of your client or individuals your client knows socially could likewise assist you as allies in your therapy efforts.

As you counsel your clients, then, it is important to listen for any mention of potential allies in clients' lives. In the scenario, Sydney mentioned Sheri during her recounting of an imaginary "miracle story." An alert should sound when your clients mention an acquaintance: this person might be able to help (or hinder) progress toward your goals. It is a good idea to write down or record the name of a potential ally as soon

Facts about the Ally

- Personal: name, address, gender, age, profession, education
- Relational: relationship to client, how long client has known ally, frequency of contact, usual mode of contact (face-to-face, phone, email, social network)

Implications of the Relationship with the Ally

- How influential is the ally with the client?
- In what ways might the ally be helpful to progress in therapy?
- In what ways might the ally be detrimental to progress in therapy?
- How might the ally be enlisted to serve a positive role in the therapy process?
- Has the client given permission for you to share information with the ally?
- Is there good reason to have confidence that this ally will observe confidentiality as required by HIPAA regulations or by your explicit standards?

as it is mentioned. When you do decide to seek information on the potential ally, there are two aspects to consider: (1) facts about the ally and the ally's relationship with the client; (2) positive and negative implications of this relationship.

Facts about the ally are straightforward. They are not matters of opinion.

Positive and negative implications of this relationship can encompass conclusions or opinions you have arrived at based on your conversations with the client.

Using the information you now possess about Sheri's connection to Sydney, you can review the items above and imagine possible responses to each item. Once you have assembled these data and opinions, they become part of the record you keep on your clients. As you discover more about a particular ally, you can add it to the record. You should review the record regularly. Then, when an opportunity arises to enlist the ally, you will more easily recognize it.

In the case of Sydney and her assistant, Sheri, the clinician knows that their 5-year relationship, both as friends and as manager–employee, has made Sheri a trusted confidante who is strongly supportive of this therapy. With a little reflection, you should be able to envision at least three or four situations in which Sheri could be enlisted as an active ally.

Allies versus Adversaries

Individuals within your clients' Circle of Power can play one of three possible roles: they may be allies in your therapy efforts, they may be adversaries, or they may be irrelevant or neutral.

Helping and hindering

Neutral members of your clients' Circle of Power may merit your watchfulness, because they are in the circle and therefore have influence, but the allies and adversaries warrant special attention. Allies are likely to help your efforts; adversaries could become a hindrance. Being proactive about these individuals is usually better than remaining passive.

The first thing you should realize is that these individuals do not necessarily view themselves as either your allies or your adversaries. *Ally* and adversary are your designations, based on the impact these individuals are likely to have on your clients as you and they work to achieve their goals. Those you have determined to be adversaries, for instance, do not necessarily think of themselves as such. Quite possibly, they see themselves as sincerely supportive of your clients' best interests.

> Adversary: An individual who has a negative influence or who is not supportive of a client's efforts in the therapy process.

You will come up against numerous examples of the "undeclared adversary" throughout your career. The reasons could be cultural; for example, a parent may believe that his daughter, an individual who is hard of hearing, should not wear visible hearing aids or use sign language because she would be ostracized if she did so. Peer pressure might be a factor. A good friend may warn an individual who stutters not to speak in front of peers for fear of bullying. In both of these cases, the well-intentioned father and friend have unintentionally made themselves adversaries advising the opposite of what you and your clients have prescribed.

Adversaries, however, may be well aware that their advice puts them in direct opposition to what you and your clients are proposing in therapy. Even so, you should not view these individuals as enemies; they simply have a different idea of what is best for your clients. You may be able to win them over; you may be able only to lessen their influence. No matter what, it is risky to ignore them.

Turning adversaries into allies

Winning over adversaries, turning them into allies, is usually an excellent objective to pursue. If you succeed, they become part of your Circle of Power as well as that of your clients. You have two ways to win over adversaries, direct and indirect. The direct method is to interact personally with the adversaries, hear them out, and convince them to become supportive of your goals and techniques. The indirect method relies on the clients, or others, to make an appeal to the adversaries. You can counsel your clients on the best way to approach an adversary, but you play a secondary role when you opt for the indirect method.

If you decide to use the direct method, you must contrive a way to meet with the adversary. This meeting may be easy to set up, as with the parent of a client who is a minor or the caretaker of an individual with dementia. In other cases, the meeting may not be so easy to arrange; the adversary might be your client's schoolmate or soccer coach, someone with whom you would not ordinarily come into contact. In any case, you must make a judgment. Are the stakes high enough to justify a meeting? If so, you and the adversary should meet. At this point the adversary becomes a potential ally. Later in this chapter, you will examine the step-by-step Interaction Process Model for preparing and conducting a successful meeting.

Constructing the Circle of Power

Meeting with a potential ally and devising an individual plan with that ally is one part of the larger reality we are calling the Circle of Power. Because potential allies are influential with the client—that is why you may be enlisting them to help you—they are already in your client's Circle of Power. If you succeed in enlisting their support, they become part of the Circle of Power that surrounds you and your client. You must never lose sight of this bigger picture.

Choosing who will help

Enlisting an ally is work and it is time-consuming. Choose these allies carefully. Make sure that their assistance will be worth the effort it takes to enlist them.

Factors in Choosing an Ally

- Their relationship with the client is so influential that the help they might provide is really significant.
- They have special knowledge or skills that make them ideal prospects to help the client make genuine progress in a particular area.
- They possess the ability and willingness to maintain required confidentiality and to honor the privacy rights of clients.
- They could become adversaries, and having them as allies instead is preferable, so much so that enlisting them is well worth the effort.

Constructing a visual representation of the Circle of Power may help you decide whom to enlist to help you in the therapy process. Refer to **Figure 7-2** for an illustration of a Circle of Power. Have clients indicate roles that potential allies play in the lives of the clients (e.g., mother, father, daughter, son, grandfather, friend, student, manager, teacher). Draw lines from the main circle and place the label of each role in a separate box. Have clients indicate the names of people they interact with within each role (e.g., role of mother will include names of children, role of student will include names of teachers and classmates). Spend time with your clients discussing who they believe are allies and who are potential adversaries within each role. Individual names can appear under different roles and may be perceived in one role as an ally and in another as an adversary. Individuals within a particular client's inner circle who you may want to enlist to help you should become obvious during this exercise.

Deciding how and when they will help

Occasionally, you will employ particular allies throughout the entire course of therapy. People within the innermost Circle of Power or people who are a constant

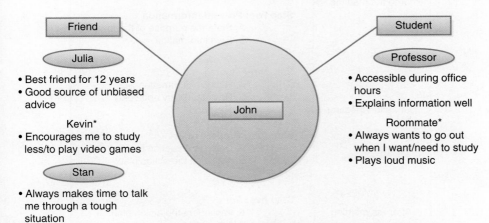

FIGURE 7-2 Constructing a Circle of Power. Creating a circle allows clients to identify the individuals they interact with in the various roles in their lives. After identifying individuals, clients can assess whether each individual is an ally, adversary, both, or neither. Circle the ones you believe are allies (supportive of your efforts) and put a star next to those who may potentially be adversaries (not supportive of your efforts or who cause some strain or turmoil in your efforts).

presence in your client's life might become such long-term allies. Their roles may change as therapy progresses, and the roles must be updated accordingly.

Other allies may enter the picture for a brief time and for a specific reason. A school counselor may be enlisted to guide your high school client through the college admissions process; a choir director may be ideal for helping a client practice a voice technique; a work colleague may be a suitable observer of your client's interactions with customers. Once you ascertain how particular allies can best provide benefit to your client, you should carefully select "insertion times," the moments when the allies actually provide the help to the client.

Once you have determined how and when an ally will assist you, you can use the following Interaction Process Model to make it happen.

The Interaction Process Model

Soon after you have decided to enlist a particular person as an ally in your efforts with one of your clients, you will want to meet with them. The Interaction Process Model (**Figure 7-3**) provides you with a procedure to guide you to a successful meeting. The model begins with careful preparation before the meeting and culminates in a sensible long-term monitoring process after the meeting. Allot enough time to achieve your goals, and make sure the goals are worth the time you are setting aside.

Step One: Prepare to Meet the Individual
A. Collect Data

> **Interaction process model:** A five-step procedure serving as a guide to a successful meeting. The steps are: (1) prepare, (2) present information, (3) listen, (4) prepare to act, and (5) act.

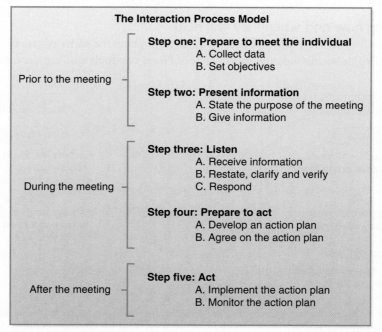

The Interaction Process Model

Prior to the meeting
- **Step one: Prepare to meet the individual**
  - A. Collect data
  - B. Set objectives
- **Step two: Present information**
  - A. State the purpose of the meeting
  - B. Give information

During the meeting
- **Step three: Listen**
  - A. Receive information
  - B. Restate, clarify and verify
  - C. Respond
- **Step four: Prepare to act**
  - A. Develop an action plan
  - B. Agree on the action plan

After the meeting
- **Step five: Act**
  - A. Implement the action plan
  - B. Monitor the action plan

FIGURE 7-3 The Interaction Process Model. Once a client gives permission for the clinician to contact a potential ally, this model provides guidelines on how to appropriately prepare for, conduct, and execute the plan established in a meeting.

Sheri, Sydney's Adm. Asst.
- Sydney says, trusted friend, ally, supportive of therapy, able to maintain confidentiality...
- Sydney's mother says, Sheri is aloof, overly protective of Sydney...
- Sydney's boyfriend says, Sheri is friendly, outgoing, protective of Sydney...

Before the meeting, find out all you need to know about the potential ally and that person's relationship with your client. Your client is an important source of this information, as are other people in your client's Circle of Power. Those people can give you a useful perspective not necessarily shared by your client. The data you gather should fill you in on suggested ways to form a positive connection to the potential ally and ways to avoid alienating the ally. The information could even provide ways that the ally might be enlisted to help as well as give you clues to the ally's willingness to observe your standards, especially confidentiality.

The point of collecting data is to learn all you can before you meet the potential ally, so you plan effectively and avoid missteps. Here is a fairly typical, though abridged, set of notes on data about an advocate gathered by a clinician.

With information from various sources, you can plan a meeting with more clearly defined outcomes and fewer surprises.

B. Set Objectives and Standards

In preparation for the meeting, you should identify your objectives and the standards that must be observed. In this case, you should be clear in your own mind just what you hope to accomplish by meeting with this potential ally. Are you going to ask for help in some direct way? Are you simply soliciting support in a general sense? Or are you planning to give the potential ally information that could make the ally more sympathetic to the therapy goals? Will this information require the ally to observe confidentiality? Whatever you wish to achieve, make your objectives as specific and comprehensive as you can. You may need to adjust them later, but go into your meeting with a clear set of goals and standards.

Step Two. Present Information
A. State the Purpose of the Meeting

When you ultimately meet the potential ally and have exchanged the usual small talk, say something like, "I'd like to tell you why I asked to meet with you. I know you are close to [client], and I would greatly appreciate it if you could help us." Then state, as concretely as possible, your objectives and standards for the meeting. You might say, for example, "There are three things I'd like you to do to help us."

B. Give Information

After stating your objectives and standards, give whatever information is necessary for the potential ally to understand what is expected and how each objective is to be achieved. At this point, try to avoid discussions about the value of the objectives. If you are challenged, you can say, "I see you have an issue with this objective, and I want us to talk about that, but right now, I want to make sure you have a full understanding of what I'm asking for." Make sure the ally expresses an explicit willingness to observe the standards you have established.

Step Three. Listen
A. Receive Information

Once you are sure that the potential ally understands what you and your client are trying to accomplish, you are in a position to hear what the ally has to say. Be patient and allow the ally to air all thoughts and feelings.

B. Restate, Clarify, and Verify

As you continue the interaction, you can use a number of techniques to achieve a full understanding of what the potential ally thinks and feels about the process. The Responsive Listening Model depicts exactly what you ought to be doing at this stage in the meeting process. You should use techniques such as paraphrasing and questioning to determine whether the ally fully understands what to do to help and whether the ally will maintain a strong commitment to helping you. You will also have the opportunity to correct any misunderstandings that otherwise might have gone unnoticed.

Practical matters will also arise at this point. For example, the ally's own schedule may not permit the ally to perform a given task at a particular time. Issues like this are ironed out before you are in a position to formulate a response.

C. Respond

Your next task in the meeting is to formulate your response based on the information you have received from the potential ally. Responding is in effect a review when you evaluate the situation and then formulate your reaction. This is a creative process of integrating your objectives with the ally's attitudes, feelings, and availability to reach the doable goals you will finally agree to accomplish.

You make clear to the ally once again what you want the ally to do, with whatever modifications you might have made after listening thoroughly. You reiterate your standards. You answer as best you can any objections or problems the ally has, and you express your appreciation at the prospect of help.

Step Four. Prepare to Act
A. Develop an Action Plan

At this point, you and the ally move from discussion to action. Here is where you lay out with precision what the ally will do. Set time lines and ways to review the actions. The more specific and concrete the plan, the better. The plan, along with the clear standards, should be in writing, although a final draft may be emailed later.

B. Agree on the Action Plan

This step may take several rounds as you discuss the full range of actions to be taken by the ally. It is vitally important to gain explicit agreement to the entire plan and all its particulars.

Step Five. Act

This step takes place after the meeting, of course, when the plan is executed.

A. Implement the Action Plan

The expectation following the meeting is that the plan will take effect. The ally is empowered to take all the measures laid out in the action plan. The client is brought on board and fully informed about the plan. A follow-up meeting to provide focus and clarity might include you, the ally, and the client. Client interactions are done in a manner appropriate to the client's age and level of comprehension.

B. Monitor the Action Plan

When you monitor, you and the ally agree to a periodic review of the action plan. No plan is complete without a means to measure progress on a continuing basis. You can adjust the action plan as conditions change and ensure that the plan is being carried out. This ongoing review in fact becomes a part of your overall plan to achieve your clinical goals.

Reciprocity: Helping allies

A solution-focused approach never loses sight of the clear and defined benefits of the actions you take. If you enlist an ally to assist you with a particular client, beneficial results should flow in two directions, from the ally to you and your client as well as from you and the client back to the ally. This type of mutual benefit is called reciprocity. This does not mean you start to do therapy with allies, although your interactions with allies might be one of the benefits they experience. Reciprocity simply means that you and your client do not just take from allies; you find ways to give as well.

Sydney's associate Sheri can potentially help in a variety of ways. What good might accrue to Sheri for all her efforts? Well, if Sydney becomes more fluent, Sheri will certainly benefit in the workplace during her daily interactions with Sydney. Sheri should also be made fully aware of the significant value she is bringing to the therapy process. For many allies, knowing that they are being helpful is in itself rewarding.

Although identifying the benefits for allies requires thought and even creativity, some benefits are obvious and need only be made explicit. Kaching is Shen's wife. Shen depends on her to make phone calls for him. He has been ashamed to speak on the phone since dysarthria has made his speech increasingly less intelligible. Kaching will be relieved of this responsibility if she and the clinician successfully assist Shen in overcoming his embarrassment at using the phone. This clear benefit to Kaching should be included in your goal setting as you tackle this difficulty.

There are other instances when the benefit to the ally may not be readily apparent. If Kaching receives a strong sense of purpose by making phone calls for Shen, then she might perceive the removal of that responsibility in a negative way. Although the ultimate benefit may generate a sense of freedom for Kaching, she may have difficulty letting go initially. As a clinician, you should stay in touch with the motivations of both clients and allies to ensure ongoing success in therapy.

> Reciprocity: A situation in which beneficial results flow in two directions, for instance, from ally to client as well as from client back to ally. The benefits are mutual.

Counseling Allies Along with Clients

Some allies bring problems of their own into the clinical setting, and these problems could have an impact on progress made in therapy. One example is Juliana, the mother of David, a 4-year-old boy with autism, whom you have been treating. One day, Juliana approaches you and admits that she was on a prescribed medication during the first trimester of her pregnancy with David. She claims that she did not know that she was pregnant at the time and is extremely worried about the possible effects of the medication on David. She is deeply aggrieved and asks you whether it is her fault that her son has autism.

Although it is not your job to counsel Juliana in regard to her anxieties, she will become an integral part of your counseling process with David. She may require individual counseling with a licensed psychologist, and you might advise this. Juliana has intense feelings about taking a prescribed medication before she knew she was pregnant, and those feelings will play a part in the successful inclusion of Juliana in David's therapy.

Understanding the Nature and History of this Client–Ally Relationship

There are at least two relevant factors about Juliana's relationship with David. First, she is his mother; she is living with him and raising him. She cares about him and has a major impact on his life. There is definitely a history between the two. The medication she took during pregnancy is also part of that history and another relevant factor. Knowing that she took the medication affects many of her feelings and attitudes about David and his autism. Juliana will almost certainly be enlisted as an ally on David's behalf, and her feelings about the medication she took is an aspect of their history that cannot be ignored.

Every ally has a history with the client, and understanding the impact of that history is indispensable in creating a plan for inclusion of the ally as someone who will help your clients succeed in achieving the therapy goals.

Making the Ally Instrumental in Goal Attainment

Once you grasp the significance of the nature and history of the ally–client relationship, you are in a position to offer the ally a role in your clients' progress. As you have seen, you do this by clearly identifying how you expect the ally to help, by gaining agreement from the ally to provide help, and by imparting to the ally what the ally needs to render that help. You will also become aware of possible obstacles to a successful alliance.

Juliana's guilt might obstruct progress with David in a number of ways. She might be too protective, too hesitant about providing needed structure. You may have to help Juliana see the low probability that the medication she took has anything to do with David's autism. This very information might be one of the reciprocal benefits to the ally that we discussed earlier. In fact, you may become convinced that this is a critical piece of data that must be given to Juliana as part of the information she needs.

Cautions When Dealing with Allies Enlisted in Therapy

- Do not try to assume a role properly held by an ally. For example, Juliana is David's parent; you are not. Attempts to replace a parent or fulfill a parent's role are inappropriate and usually doomed to failure. You cannot replace a friend, either, or an athletic coach, or any of the allies functioning in the life of your client.
- Do not seek to undermine the relationships your clients have with others. Yes, the behavior of allies will change in some respects as they participate with you in helping your clients, but it is inadvisable to go beyond those changes and seek to "fix" or alter other aspects of the relationship between your clients and their allies.
- Be careful of cultivating a separate relationship with the ally. Such a development may be innocent or not so innocent, but you should guard against jeopardizing the trust and progress you are seeking with your client.
- Counsel the ally only when the counseling is related to your clinical work with your client. This does not mean the ally cannot benefit from your interactions; the benefits of reciprocity have been affirmed. What this principle maintains is that you cannot counsel an ally unless the counseling is relevant to your therapy.

When the allies' issues are relevant to therapy or to the successful treatment of your clients, then you may be called upon to counsel them. You may need to help Juliana see that her feelings about what happened early in her pregnancy are affecting her interactions with her son and hindering progress in David's therapy. If she is being overprotective, your counseling could help her see the benefit of letting go, at least a little.

Recognizing the Limits of the Clinician–Client–Ally Triangle

This chapter encourages you to focus on your clients' Circle of Power and enlist allies to assist you in achieving the goals you set during therapy. As important, even critical, as the Circle of Power can be, you must recognize and respect its limits. If you transgress these limits or pretend they are not there, you can thwart progress and possibly alienate your clients. Here is a list of principles to help you see these limitations and avoid "stepping out of bounds."

Counseling in Groups

The Circle of Power may extend to a literal circle, the one formed by the participants in group sessions. These sessions may take the form of group therapy or groups that meet for mutual support.

Group Therapy

As a clinician, you will sometimes find yourself working with clients, and possibly their allies, in groups rather than individually. Schools often mandate group therapy, or you may find it advisable to do therapy in groups. Such groups provide clients with a fresh source of potential allies: each other (Metcalf, 1998).

Every therapy group takes on its own character or "personality." Acquaintances and friendships form, and animosities may develop as well. During the sessions, you will see opportunities to cultivate useful alliances. These alliances may develop along the same lines as the others we have discussed in this chapter, and you might follow the same planning process in taking advantage of them.

The allies may simply help each other during the group sessions, under your facilitation. Such mutual assistance might arise spontaneously during a session, or you may plan it. The point is, group therapy provides occasions to take full advantage of the opportunities inherent in the Circle of Power. Individuals in groups can help one another achieve therapy goals. In fact, peers can be more influential than clinicians in helping clients gain an important perspective they may be missing. Peers have also been shown to reinforce undesirable attitudes and behavior in certain circumstances (Dishion, McCord, & Poulin, 1999). You must be a watchful and wary observer of peer influence.

Counseling Families

Heejoung Kim (2006) discusses how a strength-based approach such as solution-focused therapy is beneficial to families dealing with all types of issues. The goal is to encourage family involvement in the therapy process by directing the family's attention toward a future when the problem will be effectively managed. Successful coping strategies used by the family in the past are helpful in creating therapy goals. Counseling can reduce family conflict and foster family cohesion and positivity.

All family members do not have to be present during family counseling sessions (Kim, 2006). Sometimes it is advantageous to see family members separately—each person has the opportunity to express an unfiltered view of the situation and provide you with suggestions for change (Murphy & Duncan, 1997). Working primarily with just one member of a family can be as effective as working with several members. Changing the family's perspective can occur through a behavioral change in one member (Berg, 1994; Corcoran, 1998; de Shazer & Molnar, 1984; Williams, 2000).

Support Groups

As you counsel, you may also advise individual clients to join support groups. These are groups of individuals with issues common enough to benefit from discussion and interaction. Individuals who are deaf or who stutter often find relief and lowered anxiety in group settings where they can disclose their apprehensions to others like themselves. Support groups are allies by design. The whole point of a support group is to build alliances. Get to know the support groups in your area so you can select those that will be most helpful to your clients. Many clinicians start their own support groups, and this is an option you might consider.

If your clients are in a support group, be certain to monitor what is happening in the group and the effects it is having on your clients. Although most well-run support groups clearly enhance your efforts in therapy, careful monitoring can reveal the occasional case when elements of the support group question or undermine an aspect of your therapy.

The Power of the Circle of Power

As you have seen throughout this chapter, your clients' Circle of Power supplies a unique and varied array of resources that can assist you and your clients in achieving therapy goals. The Circle of Power includes the people in your clients' world who play a part in their lives, who exert influence on them. Ideally, they are the ones who care, the ones who show up, and, most important, the ones who are willing and able to help.

The Circle of Power consists of people who can serve as allies or adversaries in your efforts to achieve your therapy goals. Effective counseling identifies acquaintances, family members, authority figures, and friends who can become helpful and not so helpful players during therapy. Once identified, they and their influence can be ignored or addressed.

You address potential allies with a view to maximizing their helpfulness at the right moment. Potential adversaries are approached with a view to minimizing their deleterious impact or turning them into allies.

A final thought: your clients' Circle of Power can remain an influential part of their lives after therapy has concluded, while you, the clinician, may have left the scene. Whenever you interact with your clients' Circle of Power, remember that you are sowing seeds that can bear fruit well into the future.

Review of Key Points

- The Circle of Power consists of the people you depend on or seek out to enhance your effectiveness at whatever task or project you are doing or contemplating. Your clients' Circle of Power contains the people who can help your clients achieve the goals they set in therapy.

- Potential allies often emerge during discussions about other things. As you counsel your clients, listen for any mention of potential allies. When you do decide to seek information on the potential ally, there are two aspects to consider: (1) facts about the ally and the ally's relationship with the client; (2) positive and negative implications of this relationship.

- There are three possible roles individuals could play if they are in your clients' Circle of Power: they may be allies in your therapy efforts, they may be adversaries, or they may be irrelevant or neutral. Being proactive about allies and adversaries is usually better than remaining passive.

- *Ally* and *adversary* are your designations, based on the impact these individuals are likely to have on your clients as you and they work to achieve the therapy goals. Those you have determined to be adversaries do not necessarily think of themselves as such.

- Undeclared adversaries see themselves as sincerely supportive of your clients' best interests but in fact work against your therapy goals. Some may be well aware that their advice puts them in direct opposition to what you and your clients are proposing in therapy. It is risky to ignore them.

- If you succeed in turning adversaries into allies, they become part of your Circle of Power as well as your clients'. There are two ways to win over adversaries, direct and indirect.

- If you opt for the direct method, you must meet with the adversary. If the stakes are high enough to justify a meeting, plan the meeting. Determine precisely what you want to achieve at the meeting, and allot enough time to accomplish your aims. Use the Interaction Process Model: (1) prepare to meet the ally by collecting data, writing objectives, and setting standards; (2) present by stating the purpose of the meeting and giving information; (3) listen to receive and clarify information and then respond; (4) prepare to act by developing and agreeing on an action plan; (5) act to implement and monitor the plan.

- Choose allies carefully. Make sure that their assistance will be worth the effort it takes to enlist them.

- You use some allies throughout the course of therapy. Other allies enter the picture for a brief time and for a specific reason. Once you determine how particular allies can best provide benefit to your client, you should carefully select insertion times, the moments when the allies will actually provide the help to the client.

- The Interaction Process Model can be used as a guide to conduct a successful meeting, especially with potential allies for your client.

- If you enlist an ally to assist you with a particular client, the benefit should flow in two directions, from the ally to you and your client as well as from you and the client back to the ally. There should be reciprocity.
- Every ally has a history with the client, and understanding the impact of that history is indispensable in creating a plan for inclusion of the ally as someone who will help your clients succeed in achieving the therapy goals.
- As important as the Circle of Power can be, you must recognize and respect its limits. If you transgress these limits or pretend they are not there, you can thwart progress and possibly alienate your clients. Follow the principles that help you see these limitations and avoid stepping out of bounds.
- Group therapy can provide clients with a fresh source of potential allies: the other members of the group. These alliances may develop along the same lines as any others, or the allies may simply help each other during the group sessions, under your facilitation. Such mutual assistance might arise spontaneously during a session, or you may plan it.
- Support groups, groups of persons with issues common enough to benefit from discussion and interaction, provide allies by design. The whole point of a support group is to build alliances.
- The Circle of Power supplies a unique and varied array of resources that can assist you and your clients in achieving your therapy goals.

Practice Exercises

For this assignment, you will use the Spider Chart from the previous chapter's practical exercise to create a Circle of Power for yourself and for another individual. Your circle will comprise all the people in your life, both allies and adversaries. Under each "role," list the names of the influential people in that role. After you have listed all the people, circle the ones you believe are allies (supportive of your efforts) and put a star next to those who may potentially be adversaries (not supportive of your efforts or who cause some strain or turmoil in your efforts). It does not matter what the specific "effort" or goal is at this time; just think about these individuals in general. Then indicate briefly how each individual is either supportive or adversarial.

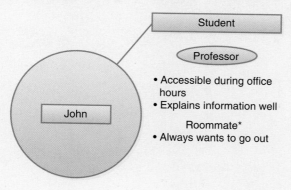

Now, repeat the process for a client you have, a family member, significant other, or a friend. Complete the wheel to the best of your knowledge.

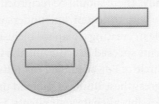

REFERENCES

Berg, I. K. (1994). A wolf in disguise is not a grandmother. *Journal of Systemic Therapies*, *13*(1), 13–14.

Corcoran, J. (1998). Solution-focused practice with middle and high school at-risk youths. *Children & Schools*, *20*(4), 232–243.

de Shazer, S., & Molnar, A. (1984). Changing teams/changing families. *Family Process*, *23*(4), 481–486.

Dishion, T., McCord, J., & Poulin, F. (1999). When interventions harm: Peer groups and problem behavior. *American Psychologist*, *54*(9), 755–764.

Kim, H. (2006). *Client growth and alliance development in solution-focused brief family therapy.* Ann Arbor, MI: ProQuest.

Metcalf, L. (1998). *Solution focused group therapy: Ideas for groups in private practice, schools, agencies, and treatment programs.* New York, NY: The Free Press.

Murphy, J. J., & Duncan, B. L. (1997). *Brief intervention for school problems: Collaborating for practical solutions.* New York, NY: Guilford Press.

Williams, G. R. (2000). The application of solution-focused brief therapy in a public school setting. *Family Journal: Counseling and Therapy for Couples and Families*, *8*(1), 76–78.

SECTION IV

The Solution Cycle
Phase Three: Envisioning the Preferred Future: "Setting Goals"

Chapter 8
Persuasion/Direction: Changing Client Behavior

Chapter 9
Readiness as Openness

This section focuses on Phase Three of the Solution Cycle: envisioning the preferred future and setting goals. Chapter 8 discusses persuasion/direction as one of the Five Intentions of Communication that clinicians can use to help clients create and establish therapy goals. These goals represent a change in the lives of your clients, an improvement aptly called the "preferred future." You and your clients have decided not to let that future unfold passively. You are going to act. You are going to affect the future, make it better. Chapter 9 addresses the impact quality of life has on clients' readiness and willingness to participate in therapy. Chapter 9 also explores the Counseling Integration Matrix, and counseling strategies are offered to optimize clients' success in therapy.

CHAPTER 8

Persuasion/Direction: Changing Client Behavior

KEY TERMS

- Behavior
- Doable goals
- Generalization
- Habituation
- Logical argument

- Maintenance
- Measurable goals
- MUSTDO goals
- Observable goals
- Pattern of behavior

- Repatterning
- Roadblocks to repatternings
- Solution-focused goals
- Time-bound goals
- Understood goals

LEARNING OBJECTIVES

After reading this chapter, you will be able to:

- Define the two types of clinical goals
- Identify and apply the elements of the MUSTDO acronym for intermediate goals
- Distinguish between a behavior and a pattern of behavior
- Clarify and apply the repatterning process leading to habituation
- Identify the key roadblocks to repatterning and how they can be removed

Setting Goals

Mario is a 62-year-old lawyer who recently had a partial tongue resection as a result of a recurrence of tongue cancer. His initial evaluation is complete and he is meeting with his clinician to set goals.

Clinician: Mario, what would you like to get out of these sessions?

Mario: This time around the cancer has really affected my life. I can't talk. People can't understand me. I thought this would be a big year for me. Now things are so bad I've started skipping Monday morning meetings at the firm.

Clinician: You're skipping them, why?

Mario: That way I don't have to participate.

Clinician: You mean talk?

Mario: Yeah, talk.

As Mario's scenario unfolds throughout this chapter, you will focus on the goal-setting process, distinguishing types of goals and their key features. Then you will examine the persuasion/direction aspect of therapy and counseling. You will learn and apply the rules of logic to convince and to change behavior. Finally, you will examine obstacles and roadblocks to goal attainment.

Defining a Goal: Therapy Goals and Counseling Goals

In your clinical experience, goals will usually come in one of two varieties. There are, first, goals that define the reasons your clients are engaging in therapy. These are therapy goals, goals that directly address remediation or improvement of the communication disorder. Second are counseling goals, those goals that support therapy progress by addressing factors such as attitude, motivation, emotion, and self-perception. In this chapter you will examine the most effective ways to set goals throughout therapy. You will see that all such goals—those related to remediation and improvement as well as those related to counseling—are solution focused.

When the clinician asked Mario what he would like to get out of therapy, he alluded to speech improvement goals and a possible counseling goal. The speech-related goal will probably focus on increasing his intelligibility because he "can't talk." One potential counseling goal is to address his avoidance of important company meetings and the reasons he is withdrawing. With these thoughts in mind, the clinician continues.

Clinician: So, one of your goals, I guess, would be to be able to talk so others can understand you.

Mario: Yes. I want to be able to talk clearly again.

Clinician: We'll make that a goal then.

Mario: Absolutely.

Clinician: That will be one of our long-term goals.

Mario: Fine. That works for me.

Clinician: We're going to take this step by step, Mario. There are particular sounds that are hard for you. We may work on these sounds one at a time until you master each of them in your everyday speech. OK?

Mario: OK.

Long-Term Goals and MUSTDO Goals

The clinician and Mario are formulating an ultimate goal, one of the end results of a successful therapy process. Such a long-term goal expresses the purpose of therapy. In a business setting such a goal would be called "the mission," the purpose for which a particular organization exists. In a similar sense, Mario's long-term goals, which include regaining intelligibility in speech, constitute the "mission" of therapy, the reason this therapy is taking place at all.

Without a clear statement of the ultimate mission or the long-term goals, it is hard to imagine how therapy can proceed in a sensible, positive direction. If your goal is to reach a geographic destination, say, your friend's house, you will not be able to take the first step if you have no idea what the address is. When you input that address into a GPS navigation device, chances are the first graphic you see is a map with the destination clearly highlighted, perhaps blinking. The GPS device must identify the goal before it can begin directing you toward it.

In Mario's case, without establishing and clarifying the goal of intelligible speech, the clinician has no way to determine what the therapy process will be.

Once the long-term goals are clarified, you and your client can plan out the steps necessary to achieve those goals. The plan will probably not be complete at the beginning of therapy because you learn things along the way that will cause you to rework the plan. With the information and data you possess at the start of therapy, however, you can establish intermediate or short-term goals that propel you to the long-term goals. These intermediate objectives can be described as MUSTDO goals.

MUSTDO goals are goals you "must do" to get to the long-term goals (see **Figure 8-1**). Some of them relate to remediation and improvement, and some of them are counseling goals. They reflect the primary tasks and activities that must be accomplished to achieve therapy aims. MUSTDO goals must be done completely, not partially.

In the case of Mario, whose partial tongue resection affected his speech and his willingness to go to meetings, the clinician should work to establish MUSTDO goals that will pave the way to his long-term goals. These goals can address sound production as well as such issues as Mario's fear of attending meetings.

> **MUSTDO goals:** Intermediate goals seen as requirements for meeting longer-term goals. MUSTDO is an acronym describing this type of goal: measurable, understood, solution focused, time bound, doable, and observable.

Clinician: We're going to take this step by step, Mario. There are particular sounds that are hard for you. We may work on these sounds one at a time until you master each of them in your everyday speech. OK?

Mario: OK.

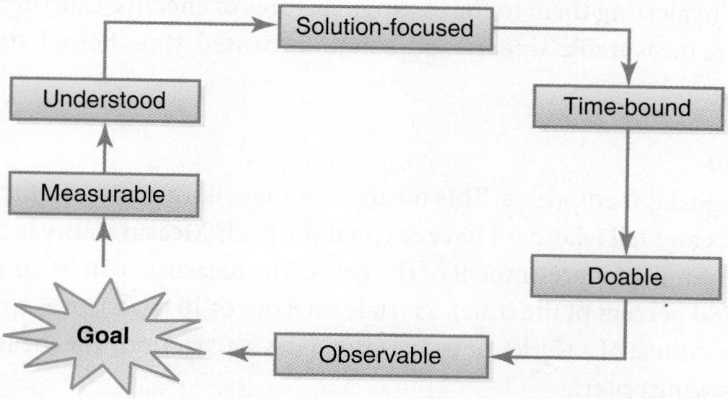

FIGURE 8-1 MUSTDO Goals. The MUSTDO criteria are vital to consider when creating and assessing a client's individual goals.

Clinician: First, though, we probably should tackle your difficulties in situations where you might be called on to speak.

Mario: Like those Monday meetings?

Clinician: Yes, exactly. What happens just before the meeting? Have you already decided not to attend?

Mario: No. The last few Mondays, I went to work figuring I would show up at the meeting. Then I'm sitting in my office just before. My heart starts racing; my hands are shaking. It's not just about speaking then. I don't want to be seen in that condition.

Clinician: Because you—

Mario: Because I'm a mess. I can't make myself leave the office. It takes fifteen minutes just to calm down.

Clinician: How do you feel about missing those meetings?

Mario: Lousy. I had a hand in starting weekly meetings because I thought, still think, communication is important. Now I've missed three in a row.

Clinician: Let's work on getting you back attending them. The first thing we have to do is find a way to keep you calm before the meeting. It looks like you are experiencing some kind of anxiety attack.

Mario: Whatever you call it, I don't have control over it.

Clinician: Do you have episodes like this in any other situation?

Mario: No, this is new. I mean, I'd get butterflies before a court appearance, but I thought of myself as pretty fearless. I was prepared and I felt capable. Just the opposite of what's happening now. I feel totally unprepared, frazzled, like an idiot.

Clinician: All because you might have to talk during the meeting.

Mario: In front of my peers, yes.

Mario and his clinician are in the process of setting a MUSTDO goal, a goal they both believe is essential to the ultimate success of therapy. MUSTDO is also a useful acronym alerting them to the essential features of effective short-term goals. These goals are measurable, understood, solution-focused, time-bound, doable, and observable.

Measurable

A MUSTDO goal is measurable. This means that there is an answer to the question: How, exactly, can I tell whether I have reached the goal? Measurability is often framed as a key requirement for attainment of the goals. The measures can be composed as percentages (80 percent of the time), as trials (in 8 out of 10 trials), over time (in 3 settings over the course of a week), or to the clinician's satisfaction. The measures should meet the following criteria.

Mario wants to speak clearly enough that people understand him without difficulty. A likely MUSTDO goal is that Mario participate in group settings, like that Monday

Measurable goals: Goals that meet the following criteria: they describe what it means to reach the goal; they may be quantitative (what things are to be accomplished?) or qualitative (how well will those things be accomplished?); an outside person, properly briefed, can use the measure to confirm goal attainment with certainty.

Criteria of a Measurable Goal

- They describe what it means to reach the goal.
- They may be quantitative (what things are to be accomplished?) or qualitative (how well will those things be accomplished?).
- An outside person, properly briefed, can use the measure to confirm goal attainment as well as you or your clients can.

meeting, where he can practice speech and gauge improvement. This is clearly a therapy goal with a strong counseling dimension. How can you determine its accomplishment? How do you measure its attainment? Mario has episodes of great anxiety before the Monday meetings, so the clinician may decide the best first step is to reduce the anxiety enough that Mario is able to be present at the meetings, whether he talks or not.

Clinician: If you didn't have to talk during those meetings…

Mario: I don't know, if I could just sit there, I guess it wouldn't bother me. But that's not how those meetings work.

Clinician: Well, let's see. Maybe we can find a way for you to show up at the meeting and not have to speak or not be expected to speak.

Mario: How could we do that?

Clinician: OK, who is the highest-level person at those meetings?

Mario: My boss, Julia.

Clinician: What if you went to Julia privately and told her the situation?

Mario: Well, she knows about the cancer and the tongue surgery. Everybody does.

Clinician: Good. You could tell her that you find it difficult to participate in open meetings right now, but you'd like to attend. Ask her whether it would be all right if you participated by listening but, for the time being, you didn't speak. You could work out with her how she would couch this to the group so no one would expect you to chime in.

Mario: I guess I could arrange that.

Clinician: OK. So, here's what we're trying to do. We're trying to get you back to attending the meetings with everybody being OK with you not speaking. We also want you not to experience all that anxiety before the meetings, so we want your heart rate to stay normal and your hands to stay steady. Right?

Mario: Yep.

The goal is measurable. Mario and the clinician know what it means to accomplish it. There are several measures: (1) Mario shows up at the meetings; (2) other attendees do not expect him to speak; (3) his anxiety symptoms abate.

In this situation, you may think that getting Mario to the meeting but having him remain silent does nothing to promote his long-term goal of intelligible speech. However, you need to take Mario's feelings, his anxiety about the speaking situation, into account. If he continues to avoid the meetings, his anxieties about speaking may only increase, possibly extending into other speaking situations. Integrating a cognitive behavioral approach, as expounded by Albert Ellis, into your solution-focused therapy prescribes that you systematically get your clients into the situations they fear (Ellis & Dryden, 2007). So, by setting a short-term goal of having Mario initially attend meetings, but not talk, you are making it more likely that he will eventually talk at those meetings as well as in other speaking situations.

Understood

A good set of measures is understandable. That is the second aspect of a MUSTDO goal: it is understood by you and by your clients. The goal must not only be understood; you and your clients must understand it in the same way. Both of you know what the goal means and what the world will look and feel like when the goal is achieved. A high level of listening is required to achieve this degree of mutual understanding. If you fail to achieve understanding, you and your clients run the risk of going down separate paths to accomplish different versions of the goal.

Understood goals: Of goals formulated by a therapist and client. Fully comprehended by both parties. The goal must not only be understood but also therapist and client must understand it in the same way.

From the scenario as it has unfolded so far, the clinician can be pretty sure that the MUSTDO goal is well understood by Mario and by the clinician. Notice that the clinician ended this segment of the dialogue by summarizing the agreed upon tactic and getting a positive response from Mario. The clinician enumerates the key elements of the goal and gets a positive response, "yep," from Mario.

> **Clinician:** OK. So, here's what we're trying to do. We're trying to get you back to attending the meetings with everybody being OK with you not speaking. We also want you not to experience all that anxiety before the meetings, so we want your heart rate to stay normal and your hands to stay steady. Right?
>
> **Mario:** Yep.

Solution focused

Of course, MUSTDO goals should be solution focused. They should seek to solve a problem or answer a need. There are no "stand-alone" MUSTDO goals. Each of these goals is linked to a long-term goal—what you are trying to accomplish in therapy. That link is the reason you bother putting time and effort into achieving the MUSTDO goal. Solution focus is what gives this goal its importance. It is "wired into the circuit board" of the therapy. In the scenario, Mario may have a reason to question the solution focus.

Solution-focused goals: Of a goal, seen as improving a situation or solving a problem.

> **Clinician:** Great. You know what we're going to do.
>
> **Mario:** I understand, yes. But, really, what's the point? I'll be at the Monday meetings, but I won't be speaking. I'll just be sitting there.
>
> **Clinician:** One step at a time, Mario. You have developed a dread of even attending those meetings, and maybe this dread will crop up in other situations. Right now, what we want is for you to be in a position to speak in a real-life setting, even if, at this moment, you just show up.

Mario: Good point. I can't very well practice speaking to people if I'm stuck alone in my office.

Clinician: Right. What we're doing is just the first step. We're focusing on the things you can do. Steps like this are moving us in the right direction toward your ultimate goal.

The clinician has established the connection between the intermediate goal and the long-term goal. Mario now sees the intermediate goal as solution focused. The clinician has also focused Mario's attention on what he can do rather than on what he can't do.

Time bound

The MUSTDO goal is accompanied by a time or schedule for completion; it is said to be time bound. This aspect is an obvious consequence of the fact that the goal is a "must do." If you must do it, then you must do it by some time or other. It makes no sense to say, "We must accomplish this goal, but we can take forever to accomplish it." When you discuss your MUSTDO goal with your clients, you have to address the issue of time, when this goal will be accomplished. You may devise a schedule outlining the levels of progress toward the goal and the date for the attainment of each level of progress. Events may require you to change the schedule, but that fact does not make a schedule less critical.

> **Time-bound goals:** Goals scheduled to be achieved at a finite, established point.

Clinician: Right. What we're doing is just the first step. We're focusing on the things you can do. Steps like this are moving us in the right direction toward your ultimate goal. Now, today is Tuesday. Can you meet with Julia this week?

Mario: Oh, you want this to happen right away.

Clinician: Unless you see a reason to delay.

Mario: No. I can see her tomorrow. I'll tell her the situation and ask her to talk to the team.

Clinician: Fine. Then, this Monday.

Mario: I'll see how I feel before the meeting. If I'm not sweating buckets, I'll go to the meeting.

Clinician: Good. Do you think you'll be sweating buckets?

Mario: I don't really know. This anxiety was unexpected in the first place.

Clinician: Good point. Well, there are two Mondays before our next session. If you don't get to attend this Monday, make it next Monday for sure.

Mario: OK.

Goals are time bound not just because doing so assigns them a schedule of completion. They are time bound because they also provide clinicians with a schedule to assess client progress toward their goals. You and your clients should know that goals will be continually assessed at certain intervals. Having a specified time for assessment of the goal does not mean goals cannot be evaluated earlier; it just means that they will be assessed at some specified time. Evaluation of goals helps to ensure doability of the goals.

Doable

When assessing goals, you determine whether the goal is doable, whether the goal can be achieved. Doability has two elements. You should first decide whether your clients have the tools, people, resources, and support available to accomplish the goal. You then need to evaluate whether your clients are able to complete the goal given their knowledge, abilities, available time, and the authority they possess to access the people and the resources they need to get the goal accomplished.

In Mario's case, the clinician takes the time to make sure Mario sees the goal as doable, something Mario knows he can accomplish.

Mario: OK. As long as I don't have to talk.

Clinician: You don't; we're setting it up that way, and with your boss's help, there should be nothing embarrassing about it.

Mario: Right. Good.

Clinician: And you have two Mondays to work up to it.

Mario: I think it would be best if I started this Monday.

Clinician: I agree. But if you get too nervous, you can opt to wait a week.

If goals are not doable, clients resist working on them or find it difficult to make progress toward them. Clients may agree that the goals are important, even essential, but indicate that they are too busy, have other priorities, or are not invested in the goals. Other clients may fail to realize that their goals are not doable because of their inability to perform the tasks required to reach the goals. You need to be keenly aware of the difference and engage your clients in honest discussions about the doability of their goals.

Observable

MUSTDO goals should imply an action that can be detected with your senses. Successful therapy and successful counseling result in a change, an improvement, a reality that can be perceived, observed. If your clients meet the criteria for a MUSTDO goal, they do not say, "I can do it, but I can't show you." They can do it and they can demonstrate to your satisfaction that they can do it. The observable part of the written goal is often called the "do statement"; it is what your clients must do.

Observable goals should be constructed using objective terminology. Phrases like "show understanding," "demonstrate knowledge," and "decrease nervousness," although appropriate to discuss in counseling settings, are not terms likely to meet the MUSTDO criteria. Terms such as *identify*, *state*, *change*, and *display* are more objective and thus more observable. Bloom's taxonomy provides a framework for classifying goals and offers examples for appropriate objective terminology (Bloom, 1994; Bloom, Englehart, Furst, Hill, & Krathwohl, 1956).

Mario: I think it would be best if I started this Monday.

Clinician: I agree. But if you get too nervous, you can opt to wait a week. Next session, we'll start off by checking how it went. If you attend the meetings on both Mondays, great. If you attend only the second Monday, that's fine, too.

Mario: Right.

Mario's presence or absence at a meeting would clearly be observable. The clinician discussed with Mario that the goal was intended to reduce his anxiety about attending meetings. "Reduce anxiety" would not necessarily be observable terminology to use for the short-term goal. A short-term goal, such as, "Mario will attend at least one Monday meeting at work over the next two weeks," is acceptable. The goal meets all the MUSTDO criteria.

In the entire scenario with Mario, the clinician carefully moved through each of the MUSTDO criteria, making sure that the goal was measurable, understood, solution focused, time bound, doable, and observable. In the real world, you might not consider these criteria in this exact order; the scenario is designed to illustrate the kind of conversation you might have when meeting each of the criteria. The important task is to see that each MUSTDO criterion is met (see **Figure 8-2**). Then the short-term goal is established and ready to be acted on.

The following are some scenarios with long-term and associated short-term goals.

Scenario 1: Jim is a 57-year-old man who has been attending voice therapy for 1 year to treat his voice disorder caused by a unilateral vocal fold paresis and associated muscle tension dysphonia. Despite being enrolled in therapy for a year, Jim has made very little progress in changing his high-pitched, strained vocal quality. He has inconsistent attendance, blames his lack of progress on his clinician and personal situations,

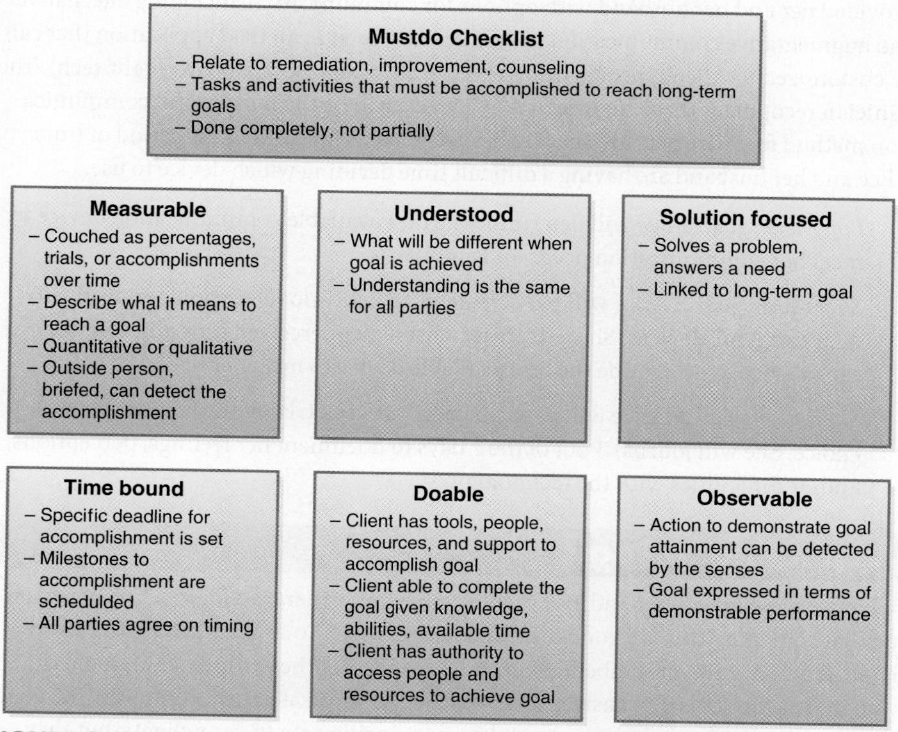

Mustdo Checklist
- Relate to remediation, improvement, counseling
- Tasks and activities that must be accomplished to reach long-term goals
- Done completely, not partially

Measurable
- Couched as percentages, trials, or accomplishments over time
- Describe what it means to reach a goal
- Quantitative or qualitative
- Outside person, briefed, can detect the accomplishment

Understood
- What will be different when goal is achieved
- Understanding is the same for all parties

Solution focused
- Solves a problem, answers a need
- Linked to long-term goal

Time bound
- Specific deadline for accomplishment is set
- Milestones to accomplishment are scheduled
- All parties agree on timing

Doable
- Client has tools, people, resources, and support to accomplish goal
- Client able to complete the goal given knowledge, abilities, available time
- Client has authority to access people and resources to achieve goal

Observable
- Action to demonstrate goal attainment can be detected by the senses
- Goal expressed in terms of demonstrable performance

FIGURE 8-2 MUSTDO Checklist. This checklist of items will help to ensure clients' goals meet the MUSTDO criteria.

and often reports to his clinician that he has not practiced his techniques at home. Jim speaks openly about being frustrated with his lack of progress and he "wishes he had a magic pill to fix his voice." Whereas Jim's desire to experience a vocal improvement is very real, his commitment to the therapy process is absent. His lack of ownership of his goals and lack of motivation to participate in voice therapy activities and techniques create a significant obstacle that his clinician must address before Jim can make any real progress in therapy.

Long-term goal: Jim will demonstrate ownership of his short-term therapy goals by meeting the criterion for each goal over three consecutive sessions.

Short-term goal 1: Jim will participate in writing two short-term therapy goals in the next session.

Short-term goal 2: Jim will state three ways he actively pursued changing his voice throughout the week at the beginning of each session across three consecutive sessions.

Scenario 2: Alice is an 82-year-old woman recently diagnosed with amyotrophic lateral sclerosis (ALS). Since her diagnosis, Alice has had significant difficulty articulating consonant sounds, which makes her speech hard to understand. She writes notes to her family to communicate with them but knows that the motor abilities that allow her to write will deteriorate as her disease continues to progress. Her clinician recently provided her and her husband with options for communication, including alternative and augmentative communication (AAC) devices, such as an iPad application that can be customized to Alice's specific needs (high-tech) and a picture board (light-tech). The clinician recognizes that a high-tech AAC device will be the most useful communication method for Alice because she will be able to use it for the longest period of time. Alice and her husband are having a difficult time deciding which device to use.

Long-term goal: Alice will determine the best available communication device to meet her communication needs and abilities.

Short-term goal 1: Alice will participate in an educational session pertaining to ALS and AAC devices. She will create a list of her perceived pros and cons for each device to determine the best available device to meet her needs.

Short-term goal 2: Alice will participate in a 1-week trial of the device of her choice. She will journal 3 out of the 7 days to document her feelings, perceptions, and/or difficulties with the technology.

Appealing to Logic

Behind every goal you set and every tactic you employ there is a logic, a line of reasoning that contends "this is a good idea, and here is why." Your MUSTDO goals always have the best arguments embedded in the six aspects of the acronym. This logic is what makes the goals persuasive, goals the client is motivated to accomplish. The goals provide the raw material for you to make a convincing case to your clients, but they are not in themselves enough.

In the dialogue above with Mario, the clinician indicated that the goal of attending Monday meetings was solution focused (the *S* of MUSTDO) when the clinician said, "Right now, what we want is for you to be in a position to speak in a real-life setting, even if, at this moment, you just show up." The clinician is proposing a reason, a logical argument for attending Monday meetings, even if Mario does not speak there.

Presenting a Logical Argument That Is Heard

You must not only present your case for the goal but also present your case in a way that your clients can hear and accept. The age and cognitive ability of your clients are two critical factors to consider in building an acceptable, logical argument. You must use language and concepts they fully comprehend. You must use arguments that make sense to them.

> Logical argument: A pattern of reasoning that correctly uses accepted rules of logic to support the conclusion being asserted.

Suzette, a bright 8-year-old, had been dealing with swallowing issues related to an enlarged thyroid when it became evident she had to have surgery to remove the malfunctioning organ. After her pre-op visit, she had this conversation with her speech-language pathologist.

Suzette: I don't think I want to have this operation.

Clinician: Why?

Suzette: I don't want anyone taking something out of my body.

Clinician: You don't?

Suzette: No. It's my body. I don't want something taken out of it.

Clinician: It sounds like you are afraid you won't have your whole body if the doctor takes out your thyroid.

Suzette: That's right. There will be a part of me that won't be there anymore.

Clinician: But your thyroid is a part that isn't working.

Suzette: I know.

Clinician: The doctor is taking it out because it isn't working.

Suzette: I know.

Clinician: Everything else in your body is working fine. I promise you the doctor will not take out anything that is working fine. The doctor will take out only what isn't working. Only the thyroid. You will still have your whole body except what isn't working.

Suzette: Can I keep the thyroid?

Clinician: You mean after it's taken out?

Suzette: Yeah, can I have it to keep?

Clinician: They don't keep thyroids once they are taken out. How about if I get you a picture of it? Would that be OK?

Suzette: Yeah. I'd like that.

The logic embodied in this conversation is compelling, yet this may not be a discussion you would have with a 30-year-old. It is suitable for an 8-year-old with an 8-year-old's level of maturity and an 8-year-old's fears. The clinician used arguments that made complete sense to Suzette. They were geared to her age, intellectual capacity, and maturity.

Distinguishing Logical from Illogical

No matter the client's age, a persuasive argument does begin with making sure your case is logical and not illogical. If you pose a classically illogical argument, do not be surprised when your clients call you on it. Marisa is an adult client who is hard of hearing. She has recently been fitted for hearing aids, which she has been wearing now for 3 weeks. In the following dialogue, Marisa and her clinician are discussing issues Marisa is having with her hearing aids.

> **Marisa:** They are fine when I am alone with someone or watching TV. When I am in a crowd, like the wedding reception I attended last week, I have a lot of trouble hearing people talking to me. The background noise really gets in the way.
>
> **Clinician:** Then, we'll need to find a way to get away from all background noise.
>
> **Marisa:** No. Not really.
>
> **Clinician:** You mean you don't want to find a way to avoid background noise?
>
> **Marisa:** No, that's not what I mean.
>
> **Clinician:** Well, do you want to avoid noise or not?
>
> **Marisa:** I know that I can't avoid all noise. I just want to find a way to make sure I can hear people I'm talking to despite the background noise.
>
> **Clinician:** Oh.

You should be able to determine what went wrong in the dialogue above. The clinician drew an illogical conclusion from Marisa's premise that "The background noise really gets in the way," inferring that Marisa wanted to avoid all background noise. What Marisa was trying to transmit was that she needs a way to manage her hearing in situations with background noise. Removing her from all background noise was not a necessary step, but that is precisely what the clinician thought was the logical course of action. In the scenario, Marisa was able to correct the clinician's mistake immediately.

One way to make sure you proceed down a logical path in conversations with your clients is to clarify with your clients' their key words and phrases. To identify key words in an ongoing conversation, you need to pay close attention. In the revised scenario below, see how the clinician clarifies what Marisa is trying to say.

> **Marisa:** They [my hearing aids] are fine when I am alone with someone or watching TV. When I am in a crowd, like the wedding reception I attended last week, I have a lot of trouble hearing people talking to me. The background noise really gets in the way.
>
> **Clinician:** When you say, "background noise," what are you referring to?

Marisa: Music, other people talking and shouting nearby, things like that.

Clinician: Well, background noise is hard to avoid.

Marisa: Yeah, I realize that. I'm wondering if there is a way to make sure I can hear people I'm talking to despite the background noise.

Logic worked against Marisa's clinician in the first of the scenarios. In the revised example, however, the clinician was able to identify a key word, obtain an appropriate definition, and then work with Marisa to devise a logical way to proceed. You can make logic work for you as well. Clients often have a seemingly instinctive appreciation for logically sound lines of reasoning (Nelson, 2005). As you set MUSTDO goals and work with clients through the criteria of the acronym, you can generate a case that is truly compelling.

Clinician: OK, Marisa, during the past two weeks you found yourself in a situation where the background noise interfered with your hearing.

Marisa: Yes. Twice. The noise made it hard to hear the person who was talking to me.

Clinician: What did we agree that you would do when that happens?

Marisa: We decided that as soon as I noticed the problem, I would suggest to the other person that we move to a place where there wasn't so much noise. You said taking charge of my listening environment would make it much easier to converse.

Clinician: How did it work out?

Marisa: The first time it was great. I was with my sister, and I said, "I can't hear with all this noise; let's go to that corner." We moved and I heard her just fine. The other time was that same night, a little later. I was in a group then, and it was harder to speak up and tell everyone to move just for me.

Clinician: So, what do you think? We set a goal that you would take charge of your listening environment, and in one instance our strategy worked better than in the other.

Marisa: Yeah, I think I'm getting the hang of it for the most part.

Marisa confirmed that the clinician's logic was sound, and she was persuaded that "taking charge of her listening environment" was a good idea. Even so, she found herself hesitant to speak up in a group setting. Strong logic helped, but something more than logic was needed for Marisa to overcome her difficulty in asking a group to relocate "just for her." Obtaining agreement from clients that they are committed to the process may also help maintain momentum when barriers arise during the therapy process.

Creating Agreement

Agreement means that clients make a firm commitment to do what it takes to achieve the goal. They will spend time, energy, and focus on the goal until the goal is met. Even experienced clinicians and counselors can sometimes do an inadequate job of getting explicit agreement to any goal. It is not enough that clients accept the goal as a "good idea" or something that they feel would be nice to attain. Clients have to understand the goals, agree to the process, and commit to change. In the dialogue above, it may seem to you that agreement has been reached. Indeed, many would stop at this point. In fact, the agreement process has just begun.

Consider these additions to the dialogue. Notice how the clinician explicitly states the process and confirms agreement with the client.

Clinician: So, what do you think? We set a goal that you would take charge of your listening environment, and in one instance you did.

Marisa: Yeah, I think I'm getting the hang of it for the most part.

Clinician: So, you are willing to make a big change in the way you communicate, right? You are going to stop allowing a conversation to go on if the background noise is getting in the way of your ability to hear. Instead, you will take charge by moving to a place where the noise is not intrusive. And you'll do this from now on.

Marisa: Yes. When I can do it without making a scene, like in a big group.

Clinician: That's OK for now. We'll work out some strategy for larger groups. You know that by stopping a conversation and moving, you are breaking a strong habit and forming a brand new one.

Marisa: I know. It's hard, but I will do it.

Clinician: I think that's great. If you do what you say, you will definitely decrease the problems you have with your hearing aids in large noisy rooms. Now, if it's OK with you, we'll check every session to see whether you are successful in changing this habit. And we will begin to see whether we can create better listening conditions in every situation.

Agreement here refers to the understanding that the client will invest the time, energy, and focus on the accomplishment of a goal as well as the steps that must be taken to achieve the goal. The clinician accepts where the client is in the process of therapy by validating that some speaking environments are still more difficult to take charge of than others. Marisa explicitly states agreement as well as her willingness to participate in the monitoring process established by the clinician. The client is well on her way to changing behavior.

Behavior and Patterns of Behavior

Behavior: A discrete action a person does.

Every goal set by you and your clients involves the creation of change in the lives of clients. All therapy goals, even many counseling goals, signal a change in behavior or a pattern of behavior. The distinction between a behavior and a pattern of behavior is like the difference between a patch lying on a table and the same patch sewn into a patchwork quilt. One is a piece of cloth with a particular form. The second is a piece of cloth that is part of a pattern.

Pattern of behavior: A connected series of actions.

For our purposes, a behavior can be viewed as a thing done or doable by a person. It may be fairly simple, such as taking a step. Or it may be more complex, such as brushing your teeth or singing a song. *Behavior* is actually a malleable concept;

brushing the teeth can be called a behavior, and swiping the toothbrush once over the front teeth can also be a behavior. Singing one note and singing an entire phrase can both be termed "behaviors." Having a flexible notion of behavior is useful. It gives you the opportunity to define a behavior in a fairly broad manner.

A pattern of behavior is behavior that is a recurring part of your life and practices. Brushing your teeth is a behavior. Brushing your teeth nightly is a pattern of behavior. Making a sibilant /s/ sound is a behavior. Making an /s/ sound in everyday speech when appropriate is a pattern of behavior. In speech-language pathology and audiology, turning a behavior into a pattern of behavior is what is called maintenance and generalization (Ingersoll & Wainer, 2013). These terms have long been associated with classical and operant conditioning.

Maintenance occurs when a desirable behavior is elicited regularly. An example is producing the /s/ phoneme correctly in appropriate word positions during therapy. Generalization occurs when the correct behavior is elicited in a variety of situations. Producing the /s/ sound appropriately outside therapy is an instance of generalization.

In the scenario featuring Marisa, she is learning to assert her listening needs during conversations in specific situations in which she must move to hear better. If Marisa does this every time she finds it difficult to hear because of background noise in one-on-one conversations, she is maintaining the behavior. If she then extends this assertiveness to group settings or other appropriate venues, she is generalizing.

> **Maintenance:** A state of affairs where a desirable behavior is elicited regularly.

> **Generalization:** A state of affairs where the correct behavior is elicited in a variety of situations.

Repatterning Behavior: A New Way of Doing It

The term repatterning refers to the entire maintenance and generalization process. An old habit, in some cases a complex one, is replaced with a new set of behaviors. Repatterning is done intentionally and consciously. Marisa can be said to be repatterning the way she conducts conversations. In a counseling setting, the repatterning process is subtle, because it relates to such matters as motivation, attitude, and emotion.

> **Repatterning:** The total process of maintenance and generalization.

Breaking with the old way

Raffi is a 54-year-old corporate accountant. He has stuttered for as long as he can remember. He had therapy as a teenager, but it had no lasting effect. His encounters with the impatience and ridicule of others discouraged him from trying to become more fluent, and he found a job where his interaction with others is highly limited. Now, Raffi has been told by management that, to advance in his position, he must deliver more internal presentations to upper management. Nick, his speech-language pathologist, comes to realize that Raffi's perception of others' attitudes toward stuttering derives from experiences that took place 30 years ago.

Clinician: So, when you were in high school, the other students made fun of you?

Raffi: Yes. Even those who weren't unkind were frustrated with me when I stuttered. I guess it wasn't considered cool to wait me out. They'd tell me to calm down or "take a breath, man." You know how well that worked.

Clinician: Yes. Do you think you'll meet the same attitudes today?

Raffi: Why wouldn't I?

Clinician: It's been thirty years since those experiences. Studies show there has been a big change in attitudes toward disfluencies.

Raffi: Studies? Pardon me if I don't trust your studies.

Clinician: I don't blame you, but I will be emailing some of the data to you. Take a look at it, why don't you. I can also tell you that in my own experience over the years, I've seen a definite change in people's attitudes. And, don't forget, Raffi, you're not dealing with high school students now.

Raffi: No, adults are different. They're more subtle, but they can be just as bad as kids.

Clinician: There will be challenges, that's for sure. The question is, do you want this promotion?

Raffi: Yes. I've more than earned it.

Clinician: Well, the job requires that you give presentations. You are not up against high school students who are less knowledgeable and less mature. We'll talk about the subtle ways adults show their negativity. We'll develop strategies to address that and get past it. Meanwhile, we'll be working on the goals we set last session for improving your fluency.

Nick, the clinician, knows the value of repatterning Raffi's expectations about how people will react to him. Raffi's current attitude is demotivating and will get in the way of the progress he can make in therapy. Seeking to move Raffi away from his old way of thinking, the first step in repatterning, Nick begins by presenting information.

Experienced clinicians know the importance of assuring that they have informed clients. Nick is aware of this factor as he shares information about changed attitudes toward stuttering, both research data and Nick's own experience. Nick uses this information to help Raffi begin the process of breaking with his old way of viewing the attitudes he is likely to encounter when he stutters. The scenario illustrates that information like this is not always completely persuasive. It is, however, an excellent starting point for helping the client begin the repatterning process.

After presenting the information, Nick's next move is to assure Raffi that any challenges he encounters from others will be identified in therapy and addressed. You may be called upon to use several measures to help your clients break an old pattern, and you may have to revisit the process repeatedly. The expression "old habits die hard" is all too frequently very true.

Learning the new way

As the old pattern breaks down, it is replaced by a new mode of behavior. The processes of extinguishing an old pattern and establishing a new one are often simultaneous. The new pattern itself is frequently the cause of the old one's disappearance. A new way of brushing your teeth or swinging a golf club replaces your previous technique as you practice the new method and become familiar with it. In these cases it is difficult to see the difference between breaking the old pattern and forming the new one.

Although attitude change can occur in this manner, you may need to view it as a two-step process of extinguishing the former attitude and then inculcating the new one. Nick may need to convince Raffi that his fears about the attitudes of others are not well founded before he can proceed to foster a different set of expectations. Once the new attitudes are "seeded," you and your clients must strive to nurture them and give them permanence.

Habituation: Making the new way the client's way

Habituation is the term frequently used to denote the process of making a new pattern permanent. When you brush your teeth or swing that golf club the new way every time without thinking about it, habituation has occurred. Repatterning is complete. If Raffi comes to be convinced that other people's attitudes about his stuttering are much more positive than he previously believed, he now thinks differently about those attitudes. Nick can conclude that the repatterning is a successful counseling outcome. Raffi now thinks habitually that other people will greet his disfluency with more patience and understanding than he previously believed.

With Raffi, as well as with the earlier example of Mario, short-term goals have been established. If those goals are achieved, Raffi will have more positive expectations about the attitudes of others toward his disfluencies. Mario will be comfortable attending business meetings. Their long-term goals have not been met, of course, but attainment of these intermediate, MUSTDO goals denotes real progress as specific obstacles are removed.

> **Habituation:** A term frequently used to denote the process of making a new behavioral pattern comfortable and permanent.

Common Roadblocks

These outcomes, positive as they are, must be put in perspective. Raffi's fear of public speaking may have more than one cause, and new patterns have a way of slipping back toward the old. Mario is attending meetings, but not yet speaking, so there may be challenges ahead. Marisa is still hesitant to improve her listening environment in any situations but one-on-one conversations. As you move forward in the therapy process, you need to be aware of old and new roadblocks that may hinder successful and long-lasting repatterning of attitudes, emotions, and motivations.

Determining Roadblocks

Roadblocks to repatterning tend to arise in three places. You might experience an obstruction in your efforts to break an old pattern, or there could be difficulties in forming an enduring new pattern. Finally, your clients might slip back toward the older pattern after you have concluded that repatterning has been successful, a situation known as relapsing.

Below are some common roadblocks to successful repatterning in counseling.

As a clinician, you must be aware of these possible roadblocks every time you embark on the repatterning process. When you detect that one has arisen, discuss it with your clients, and seek an agreement to address it.

> **Roadblocks to repatterning:** Complications that obstruct the path to maintenance and generalization. Obstructions can arise in efforts to break an old pattern, or difficulties might be encountered in forming an enduring new pattern. A person might slip back toward the older pattern after repatterning has apparently been achieved, a situation known as relapsing.

Brainstorming Strategies

When you meet a roadblock and define it, you may then want to brainstorm strategies for addressing it. The most useful strategies are the ones that fit in with your therapy

Roadblocks to Repatterning in Counseling

- Clients simply do not accept the argument that the old pattern is flawed and needs changing.
- Clients believe the old pattern is problematic, but they are unwilling to go to the trouble of making the change. They are "comfortable with the uncomfortable."
- Clients are indecisive, expressing a desire to change in one session and seeming to lose interest in changing during the following session.
- Clients do not commit fully to the practice or regimen necessary to repattern. This lack of commitment can show itself at any point in the repatterning process.
- Clients do not have a clear idea of what the repatterning consists of, what it looks or feels like.
- Clients seem to have habituated, but they begin to slip back toward the old pattern. This relapse can be gradual or more sudden.

goals and maintain the progress you are making in meeting those goals. At the onset of a brainstorming session, allow clients to be open to all possibilities, even their wildest thoughts and notions. Do not judge any strategy or remedy. Judgments can restrict the brainstorming session. There will be several possibilities from which you will then select the most suitable.

You may agree that the roadblock must be removed immediately or there will be serious consequences. Let us say that Nick and Raffi determined that Raffi's conviction about other people's attitudes toward his stuttering would totally undermine progress in achieving his goals. In that case, Raffi's conviction must be removed. This is a roadblock that cannot be allowed to stand in the way.

You may decide that the roadblock can be sidestepped for the time being or that a partial solution is acceptable. Perhaps Raffi does not accept the premise that people's attitudes toward stuttering have really changed over time, and Nick, the clinician, cannot convince him otherwise. Instead of focusing on that obstacle, Nick and Raffi decide to take a few sessions to improve Raffi's presentation skills and then take stock of where they are. If Raffi's confidence has gained traction during these sessions, perhaps the roadblock will not present as much of an obstacle to progress as before. You might even conclude that it is not worth the trouble to try to remove this roadblock at all, and then your strategies will be geared to making therapy progress without taking the time to address the roadblock.

Action Planning for Removing Roadblocks

If you find it necessary to remove the roadblock so that you can make therapy progress, you cannot pretend otherwise. You and your clients must put together a workable action plan to get past the roadblock and see that it does not create an obstacle in the future.

Changing client behavior is challenging but possible and rewarding. Existing patterns constitute your clients' lifestyle; these patterns and habits get them through each day. The existing patterns may have "worked" for the clients, and clients are comfortable with them. It can take a great deal of convincing and a great deal of effort to make a change in such a key part of a person's daily life. Even small changes can be exasperating. Try storing your wallet in your left pocket if you habitually place it in the right one. Or hanging your purse on your right shoulder if you typically put it on your left. Repatterning where you place your wallet or purse is definitely a challenge.

Repatterning an attitude, a belief, an emotion, or a motivation is all the more difficult. Make sure the repatterning is worth the effort. If it is, commit fully to the process. We humans may find that change is tough, but our belief in progress makes change not only possible but desirable. As a clinician you play many roles with your client. Change agent is among the most important.

Review of Key Points

- This chapter covers the goal-setting process, distinguishing types of goals and their key features, the persuasion/direction aspect of therapy and counseling, and changing behavior.
- The two types of clinical goals are (1) therapy or purposive goals and (2) intermediate and counseling goals.
- Intermediate goals are MUSTDO goals: measurable, understood, solution focused, time bound, doable, and observable. They are goals you "must do" to get to the purposive goal.
- Some MUSTDO goals relate to the therapy strategy you are employing and some of them are counseling goals. They are within the power and capability of clients to achieve, and they reflect the primary tasks and activities that must be accomplished to achieve therapy aims.
- Behind every goal you set and every tactic you employ there is a logic, a line of reasoning for you to make a convincing case to your clients.
- Make sure your case is logical and not illogical. Clients often have a strong appreciation of a logically sound line of reasoning.
- Agreement means that clients make a firm commitment to do what it takes to achieve the goal. They will spend the time, energy, and focus on the goal until they reach it. It is not enough that clients accept the goal as a "good idea" or "nice to attain."
- Every goal set by you and your clients involves the creation of change in the lives of clients. All therapy goals, even many counseling goals, signal a change in behavior or pattern of behavior.
- Behavior can be viewed as a thing done or doable by a person. A pattern of behavior is behavior that is a recurring part of a person's life and practices.
- Maintenance occurs when a desirable behavior is elicited regularly in the presence of a specific cue (or stimulus). Generalization occurs when that behavior is elicited in the presence of different cues when the behavior is appropriate.
- The term *repatterning* refers to the entire maintenance and generalization process. An old habit, in some cases a complex one, is replaced with a new set of behaviors. Repatterning is done intentionally and consciously.
- In a counseling setting, the repatterning process is often more subtle, because it relates to such matters as motivation, attitude, and emotion.

Practical Exercises

For this assignment, read the scenarios and for each client create one long-term goal and two short-term goals that meet MUSTDO criteria.

1. Caroline is a 10-year-old girl who was diagnosed with congenital hearing loss. She has worn hearing aids for years but has been wearing them less and less often at school this year. Caroline's parents realized she had stopped wearing her

hearing aids when her grades began to drop. When they asked Caroline about it, she told them that she was embarrassed to wear her hearing aids in front of her friends and that she felt different wearing them.

2. Jacob is an 8-year-old boy who has difficulty with reading fluency and comprehension. He has been attending speech therapy once a week for 3 months. Within each session, Jacob makes great progress, but he rarely retains therapy strategies from week to week. Jacob's mother, Michelle, brings him every week but sits in the lobby during every session despite the clinician's requests for her to participate. She says that she does not need to know what he is working on as long as it is helping him. Recently, Michelle has been concerned that she is not seeing improvements in Jacob's reading ability at home and does not understand why therapy is not helping.

REFERENCES

Bloom, B. (1994). Reflections on the development and use of the taxonomy. In L. W. Anderson & L. A. Sosniak (Eds.), *Bloom's taxonomy: A forty-year retrospective* (93rd yearbook of the National Society for the Study of Education, pp. 1–8). Chicago, IL: University of Chicago Press.

Bloom, B. S, Englehart, M. D., Furst, E. J., Hill, W. H., & Krathwohl, D. R. (1956). *Taxonomy of educational objectives: The classification of educational goals. Handbook I: Cognitive domain.* New York, NY: David McKay.

Ellis, A., & Dryden, W. (2007). *The practice of rational emotive behavior therapy* (2nd ed.). New York, NY: Springer.

Ingersoll, B., & Wainer, A. (2013). Generalization and maintenance. In F. A. Volkmar (Ed.), *Encyclopedia of autism spectrum disorders* (pp. 1419–1423). New York, NY: Springer.

Nelson, H. E. (2005). *Cognitive-behavioral therapy with delusions and hallucinations: A practice manual* (2nd ed.). London, UK: Nelson Thornes.

CHAPTER 9

Readiness as Openness

KEY TERMS

- Counseling Integration Matrix (CI Matrix)
- Quality of life

LEARNING OBJECTIVES

After reading this chapter, you will be able to:

- Define quality of life and list ways perceptions about quality of life affect clients and their commitment to therapy goals
- Describe and use the Counseling Integration Matrix to assess client's commitment to therapy
- Explore strategies for counseling clients in each of the four quadrants of the CI Matrix
- Explore ways to optimize the use of allies in each of the four quadrants of the CI Matrix

This chapter focuses on how you can determine your clients' readiness or willingness to change.

Discontent with the Old Way

Individuals who have communication or related disorders realize at some point that the way they express, hear, or understand language, the way they speak or voice, the way they chew or swallow is different or has changed. Except for the smallest of children, your clients will not only recognize this difference but may become frustrated, dissatisfied, or unhappy with their current state. Their willingness to change their current state depends on many factors. Chief among these is the impact of their disorder on their quality of life or the attainment of their goals.

> Quality of life: A person's assessment concerning how close he or she is to an acceptable level of perceived happiness and satisfaction in his or her day-to-day condition.

Dysfunctions of the Current State

Dissatisfaction with their current state may be the initial feeling your clients have, but dissatisfaction alone may not be persuasive enough for clients to want to change. It can be the reason they initially come to therapy, but it's not what keeps them there. Once clients realize that there is real work involved in remediating or improving a communication, hearing, or swallowing disorder, accepting what is only "dissatisfying" is easier to do. "I can live with my voice this way. I have for this long already." "I don't really stutter all that much." "I can hear people alright. Some situations are hard, but not too many, and I can live with that." Excuses abound for why clients do not want to put forth the effort to make change.

Excuses fade and clients tell a different story when dissatisfaction becomes unacceptable. This usually happens when the problem affects their lives. They stop answering the phone because they are not sure what voice will come out. They order the honey ham hoagie when they really want the buffalo chicken wrap because they do not stutter on the /h/ phoneme. They do not participate in family discussions because they really cannot hear what others are saying. When the problem impinges on their social life and begins to affect their overall quality of life, clients often become more willing to invest the time and energy it takes to make substantive changes through therapy.

Assessing Clients' Quality of Life

Once you have established your clients' desire to change, you can use a variety of counseling techniques to assess your clients' willingness to change. Merely participating in therapy will not make change happen. Clients, first, have to want to change. Then, they have to be willing to put forth the effort to practice what they are changing more often than they practice the pattern that causes their communication, hearing, or swallowing problem. They have to answer the phone using their voice strategy. They have to use a strategy learned in therapy to help them say the /b/ phoneme in *buffalo chicken* so they get the sandwich they want. And they have to wear their hearing aids so they can be part of the discussion.

There are ways to determine how much a disorder influences your clients' quality of life. One way is to simply ask them how much their issue is affecting their life, perhaps through informal discussion. A nonstandardized method often used with clients who stutter is the "Three Wishes Task." In this task you have your clients imagine that a genie has appeared and granted them three wishes. What, you ask, would their top three wishes be? If clients mention that they would wish for their stuttering to go away, then you can assume that the disorder affects their life. If remediation of their stuttering is not one of their three wishes, then you might determine that their disorder does not have a great impact on their quality of life.

You can also obtain quality of life information through a standardized format such as the "Voice Handicap Index" for voice (Rosen, Lee, Osborne, Zullo, & Murry, 2004), the "Overall Assessment of the Speaker's Experience of Stuttering" (OASES) for people who stutter (Yaruss & Quesal, 2006), "Communicative Activities of Daily Living" for adults with cognitive and language disorders (Holland, Frattali, & Fromm,

1999), and the "Pediatric Quality of Life Inventory" for children with speech and language disorders (Varni, Seid, & Kurtin, 2001). These are only a few of many standardized instruments clinicians can use to determine how much clients' disorders affects their quality of life.

The Counseling Integration Matrix

Sometimes quality of life measures indicate the obvious need to begin therapy, sometimes not. When a clear and pressing need is evident, most clients exhibit a firm willingness to do whatever it takes to improve. Some clients, however, are less willing to commit to change even though their quality-of-life measures indicate a real need for therapy. Then there are cases when quality-of-life measures do not indicate an obvious need for therapy. Most commonly a low impact on quality of life relates to a low willingness to change, although there are less frequent situations when clients have a high willingness to change despite the low negative impact on their life. All of these different client situations are illustrated in the Counseling Integration Matrix, or CI Matrix, depicted in **Figure 9-1**.

The CI Matrix provides a useful model that encompasses the negative impact of a disorder on a client's quality of life set against the client's willingness to make the changes recommended through therapy. It is called the Counseling Integration Matrix because it provides guidance on the kinds of counseling strategies recommended in various circumstances. The CI Matrix reveals four client states, starting with the upper right quadrant and moving counterclockwise through the other quadrants to the lower right quadrant. These quadrants provide you with insight into your clients' need for

Counseling integration matrix (CI Matrix): A useful model that encompasses the impact of a disorder on a client's quality of life set against the client's willingness to make the changes recommended through therapy. The CI Matrix reveals four client states: high negative impact on quality of life with high willingness to change (high-High); high negative impact on quality of life with low willingness to change (High-Low); low negative impact on quality of life with low willingness to change (Low-Low); low negative impact on quality of life with high willingness to change (Low-High).

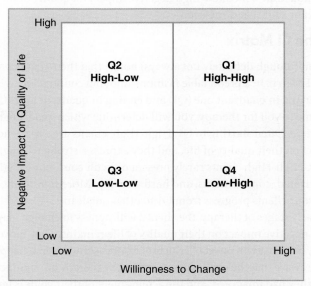

FIGURE 9-1 The CI Matrix. The Counseling Integration Matrix is used to identify the quadrant a client occupies during the therapy process. Quadrants are defined in terms of willingness to change and degree of negative impact on quality of life the communication problem has.

therapy, their openness to the idea of therapy, and their willingness to put forth the sustained effort required by therapy. Without these insights you may have great difficulty selecting counseling strategies that work for your clients and their Circle of Power.

The upper right quadrant (Q1) depicts "High-High" clients, who are experiencing a high negative impact on their quality of life and a high willingness to change. This condition is unsurprising. Clients who do not feel good about their quality of life are usually willing to make changes through therapy. The upper left quadrant (Q2) contains "High-Low" clients, who are experiencing a high negative impact on their quality of life and have little willingness to make changes or meet therapy goals. You will be likely to use a number of counseling strategies with High-Low clients.

The lower left quadrant (Q3) portrays "Low-Low" clients, who feel that their quality of life is relatively unaffected by their disorder and who are simultaneously experiencing a low willingness to make changes. This is a logically consistent state of affairs, because people content with their lives might not be all that interested in changing. The lower right quadrant (Q4) depicts "Low-High" clients, who feel very little negative impact on their quality of life though they possess a high willingness to make changes and meet therapy goals.

Wide variations can exist among clients in the same quadrant. For example, clients in a given quadrant are not necessarily at the same point in therapy. Clients can also move from one quadrant to another during the therapy process. Clients in a particular quadrant are alike in one respect: the impact of their disorder on their quality of life is similar, as is their willingness to address their disorder in therapy. Remember though that the quadrants each represent a spectrum of negative impact versus willingness to change within their respective quadrants. A client who is primarily in quadrant 3 may demonstrate a medium-high negative impact on quality of life placing them closer to quadrant 2 for that dimension.

Clients in the CI Matrix

Clinicians often (though definitely not always) notice that their clients progress through the CI Matrix in a predictable fashion—moving counterclockwise through the matrix, starting in quadrant one (Q1) and ending in quadrant four (Q4). When clients first come to you for therapy, you will determine which quadrant best describes their current state. Often starting in Q1, High-High, clients are experiencing a strong negative impact on their quality of life, and they express a strong willingness to make improvements. High-High clients rarely present difficult counseling challenges. They tend to be motivated, conscientious, and hard working. More significant challenges often arise as your clients progress from Q1 to other quadrants.

In these early stages of therapy, the clients' willingness to change may decrease while the high negative impact on their quality of life remains. They move from Q1 to Q2, which may be seen as an onset of reluctance or resistance. What happens is that the clients become aware that the challenges presented by therapy are significant, progress is slower than they had imagined, and the achievement of their goals is farther off than they had at first foreseen. These frustrations can result in a significant lowering of your clients' willingness to change.

Meanwhile, because their disorder has not improved much, its impact on their quality of life is still high. These clients require a good deal of solution-focused counseling targeted at encouraging them, keeping their goals well defined and unobstructed, and helping them to see incremental improvements clearly.

If counseling is successful, the High-Low Q2 clients will start to see the negative impact on their quality of life decrease as real improvements take hold in their world. They will begin to move from Q2 to Q3, Low-Low. In Q3, the work is hard, perhaps at its hardest because the repatterning process is reaching a critical phase with new habits replacing old ones and the changes creating a whole new reality.

Willingness to change may remain low for Low-Low Q3 clients. The counseling goals here include convincing clients that it is worth seeing therapy through; they have come so far already. You listen for indications of positive effects of the improvements that they have worked to achieve, and you highlight these effects. You help the clients envision the preferred future toward which they have been journeying, and you paint the clearest possible picture of that future as it draws ever closer.

When clients begin therapy in Q3, however, the situation may not be quite so promising. These clients come to you feeling that their disorder is not adversely affecting their lives, and, perhaps because of that feeling, they are not all that desirous of working at improving. Your counseling challenge now is to help them see the negative effects of their disorder and provide reasons for them to want to change. If you cannot accomplish that, therapy may not be productive, at least not at this time.

In any case, if you succeed in getting Q3 clients "over the hump" of resisting the permanent change or repatterning toward which you have been working, you will begin to see progress toward Q4, Low-High. Because of the improvements, clients continue to experience a relatively low impact on their quality of life, but their willingness to change rises again. The difference now is that the change is at hand, not at some distant point in the future.

Q4 represents the new reality, the future which therapy was designed to create. You counsel to reinforce this highly desirable state of affairs. You stress the benefits of repatterning, and you put in place the elements of maintenance and generalization. The best outcome is permanent change. So, no matter where your clients start out in the matrix, one of your long-term goals is always to progress to Q4, low negative impact on quality of life and high willingness to change.

Each of the following scenarios illustrates a specific version of a client who falls within a particular quadrant in this matrix.

The first scenario describes a High-High client who would fall within Q1 of the matrix, high negative impact on quality of life and high willingness to change. These individuals' lives are so affected by their disorder that they are willing to work hard to improve their situation. They are usually easy to work with and are motivated to come to therapy. High-High Q1 clients are also compliant with the generalization of their techniques to home practice. When you treat clients like this, your action plan may seem to write itself. The work is hard, but they do what is necessary to show improvement, and usually show it rather quickly. If therapy is their only option because the other options are unacceptable to them, then their willingness to change will be even stronger.

Rasha, a 51-year-old marketing analyst and mother of three adult daughters, was diagnosed with a vocal fold scar following an upper respiratory infection. She is initiating therapy after learning from her ENT that she is not a candidate for surgery. Her clinician is a certified speech-language pathologist.

Clinician: It looks as if you have investigated other options before coming here.

Rasha: Certainly. The scarring resulted from an infection of my vocal folds; I was told that surgery could do nothing to correct it.

Clinician: I notice a roughness in your voice.

Rasha: Yes, that's the way it is now. It is worse early in the morning and after I have used it for a few hours.

Clinician: Wow, it must be difficult for you. How long have you had the scarring?

Rasha: A little over a year.

Clinician: So, you waited a while.

Rasha: Yes. I didn't think it was a problem initially.

Clinician: Then?

Rasha: Well, then, my daughter—I have three—my oldest comes to my house and sits and asks me why I haven't been answering her phone calls.

Clinician: You weren't answering her calls?

Rasha: I wasn't answering calls at all, hardly. All my daughters noticed it. My oldest took it upon herself to approach me about it. At first I told her she was wrong, that I wasn't letting calls go to voice mail, as she said.

Clinician: Was that how you saw it?

Rasha: Yes. I actually got a little angry at her, defensive, I guess.

Clinician: You denied that you were avoiding the phone.

Rasha: Yes. Denial is exactly the word.

Clinician: But your daughter convinced you.

Rasha: She finally asked me if I really wanted all three of them to come over and tell me about it. That's when I gave in.

Clinician: Gave in?

Rasha: That's when it hit me like a ton of bricks. I was avoiding talking on the phone, not just with my family; it was affecting my work, too. I'd avoid taking calls and making calls I knew I had to make.

Clinician: Anything else?

Rasha: I was becoming a sort of recluse. I'd stay in my office at work just to avoid talking.

Clinician: Why did you avoid talking?

Rasha: I just thought I sounded terrible, like a baritone with a bad cold. People used to compliment me on my speaking voice. I was actually ashamed, I am ashamed, and with my daughter's help I realize now that it is affecting every area of my life.

Clinician: In my experience, people with scarring like yours never get back their original voice, not completely.

Rasha: I'm not looking for that. I want my voice to be stronger, better sounding, and more resilient through the day.

Clinician: Those are three goals we can almost certainly achieve.

Rasha: Really?

Clinician: Really.

Rasha: I'd do anything...

Clinician: Being motivated is important.

Rasha: I think I'll be your most motivated client.

Clinician: It sounds like you may be right. What we'll do first is set long-term goals based on what you want to achieve and what we determine is possible. Then we will establish an action plan to meet those goals. That plan will consist of shorter-term goals that will move us toward the big goals.

Rasha: That is pretty much what I was expecting.

Clinician: It will take time, and there will be moments of frustration, I'm sure.

Rasha: Nothing is worse than living with this. I'll take all the time needed.

Clinician: In that case, Rasha, there is every reason to believe that you can significantly improve.

Rasha: When do we start?

One of the long-term goals for High-High clients, those who begin therapy in Q1, is to progress through therapy and move closer to Q3 or Q4, where their disorder does not have such a negative effect on their quality of life. Your utilization of counseling strategies will subside as the negative impact on your clients' quality of life decreases, as long as they continue to make progress toward their specific therapy goals. You will also continue to evaluate your clients' progress to determine whether your goals are still in line with theirs.

Rasha clearly falls into Q1. It took some time for her to realize the negative effect her voice disorder was having on her quality of life; however, once she received the diagnosis and recognized its effects on her, she was ready and willing to do whatever it would take to make improvements to her voice quality.

A high negative impact and a high willingness to change do not always equate to success in therapy. You may encounter High-High clients who simply do not believe in the effectiveness of therapy as a path to change. These clients may show up in your clinic and immediately claim they do not believe therapy will help them. Their placement on the C-I Matrix is irrelevant until you can reach agreement on the efficacy of engaging in therapy.

Some High-High clients take the opposite stance. They fear any other options and therefore only want therapy, and in very few cases, therapy may not be proven to be effective or may not be the best option. For example, a client with spasmodic dysphonia may resist Botox injections, though the most effective treatment for this voice disorder is those injections. With clients who have spasmodic dysphonia, even their willingness to do therapy will not result in an improvement in their voice.

You can run into a similar problem if behavioral therapy is your clients' only option because clients will continue to decline as their disease progresses. Examples include clients with amyotrophic lateral sclerosis and clients with Alzheimer's disease. In these cases, your clients' high willingness to participate in therapy will help in the process of meeting goals, though their gains may be slowly achieved. You may even reach a point when therapy is no longer a useful option.

Similar to Q1 clients, High-Low clients' quality-of-life measures indicate an obvious need for therapy. These clients, however, exhibit a low willingness to change. These individuals fall in Q2 of the matrix, high negative impact on quality of life and low willingness to change. Ironically, their willingness to change decreases because the impact their disorder has on their life is so great; achieving even small goals is daunting because of how much the disorder affects them.

Many times High-Low clients are highly motivated to come to therapy. They arrive on time for sessions and participate in the activities conducted in therapy but often are unwilling to practice the strategies outside of therapy that are needed to effect improvement. Sometimes it is even difficult to get these clients to participate in lesson activities during their sessions. These individuals often associate themselves so closely with their disorder that they cannot see how change will make a difference; change then becomes overwhelming and almost unimaginable.

Take, for example, Micah, a college student who has had therapy in the past for his stuttering.

Clinician: You don't seem very enthusiastic. This goal setting appears to drain off your energy.

Micah: I've been in college for almost two years and nothing much has happened. I don't know why, but I just thought my speech would improve and I would be cured once I went to college.

Clinician: So, something about the move to college made you feel your stuttering would go away.

Micah: Yeah, like the problem was a kid's problem, and now I'll be in college and not a kid, and so my speech would be grown up.

Clinician: Would your life have been better if that had happened?

Micah: Sure. I've gone back to avoiding situations where I have to talk and even not putting up my hand in class. It feels bad and it is hurting my grades.

Clinician: So, you would like to be "cured," as you said, right?

Micah: Yes, but the idea of going through this therapy really brings me down. Besides I now realize that this is who I am. I'm a stutterer, that's me.

A client like Micah is often difficult to work with. From his past experience in therapy, he knows he can improve his speech, but he does not want to put forth the effort to make those changes happen. At this point, he wants his stuttering to go away, to be "cured." As a clinician, you will need to address these feelings, determine what may empower your client to want to change, and continue to progress through the CI Matrix.

Most likely, clients like this will continue in Q2 for a while with a low willingness to change. They may even begin to deny the impact their disorder has on their lives. The achievement of small goals, taking little steps and challenging clients along the way, may help to maintain your clients' motivation through difficult times.

Look for opportunities to address the fact that a client like Micah has apparently determined that he is not merely an individual who stutters; he now sees himself as a stutterer. He has acquired a version of ego impedance. Stuttering has become a part of his identity. In counseling Micah, you will want to help him see that stutterer is not who he is; stuttering is something he does, something that can conceivably be improved.

The following scenario depicts a Low-Low client, Anika, who falls within Q3. Clients in Q3 typically have quality-of-life measures that indicate that their disorder has little or no effect on their quality of life. Because of this, Low-Low clients have a low willingness to change and may appear to have little desire to come to therapy at all. Remember that if clients start out in Q3, you may decide that therapy is not warranted at that time. It is important, however, that you fully evaluate Low-Low clients before deciding to delay or not recommend therapy.

As clients move away from the onset of their disorder, they begin to identify themselves more with the person they have become rather than the person they were. Often, quality-of-life measures fall back to the norm regardless of therapy. This "acceptance" may be inadvertent because of how individuals naturally cope with adversity or change; they may have simply forgotten what their life was like before or may be denying how much the disorder affects them. Audiologists are all too familiar with this phenomenon in cases of hearing loss due to aging. The scenario below provides yet another illustration.

In this scenario, Anika, a 16-year-old high school junior, is meeting with her audiologist a week after her hearing evaluation. Anika was diagnosed with a unilateral, sensorineural hearing loss. The audiologist recommended that she try using a hearing aid for a week.

Clinician: So, Anika, how did the hearing aid work for you this week?

Anika: Right away I thought that my hearing aid helped me hear my teachers better.

Clinician: That's good, but I see you aren't wearing it right now.

Anika: Yeah, I realized that I could hear my teachers before. Things were fine before, really.

Clinician: OK. Why don't you want to wear the hearing aid?

Anika: I just don't think I need it. My three best friends even told me that my hearing loss never bothered them. Sure, when we walk down the hallway together I need them to stand on my right side. I also know to sit up closer to the teacher in class. But I'm used to doing that. Even with the hearing aid, I still found myself doing those things.

Clinician: Yes, as you know, Anika, the hearing aid can't restore your hearing completely, and it's only been one week. You are still getting used to things.

Anika: I know.

In this example, Anika appears to be a Low-Low client (Q3). She initially went to have her hearing evaluated by the audiologist and perhaps at that time felt her hearing had a more negative impact on her quality of life. After using the hearing aid for a week, she realized, or at least she felt, that she could hear fine before getting the aid. Anika, however, is a client you would not want to dismiss quickly. She exhibits some reluctance to using the hearing aid and may be denying that her hearing loss, or the act of wearing a hearing aid, is affecting her.

Sometimes Low-Low clients do not know the extent to which therapy can help them. They believe their disorder is something they just have to live with and cannot be changed. One counseling strategy that may be used with these individuals is information sharing. Clients are more likely to admit that they are bothered by their communication disorder if they are provided with information about their disorder. They may also be more willing to participate in therapy if they know what their options are for therapy.

Sometimes Q3 clients can be convinced that a course of trial therapy is worth their time. Be overly prepared for the first session. You will need to build rapport quickly and get straight to the heart of the issue. Low-Low clients need to be shown that therapy can improve their situation. They will then have to decide for themselves if therapy is worth the investment of their time and effort. Sometimes the hard truth is that clients have other priorities and therapy is not one of them. Be careful not to push Q3 clients too hard. When and if the time is right, clients may return for therapy.

Low-High clients, those within Q4, are the type of clients who experience low negative impact on their quality of life but exhibit a high willingness to change. These clients can be satisfied with the slow progress they are making in therapy and are willing to continue with the process, or they may be clients who do not necessarily need therapy anymore but still believe they can improve.

In the following scenario, Jessie is a client whose cluttering does not negatively impact his quality of life and who is okay with the slow progress of therapy.

Clinician: Well, Jessie, we have made progress in your rate of speech. You are using your pauses effectively, and your speech is much easier to understand.

Jessie: Yes, that's an improvement.

Clinician: It certainly is. I am wondering how you feel about the progress we've made beyond that.

Jessie: It has been slow, I think. Our exercises have worked pretty well for single sentences, but the cluttering picks up during conversation, and I haven't made much of a change in that.

Clinician: Does that concern you?

Jessie: Not much. You told me there was no deadline on my improvements. I want to keep working. If one part of my speech is better, I can get better in the rest.

Clinician: OK.

As a clinician doing therapy, you should continuously evaluate your client's progress to determine what type of Q4 client you have. Clients like Jessie may remain in therapy for quite some time; however, there are Low-High clients who have reached the final stages of their progression through the CI Matrix who are ready to be dismissed from therapy. Attempting to dismiss Q4 clients who want to be in therapy may be a difficult task. Keep good records to show clients data to support your rationale for dismissal. Encourage Q4 clients who resist dismissal to phase out of therapy. You may consider suggesting that the client lessen the weekly session time, go to every other week sessions, or take a 2-week break from therapy. These strategies help Q4 clients realize that they do have the capability to continue improving on their own. You can also offer to have a maintenance session in 6 weeks to 3 months to check in on how your client is doing.

Circle of Power in the CI Matrix

The CI Matrix is a useful tool not only for determining the counseling needs of your clients but also for understanding members of your clients' Circle of Power and the opportunities and challenges they present. People in the Circle of Power also occupy places on the matrix, and those places may be different from that of the client. The Circle of Power consists of associates, caregivers, and family members of your clients. These individuals exert influence with your clients and are often enlisted as allies. Where they are on the matrix provides helpful information about the role they will play during therapy.

Allies or caregivers in Q1 experience a high negative impact on their quality of life as a result of the client's disorder. Along with that impact, these individuals show a strong willingness to make whatever changes are necessary to accommodate the client's process of changing and doing therapy. An example is the father of a 6-year-old girl who is hard of hearing. The Q1 father finds it difficult to communicate with his daughter, and this difficulty creates a high impact on his quality of life. He is willing to do whatever it takes to assist his daughter in addressing her hearing disorder through therapy, so he has a high willingness to change. This change might entail weekly car trips to the clinic, practicing techniques with his daughter, ensuring that she inserts her hearing devices correctly and changes the batteries, and any number of other activities that will alter his life.

Q1 caregivers are often a joy to have in clinic. Individuals like the father mentioned in the above scenario are dependable. He will bring his child on time to every session, participate fully in the session if needed, and learn techniques taught within the session. He will practice and enforce strategies at home.

Because they experience a high negative impact on their quality of life, Q1 caregivers can sometimes be difficult to deal with in therapy. These allies need to be instructed not to bombard clients with constant reminders to practice and not to push clients beyond their abilities. Their overly aggressive behavior may turn a client away from therapy. Counseling becomes imperative when addressing overly zealous Q1 allies. Detailed practice schedules for home practice may guide these allies to maintain limits at home. Clarifying goals with these allies and updating them on progress toward goals also keeps them aware of the clients' current abilities.

Clients may also struggle with the therapy process if their primary caregiver resides in Q1 and they occupy either Q2 or Q3. The clients' low willingness to change works in direct contrast to their primary caregivers' high desire for change. You should always be aware of Q1 caregivers in this case. Share the CI Matrix with them. Explain where you believe they are in relation to where you believe the client to be on the matrix. Detail the strategies and goals you are working toward with the client to get the client to be more willing to change. Communication is imperative. Do not assume that the Q1 caregivers' willingness to invest time and energy in the client's therapy will translate into a positive effect for the client.

Whereas Q1 allies are usually very receptive and willing to help in the therapy process, Q2 allies often exhibit a different attitude toward clients and their goals. Q2 allies experience a high negative impact on the their quality of life resulting from the client's disorder; however, these allies show a low willingness to make changes as the client participates in therapy. Q2 allies often cancel or do not show for scheduled therapy sessions, do not help or encourage clients to practice strategies outside of the clinical setting, and do not appear to be invested in the therapy process.

An example of a Q2 ally is Andy's football coach. Andy is a 17-year-old individual who stutters. His coach is certainly inconvenienced by having to take Andy aside after practice and team meetings to make sure Andy's questions are answered and comments are received. For the coach, though, the payoff is letting Andy remain silent during practices, games, and team meetings. Now that Andy is in therapy for his stuttering, the coach is reluctant to allow him to slow down team meetings and "disrupt" games while he practices techniques to manage his stuttering. The coach is unable to see that allowing Andy to talk during practices and games would reduce the time spent on postmeeting conferences with him.

Because of their low willingness to change, Q2 allies can sometimes appear to be adversaries rather than allies. In this example, the behavior of Andy's coach does border on being adversarial. What makes the coach an ally is that he is willing to make an accommodation for Andy—he takes extra time after meetings and practices to let Andy ask questions and make comments. What places the coach in quadrant 2 is that he does not want to change his existing accommodations to meet Andy's present therapy goals.

Your counseling, in a case like Andy's, would be directed toward the client and not the ally. Andy is old enough to decide how he would like to proceed regarding his coach's unwillingness to change his habit. You would follow the client's lead in this situation. If Andy believes that it is not worth his time to address this issue directly with his coach because it is his senior year and the season is almost over, or he is fine practicing his strategies in other environments and is okay maintaining the old arrangement, then supporting his decision and moving forward with therapy is the correct course of action.

If, however, Andy is very bothered by his coach's unwillingness to change, then helping Andy to create an action plan to address his coach would be an appropriate way to proceed. His plan would most likely include a one-to-one meeting with the coach about the situation. You too might meet with the coach if such a meeting would be helpful.

If your clients are too young or unable to address a Q2 ally directly, then it is your job to be their advocate. Schedule a meeting with Q2 allies to discuss the therapy process. Be prepared to provide concrete evidence about how their involvement and participation in the therapy process will benefit the client as well as themselves. Remember, Q2 allies still experience a high negative impact on their quality of life as a result of the clients' communication disorder. If they can be convinced that therapy will not only help the client but also help them, they may be more willing to be an active participant in therapy.

There are two issues to consider with Q2 allies. The first is to be careful not to jump to conclusions that a caregiver is actually a Q2 ally. Caregivers who might appear to be Q2 allies because they do not respond to emails or do not attend therapy sessions with clients may really be Q1 allies who are highly invested but not privy to certain information.

School speech-language pathologists can succumb to this presupposition because they rarely meet with caregivers. Sending notes home in clients' folders does not ensure that caregivers receive them. Make direct contact with these caregivers to discuss a client's treatment plan. A quick call after school is probably most effective. An email may suffice if it is difficult to get in touch with the caregiver. Arranging a formal one-to-one meeting at school shows how serious you are about this client's needs. Do not assume caregivers know your intentions. You need to be clear, obvious, and straightforward.

The second issue to consider when dealing with Q2 allies is why the caregiver is a Q2 ally. Everyone has a story—working long hours, being a single parent, dealing with illness, going through a divorce, taking care of numerous children. All of these can affect a caregivers' ability to participate in therapy. Caregivers' experience with prior therapy for themselves or the client may also have an impact on the caregiver's ability to buy into or fully participate in the therapy process. Give caregivers a chance to tell their story. Be flexible and creative in determining ways to manage potential obstacles to the therapy process. Detailed homework schedules, checklists, and email reminders can be useful tools in your efforts.

Q3 and Q4 allies are experiencing little or no negative impact on their quality of life as a result of the client's disorder. Q3 allies, however, are reluctant to make any changes as the client participates in therapy, whereas Q4 allies are very willing to make those changes. A Q3 example would be the mother of Rocco, an 8-year-old who cannot accurately produce the /r/ phoneme consistently. Although the school speech-language pathologist has told the mother that Rocco needs therapy, she insists that Rocco will grow out of his speech problem. Her quality of life is not affected by Rocco's speech, and when the speech-language pathologist asks for her cooperation with recommendations, Rocco's mother tells him it isn't necessary. If Rocco's mother had welcomed the recommendations and agreed to help the speech-language pathologist in anyway she could, she would qualify as Q4. **Figure 9-2** lists some characteristics of members of the Circle of Power in each quadrant.

Again, there are variations on the characteristics of allies in each quadrant. The previous examples provide only some of the possibilities that fit the parameters of each quadrant. The interaction of clients and their allies is also significantly affected by where each is on the CI Matrix, and these effects, once understood, can provide you with great insight into the counseling strategies you will select, who will benefit from them, and how you will integrate those strategies into therapy. Allies can also move through the CI Matrix during the therapy process, occupying one quadrant and later finding themselves in another. Make sure you continuously evaluate allies' position on the CI Matrix so you can achieve a highly beneficial level of participation.

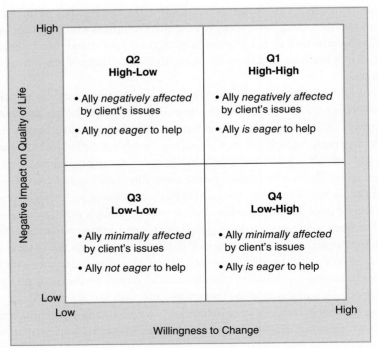

FIGURE 9-2 The CI Matrix and the Circle of Power. The CI Matrix depicts the attitudes and motivations of those who are in the client's Circle of Power. The matrix can be used to identify an ally's attitudes and feelings in relation to the client's current state.

Dealing with Allies in Different Quadrants

- In most cases the ideal quadrant is either Q1 or Q4, where the ally is willing to change to help the client meet therapy goals. Aim for one of those.
- The Q2 ally experiences a high impact on the ally's life as a result of the client's issues but is not highly motivated to help you. Your task is to persuade the ally that the negative impact will be lessened if the ally commits to helping with therapy goals; get the ally to think long term.
- The Q3 ally experiences a low impact on the ally's life as a result of the client's issues and is not highly motivated to help you. Your task is to find a way to motivate the ally to participate appropriately in the attainment of therapy goals. Look for motivators that are attractive to the ally.
- Accept that the amount of commitment the ally has is the choice of the ally. Get what you can. Don't worry about what the ally is not willing to contribute to your therapy plan.
- Monitor throughout the therapy process to see that the ally keeps to the agreements made. Respond when you discover a slackening of commitment and positively reinforce a cooperative ally.
- Don't let an ally become an adversary. The things you say to your client can get back to the ally, and criticisms might not be welcomed. Keep your relationship with the ally upbeat and positive.
- Show gratitude; make sure the ally knows the ally's help is greatly appreciated.

Here are some guidelines and recommendations for dealing with allies when you discover they occupy one of the four quadrants.

As a clinician, remember, you too are an ally of your clients and you too will be in one of the four quadrants. A good exercise is to determine which quadrant a particular client occupies and then assess where you are on the matrix. A Q3 (Low-Low) client might ultimately cause you to migrate to Q3 in your own relationship to that client. Another possibility is that a Q3 client challenges you, and you find yourself in Q1. These considerations speak to your ongoing relationship with your clients and may be worth contemplating as you engage in the therapy process with them.

Once you have decided the kind of client you are dealing with, you will be able to assess your clients' commitment to change, their motivation to stay the course and complete therapy. You must continuously evaluate how your clients' quality of life is affected by their disorder and how it is affected by the changes made through therapy. Make sure to assess your own placement on the CI Matrix because you too may change during the therapy process. You will also continue to provide opportunities for your clients to practice the strategies they are using in therapy.

Even with the most willing and motivated clients, changing a habit is hard; therefore, it is natural for clients to show reluctance or resistance toward practicing their strategies outside or even inside of therapy. The CI Matrix provides a useful starting point for recognizing where positive behavior can be reinforced and built upon and where unhelpful behavior can be reversed or extinguished. Numerous counseling strategies will present themselves as you become fully aware of your clients' level of motivation and quality of life.

Review of Key Points

- Clients' dissatisfaction with their current state and willingness to change depend on many factors, especially the impact their disorder has on their quality of life. When dissatisfaction becomes unacceptable and begins to affect their overall quality of life, clients often become more willing to invest the time and energy it takes to make substantive changes through therapy.

- You can use counseling techniques to assess your clients' willingness and readiness to change. First, clients have to want to change. Then, they have to be willing to put forth the effort to make the change permanent.

- There are informal and formal ways to determine how much a disorder influences your clients' quality of life. You can obtain quality-of-life information by asking about it or using counseling techniques to elicit the information, or you may use a standardized format for your clients' specific disorder.

- The Counseling Integration Matrix provides a useful model that encompasses the impact a disorder has on a client's quality of life set against the client's willingness to make the changes recommended through therapy; it provides guidance on the kinds of counseling strategies recommended in various circumstance.

- In the CI Matrix, the upper right quadrant (Q1) depicts "High-High" clients, who are experiencing a high negative impact on their quality of life and a high willingness to change. The upper left quadrant (Q2) depicts "High-Low" clients, who are experiencing a high negative impact on their quality of life and have little willingness to make changes or meet therapy goals. The lower left quadrant (Q3) depicts "Low-Low" clients, who feel that their quality of life is relatively unaffected by their disorder and who are simultaneously experiencing a low willingness to make changes. The lower right quadrant (Q4) depicts "Low-High" clients, who feel very little negative impact on their quality of life though they possess a high willingness to make changes and meet therapy goals.

- Clients often begin therapy at Q1, High-High. They are experiencing a strong negative impact on their quality of life, and they express a strong willingness to make improvements. High-High clients rarely present difficult counseling challenges.

- Clients may move from Q1 to Q2, High-Low, which may be seen as an onset of reluctance or resistance requiring extensive counseling They may then move from Q2 to Q3, Low-Low, as the work remains hard and quality of life improves. The counseling goals here include convincing clients that it is worth seeing therapy through; they have come so far already.

- You may then see progress toward Q4, Low-High. Because of the improvements, clients continue to experience a relatively low impact on their quality of life; their willingness to change rises again, but now the change is at hand, not at some distant point in the future. Q4 represents the new reality, the preferred future.

- The CI Matrix is also a useful tool for understanding members of your clients' Circle of Power, their allies, and the opportunities and challenges they will present. They too occupy a point on the matrix, and it may be different from that of the clients. Where they are on the matrix provides helpful information about the role they will play during therapy.

- Allies in Q1 experience a high negative impact on the their quality of life resulting from the client's disorder; they show a strong willingness to make necessary changes to accommodate the client's process of changing and doing therapy. Q2 allies experience a high negative impact on their quality of life resulting from the client's disorder but a low willingness to make changes. Q3 and Q4 allies experience little negative impact on their quality of life as a result of the client's disorder. However, the Q3 allies are reluctant to make any changes as the client participates in therapy, whereas the Q4 allies are very willing to make those changes.

- The interaction of clients and their allies is also significantly affected by where each is on the CI Matrix, and this interaction, once understood, can provide you with great insight into your counseling strategies.

- You may need to provide allies in different quadrants with different ways to best help your client. For instance, a Q1 ally may need to be reminded not to push your client too hard to practice during the week, and a Q2 ally may need to understand the purpose and importance of home practice.

- As a clinician, you too are an ally of your clients, and you too are in one of the four quadrants. That fact speaks to your ongoing relationship with your clients and may be worth contemplating as you engage in the therapy process with them.

- Once you have decided the kind of client you are dealing with, you will know whether your clients are committed to change, their resources for change are sufficient, and they are motivated to stay the course to complete therapy. Your job is to continuously evaluate how your clients' quality of life is affected by their disorder and by the changes made through therapy.

Practical Exercises

For this assignment, read each scenario, determine which quadrant of the CI Matrix best fits each individual, and explain why you chose that quadrant.

For each scenario, identify at least one counseling strategy you would use in your efforts to make progress in therapy.

For each scenario, identify at least one caution you would advise to avoid damaging your prospects for progress in therapy.

1. Ryan is a 13-year-old boy who has difficulty producing /r/ in the final position of words during conversation. He has been in therapy for 5 years and has not made much progress over the past year. He often expresses that he hates being pulled out of class and that he thinks his /r/ sounds fine.

2. Vincent is an 8-year-old boy with recently diagnosed neurosensory, bilateral hearing loss. The loss has been gradual, so he does not notice that he has a hearing problem. He says that visiting the clinician is fun, and he wants to do what the clinician tells him to do.

3. Patricia is a 63-year-old woman who has a unilateral vocal fold paresis (weakness). She says that her voice has been hoarse for 6 months and that she has difficulty talking to her elderly mother. She told her clinician she would do anything to make her voice come back.

4. Valeria is a 47-year-old female who had a traumatic brain injury (TBI) almost 20 years ago. She was diagnosed with severe spastic dysarthria and mild cognitive deficits as a result. Valeria can currently speak single words verbally but must use an iPad to communicate with longer phrases. During therapy, she expresses often that she wants to leave, and despite reminders from the nurses who care for her, she rarely practices at home.

REFERENCES

Holland, A., Frattali, C., & Fromm, D. (1999). *Communication activities of daily living* (2nd ed.). Austin, TX: Pro-Ed.

Rosen, C. A., Lee, A. S., Osborne, J., Zullo, T., & Murry, T. (2004). Development and validation of the Voice Handicap Index-10. *Laryngoscope, 114*(9), 1549–1556.

Varni, J. W., Seid, M., & Kurtin, P. S. (2001). PedsQL 4.0: Reliability and validity of the Pediatric Quality of Life Inventory Version 4.0 Generic Core Scales in healthy and patient populations. *Medical Care, 39*(8), 800–812.

Yaruss, J. S., & Quesal, R. W. (2006). Overall Assessment of the Speaker's Experience of Stuttering (OASES): Documenting multiple outcomes in stuttering treatment. *Journal of Fluency Disorders, 31*(2), 90–115.

SECTION V

The Solution Cycle
Phase Four: Creating the Preferred Future:
"Making It Happen"

This section focuses on Phase Four of the Solution Cycle: Creating the Preferred Future. The preceding sections certainly took this solution focus into the practical arena of counseling in therapy. The chapters in this section stress the practical even more. You will encounter applications, illustrations, and techniques driven by the actual experience of clinical work. You will deal with specific emotions, specific motivations, and specific points of resistance. You will learn to "practice a practice." You will confront your toughest challenges, from reducing entrenched negative emotions to helping clients face their final moments of life.

Ultimately, your mission is to set your clients on a life-long course with an improved quality of life, and this section's last chapter considers the role of counseling in achieving that mission. The tools for long-term success are presented here. Your task is to learn what they are, when to use them, and how to become highly competent at counseling your clients, their family members, and their associates.

Ultimately, your mission is to set your clients on a lifelong course with an improved quality of life, and this section's last chapter considers the role of counseling in achieving that mission. The tools for long-term success are presented here. Your task is to learn what they are, when to use them, and how to become highly competent at counseling your clients, their family members, and their associates.

CHAPTER 10

Feeling: Thoughts and Emotions, Willingness and Resistance

KEY TERMS

- Acceptance
- Anger
- Apathy
- Bargaining
- Boredom
- Bullying
- Catastrophic loss
- Denial
- Depression
- Discouragement
- Resistance

LEARNING OBJECTIVES

After reading this chapter, you will be able to:

- Identify workable techniques for counseling clients exhibiting a variety of emotions
- Assess clients' motivation and respond effectively to motivational deficits
- Counsel clients effectively when they experience trauma, bullying, crisis, or a catastrophic event

To create the preferred future, your clients need motivation. This chapter illustrates a motivational model that you can use to guide you as you counsel during the journey through therapy. You and your clients must also address emotions that can stand in the way of success, and the chapter shows how effective counseling can manage those emotions.

Stages of Grief

Elizabeth Kübler-Ross studied hundreds of clients in extreme circumstances and noted that they tended to move through five discrete stages or attitudes toward their condition (Kübler-Ross, 1969). All these stages have a direct impact on clients' motivation and on their emotional state (**Figure 10-1**). Kübler-Ross suggested that clients typically proceed through these stages in the order she indicated. Research since her groundbreaking findings has revealed a more complicated process (Konigsberg, 2011). Although many go through the five stages just as listed, many others stay in one stage for a long time or occupy two or more stages at once. Clients can revisit a

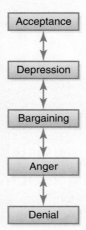

FIGURE 10-1 The Stages of Grief. There are five stages of grief. Individuals often begin in denial and continue through the stages to acceptance. These stages are not thought to be a linear process because clients and may skip over a stage and may even occupy more than one stage at a time.

stage that they once seemed to have passed through even if just momentarily. Some research suggests that many people do not experience distinct stages of grief after a devastating loss (Bonanno, 2010). They may become sad, yes, but they do not enter into a cycle of grieving with identifiable stages. Bonanno details this research indicating that humans have an innate ability to deal with loss that involves a multitude of emotions, including despair and sadness as well as joy and resiliency.

Keeping this research in mind, you do well to avoid making broad assumptions about all people dealing with a difficult loss. Even so, Kübler-Ross's stages of grief provide a useful model for clinicians dealing with their clients' emotions and motivation. Clinicians should be on the alert for symptoms of these stages and indications that clients are moving from one stage to another. Counseling can be employed more effectively with this awareness.

Denial

Denial: Often seen as the initial reaction to devastating news or trauma. When in denial, the person experiencing the difficulty simply contends that there is no problem, nothing wrong.

Stage 1 is denial. For clients suffering loss or, more specifically, loss associated with a communication disorder, denial may be the initial reaction. When in denial, the client simply contends that there is no problem, nothing wrong. This initial reaction can be useful as clients work through the powerful shock that can come with trauma or learning about a disorder. In a sense, denial can buy time for clients to gather the strength they will need to confront the challenge they are facing.

At some point, however, you must help your clients transition out of denial and admit the reality of what is transpiring in their lives. This acknowledgment is a necessary step if they are to ultimately address the trauma or disorder.

Jaylin is a 17-year-old high school senior whose unilateral hearing loss has become more profound in the past year, according to a recent audiology evaluation. Jaylin is meeting his audiologist to discuss his condition and the possible need for a hearing aid.

Clinician: We have the evaluation results, Jaylin. Let's go over them.

Jaylin: OK.

Clinician: You have hearing loss in your left ear.

Jaylin: Yes, I've had it from birth.

Clinician: Right. This assessment shows that the hearing loss is worse.

Jaylin: Worse? No way.

Clinician: [*Showing results from recent evaluation and one from a year before.*] As you see on these graphs, there is a pretty significant difference.

Jaylin: It must be a mistake.

Clinician: Well, when I noticed the results, I tested the tones two more times. The results were the same all three times.

Jaylin: I'm telling you, there's no change in my hearing.

Clinician: OK. Jaylin, when you watch TV with others, have you noticed any change?

Jaylin: Not with me. My sister complains more that I have the volume up too high, but she's always complaining about something. It doesn't mean my hearing is worse.

When speaking with clients in denial, conversations such as this one can seem never-ending and appear to be without a solution. Clients have an explanation for any change you may notice. They may blame others and may dismiss even compelling evidence. Clients in denial often seem to live in a parallel universe where the problem does not exist.

Be patient with clients in this stage. Often they are hearing the disheartening news for the first time and need some time to digest the information. Be clear and straightforward with the results of testing, your recommendations, and referrals if any. Explaining results simply using objective data, charts, or standardized results, as Jaylin's audiologist did, may help clients see a clearer picture of their problem. You might give them handouts of the information you are transmitting. Provide ample time for clients to ask questions. Denial may be long-lasting, but, when it ends, Stage 2 often begins. This chapter discusses denial in more detail later and offers ways to counsel clients in this stage.

Anger

Stage 2 is anger. This is the "why me?" stage, when clients rage at the injustice of this terrible thing happening to them. Counseling clients in the anger stage is difficult, and techniques to deal with it are presented in this chapter. Frequently, the frustration that results from lack of ownership and control is very much present in this stage. The anger sometimes emerges as envy of the "lucky ones" who are not afflicted, and that resentment might even be directed at you, their clinician, for not being able to do more. Do not be defensive in situations where clients express their anger toward you. Being defensive may make your clients more angry and frustrated. Validate their

Anger: The second stage in the classically framed stages of grief, when a person experiences fierce emotional rebellion at the terrible event.

feelings with statements like, "I realize that this is very hard for you," or "I can see that you are really angry right now." Provide your clients with ample time to talk about their anger and frustration, remembering to stay focused on your clients' objectives and goals. Many times improvement and successes toward goals can help your clients move through the anger stage. Most clients eventually realize that anger is not productive and changes nothing. Be aware, however, that anger is one of the stages that will be revisited by many clients in the course of therapy as they face new challenges or revert to old patterns.

Bargaining

Stage 3 is bargaining. Clients in this stage are looking for hope, a way to reverse what has happened, to negotiate a deal, or to get a reprieve. This stage is fraught with "what if" questions and "if only" statements. "What if I had gotten a second opinion sooner?" "If only I hadn't taken that medicine when I was pregnant." Bargaining also takes the form of a prayer that asks a higher being to make things better. In return clients promise to give up something of value or change their lives for the better.

Riya, a 50-year-old florist, recently had a right hemisphere stroke that caused difficulty with higher-level cognitive tasks. For the past several sessions, she expressed anger as she faced her cognitive challenges, but lately she has seemed more at peace with her current situation.

> **Bargaining:** The third stage in the classically framed stages of grief, when a person looks for hope, a way to reverse what has happened, to negotiate a deal, or to get a reprieve.

Clinician: During our last session, we talked about how upset you've been about the effects of the stroke.

Riya: I was angry. I think I'm past that now.

Clinician: You do seem less upset than you have been.

Riya: I have great faith that I will get better.

Clinician: Many clients find that their faith is a big help to them.

Riya: I made a promise that I will be a better person if only these thinking problems would go away.

Clinician: So, you do believe you might get better.

Riya: I would give just about anything to be better.

Clinician: Changes will occur as you recover from the stroke, Riya. You and I will work with those changes and get the most out of them.

Counseling during the bargaining phase includes letting clients know that (1) what they are going through, bargaining, is a normal reaction to their situation or a particular feeling they have at any point in time, and (2) faith and prayer can be a comfort and a help to believers.

No matter what your personal beliefs are, you should show deep respect for a client's faith, religion, and spirituality. Your special contribution to your clients' well-being derives from the realm of science, and you will proceed accordingly. Many aspects of your clients' lives can play a part in the achievement of their goals, and experienced clinicians have learned to welcome all positive influences.

Make sure, though, that the influences are positive. The bargaining stage may at first appear beneficial to the therapy process because clients who are bargaining may demonstrate characteristics of hopefulness. Be wary of statements like, "I would do anything for this to go away" and "I'm sure I'll get better if I just keep the faith." The fact is, bargaining can be an outward sign of helplessness and desperation, not optimism. When the realization is made that bargaining proves unhelpful, clients may enter into the next stage of grief.

Depression

Stage 4 is depression. In this stage, clients are dealing with the present moment, the reality of the situation. Many clients experience an emptiness for what they have lost or for what they believed would be their future. Clients in depression exhibit low energy and motivation and may become purposeless and apathetic. This stage can reach a state known as clinical depression. When you believe a client's psychological well-being extends outside your scope of practice, you should consider a referral to a licensed psychologist. The section in this chapter on discouragement provides strategies to deal with clients in this stage. Depression is a difficult stage to work through, but it must take its course so the clients can gather the strength to move to the next stage.

Acceptance

Stage 5 is acceptance. Of all the stages, this one is the target; the other four stages are negative states that clients must leave to proceed in a positive direction. This stage should not be confused with the idea that everything is "all right" or "fine." Actually, the opposite may be true. Some clients never feel that they are all right or fine with their diagnosis or deficits. What this stage does mean is that clients truly accept the reality of their diagnosis and deficits and, in the face of that reality, choose to do what they can about it.

Clients with communication disorders who reach the acceptance stage often make the decision that their condition is real, lasting, and now a factor to be taken into account as their lives progress. The movement from one stage to another denotes progress, but none of the earlier stages is an ideal long-term setting for therapy. Acceptance is not complacency or simply being immobile in the face of the loss or disorder. Acceptance is the willingness to engage in realistic therapy.

Once clients reach the stage of acceptance, they are most ready to set goals and get to work. Although some clients have more limitations than others do, no one has unlimited potential, so really their limitations are a matter of degree. Your clients and you will establish appropriate goals and plan a path to the attainment of those goals; this is the process to which all your clients commit. Your focus, as always, is on your clients' quality of life, whether to enhance it or slow its decline.

Depression: The fourth stage in the classically framed stages of grief, when a person begins dealing with the present moment, the reality of the situation. Many experience an emptiness for what they have lost or for what they believed would be their future. Those in depression exhibit low energy and low motivation and may become purposeless and apathetic. This stage can reach a state known as clinical depression.

Acceptance: The fifth stage in the classically framed stages of grief, when a person faces the reality of the situation and chooses to do what can be done about it.

Motivation to Succeed

There are a number of valid reasons to engage in counseling with your clients. One of the most important reasons is to create and sustain their motivation to succeed and to achieve the treatment goals you and they have set. The Counseling Integration (CI) Matrix is used to assess clients and caregivers in terms of two factors: their willingness to change paired with the negative impact their disorder has on their quality of life (**Figure 10-2**). The CI Matrix contains four quadrants depicting four possible states clients may exhibit in respect to those two factors. Your clients demonstrate predictable characteristics depending on the quadrant they occupy. Among these characteristics are the emotions clients may feel. Figure 10-2 gives a sampling of these likely emotions.

The emotions that appear in a given quadrant are not always consistent or similar because clients in the same quadrant can be experiencing different states. Clients in quadrant 4, for example, are always experiencing a low impact on their quality of life and a high willingness to change. They include those who have met with success in therapy and are prepared to maintain and generalize their gains to make permanent improvements. Clients like these may be "ready," "cheerful," and "stimulated." Another class of clients in Q4 might be enjoying aspects of therapy that have more to do with positive social interactions with you than with the pursuit of treatment goals. These

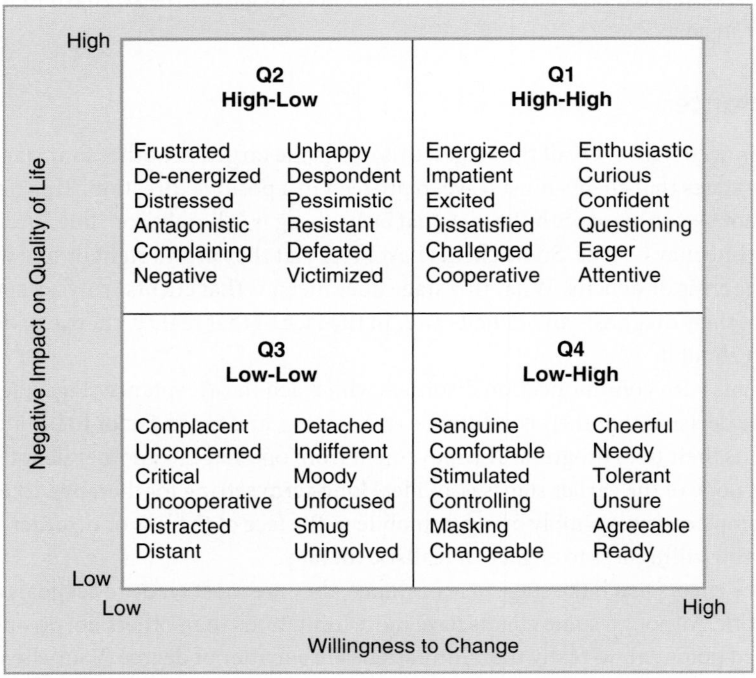

FIGURE 10-2 The Counseling Integration Matrix (CI Matrix) with Associated Emotions. The CI Matrix provides a way to assess clients' readiness for therapy based on their willingness to change in relation to their overall impact on quality of life. There are associated emotions for each quadrant in the CI Matrix.

clients may be "needy," "controlling," and "masking." A third Q4 group may want to use therapy for personal improvement even though their disorder is having little impact on their quality of life. These clients might be "agreeable," "changeable," and "sanguine."

If you are having difficulty deciding on the quadrant your clients occupy, you may find it helpful to start with an assessment of their feelings. By identifying their feelings, you may be able to determine their location on the CI Matrix, which will provide you with a better understanding of their willingness to change.

The CI Matrix is not the only indicator of the emotions your clients are feeling during a particular session. Clients may be sad or happy because of something that happened to them earlier in the day. They may be grieving a loss or celebrating a victory. They may be in a bad mood for no reason that is apparent to them or to you. To make matters even more complicated, their emotions may change during the session, sometimes for obvious reasons and sometimes inexplicably. Your task is to assess emotions accurately and counsel clients effectively to put them on track to achieve their goals. Understanding the balance of emotions that signal strong motivation is the key.

Motivation connects your clients with their goals in a focused manner. Motivation creates enthusiasm and energy, the willingness to spend time working on the goals. There are three elements in this motivational connection, and each one must be maintained and strengthened throughout therapy with constant attention and effective counseling. The three elements are (1) a sense of purpose, (2) a conviction that growth is occurring, and (3) a feeling of ownership of the goals and the process. In this chapter, you explore the power of emotion in achieving motivation and the counseling strategies you can employ to tap into that power (**Figure 10-3**).

Achieving Purpose

Merely having a goal is not enough. The goal must become a purpose; it must be seen as worthwhile, that is, worth the investment of time and hard work necessary to achieve it. A goal is an end point toward which a person actively moves. It is a destination. A purpose is a reason to act, an explanation of why a particular goal is important or meaningful. When seeking to establish purpose, you should begin with the CI Matrix and the goals of therapy. Once you have clarified your goals with your clients and determined their position on the CI Matrix, you can help clients make the purpose connection.

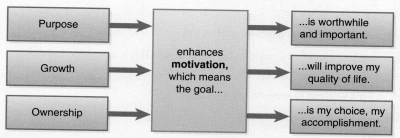

FIGURE 10-3 Motivational Balance and Achievement of Goals. Purpose, growth, and ownership must be continually assessed to maintain motivation toward clients' goals.

Anna is a 36-year-old middle school teacher who has come to therapy because in the past year she has noticed her voice tiring during the final periods of the day and especially at the end of the week. She admits she is frightened. One time her voice left her completely, and she had to shorten a class period so she could recover. She has already set a very clear goal: to learn to use her voice in such a way that it does not tire as quickly and maintains its intensity and strength longer.

Clinician: Your Voice Handicap Index indicates that your quality of life is greatly affected by your voice problem.

Anna: I won't argue with that.

Clinician: And you've told me you have a strong willingness to make the necessary changes to achieve the goal.

Anna: Yes. I can't wait to start.

The clinician has placed Anna in Q1 on the CI Matrix, high impact on quality of life and high willingness to change. The clinician can probably count on Anna being energized, eager, attentive, questioning, challenged. She may also exhibit other emotions listed in Figure 10-2. Although this is good news, the clinician will want to use counseling to help Anna make an explicit purpose connection with the goal.

Clinician: OK, Anna, let's look at that goal we are shooting for. You want to learn to use your voice in such a way that is does not tire as quickly, right?

Anna: Yes.

Clinician: Also, you want to maintain your loudness and energy for a longer period of time.

Anna: Right.

Clinician: Why?

Anna: Why? Why do I want to achieve these goals? I'm a teacher. I teach using my voice.

Clinician: So, your voice is essential to your job.

Anna: My voice is essential to who I am. I can't be who I am, a teacher, without it.

Clinician: So, your goal may be to stay louder longer, but your purpose here is to be the person you are, a teacher.

Anna: A competent and effective teacher, yes.

Clinician: Let's keep that in mind as we move along. This is more than just doing exercises to accomplish goals. We are working to…

Anna: I am working to keep my identity.

Clinician: Is that an overstatement?

Anna: No, it is not.

Clinician: I don't think so either.

When the purpose connection is made as firmly as it has been made with Anna, her motivation can be expected to become even more focused and intense. Of course, Anna is an intelligent adult professional who has grasped the notion of purpose quickly and accurately. This conversation will be different with children or adults of different cognitive ability, but you should still have the conversation at your clients' level. Help them associate the goal with the person they want to be.

Achieving Growth

Anna is now more aware of the importance of her treatment goals. The next matter she should consider is the challenge involved. As you know, change is a critical component of the therapy process. Therapy is literally senseless without it. One axis of the CI Matrix, in fact, is "willingness to change," an indication of its importance. Change, though, is not neutral. You need to clarify that your clients are making a commitment to change, but not just any change. They are committing to growth, improvement. They are not just becoming different in some way but are becoming better in some way.

Change does not imply struggle, but growth often does. No one talks about "change pains," but the term *growing pains* is well understood. Even physical growth has its discomforts as when the adolescent body adjusts to increases in height and the emergence of developmental marks of adulthood. As soon as you use the purpose connection to clarify the importance of the goal, you should use the growth connection to clarify the challenge of achieving the goal.

Anna: All right, I see how important this is. I was already a little scared, losing my voice and all, but I'm starting to get terrified.

Clinician: Let's not get terrified. Let's look at the road ahead of us, OK?

Anna: OK.

Clinician: We are going to achieve the goals we set. In others words, as we work together, you are going to make changes. You are going to improve. This is hard work, but it is not scary. You know why?

Anna: Why?

Clinician: Because you and I are going to monitor progress all along the way. We will set small, doable goals...

Anna: Benchmarks.

Clinician: Good name for them, yes, benchmarks. Bit by bit we will make progress toward the big goals. We will adjust things so you are never overwhelmed. You'll never push faster than you are capable of at a given time. OK?

Anna: I should tell you if I'm feeling overwhelmed.

Clinician: Absolutely. The important thing is not to panic, ever. We will move at your pace, but we will move toward the goals we have set. You will grow and change. You will develop skills, maybe new skills, and you will learn ways to preserve your voice that you may never have used before.

Anna: Because I didn't need them before.

Clinician: Exactly. You need those skills now because you have a problem you may not have had before. Our objective is for your voice to improve, Anna.

Anna: It'll be better.

Clinician: That's what we are after. You will work hard, and together we will achieve all the improvement we can.

Anna knows she will work hard to achieve the growth embodied in the goals she has set with her clinician. This challenge is balanced. It will not be too easy or boring. It will not be too hard or overwhelming. Continual monitoring and appropriate adjustments throughout therapy will ensure this balance.

Achieving Ownership

Anna has now connected with her treatment goals in two ways. She possesses a powerful sense of purpose and a powerful commitment to growth. One more motivational connection needs to be made. Anna needs to own the process, make it truly hers. The solution-focused approach emphasizes this critical connection. A goal can never be imposed or forced upon your clients. You work with your clients to make sure they have adopted the goals as their own. This is, in fact, their therapy, their journey, their mission.

Anna: So, what do I have to do first?

Clinician: First, we have to choose what's most important to you.

Anna: Obviously, what's important is getting my voice back.

Clinician: Yes, we can accomplish that faster if we modify your voice use for a short time. Will you be able to do that?

Anna: I'm a teacher. I have to teach.

Clinician: Right. We have to come up with a plan that meets your needs as a teacher.

Anna: What I need is the ability to teach my classes every day, but I can find times in my day to rest my voice.

Clinician: That's a good start. Now we are beginning to formulate goals that you can buy into, goals you can make your own.

Anna: Yes, I see what you mean. These are going to be my goals. They have to fit into my life.

Clinician: Right. You will own them. They'll be your goals, your choices.

When you are making the ownership connection, use ownership words like some of those in the dialogue above: *own, choose, choice, buy into, make your own.* Get agreement early on to pursue growth as a team, and check the ownership connection regularly throughout therapy. Listen for statements that may indicate that the connection is being disrupted, like "this doesn't seem/feel right to me," "it just isn't me," "I don't feel

Identifying Client Emotions

- Determine which of the four quadrants of the CI Matrix your clients occupy. Is the negative impact of their disorder high or low? Are they willing or unwilling to engage in the work necessary to change?
- Make the purpose connection by helping clients see how worthwhile it is for them to achieve their goals.
- Make the growth connection by clarifying the challenges your clients will meet in pursuing their goals. They will commit to the change.
- Make the ownership connection by assuring clients that the goals are truly theirs rather than imposed upon them. They always have choices.
- Monitor all these steps on a continuing basis and adapt your counseling activity to respond assertively when potentially detrimental changes occur. Emotions can hinder progress in therapy, and counseling can address the encumbrance once it is recognized.

like I have a choice here." Encourage your clients to address ownership issues, and listen when they do.

Steps to Determine Emotions

The steps to determining the emotions present in your clients are always the same. Generally, it is a good idea to follow these steps in the order listed below and to use the resulting information when adopting your counseling strategies.

Emotions That Hinder Progress

Motivation is a balanced state. That means that your clients can become "unbalanced" motivationally. That happens when something goes wrong with the purpose, growth, or ownership connections. Clients may have too much or too little of an emotion, too much or too little focus on the goal or task. Counseling is often a process of maintaining or reestablishing balance in purpose, growth, or ownership (**Figure 10-4**).

Addressing Apathy and Boredom

Apathy is literally a lack of feeling or emotion. When your clients become apathetic, they are getting out of balance in the purpose connection. If purpose signifies that the goal or task is worthwhile, apathy is the sense that the goal or task is worthless, not worthwhile. When this happens, as the word *apathy* implies, clients get deenergized, less willing to make an effort. There may be a lot of shrugging, sighing, and excuse making. They might procrastinate, fail to practice when they should, tune out during sessions, or do all of these.

Boredom can look exactly like apathy and result in all the same behaviors, but boredom denotes a lack of balance in the growth connection, so it has a cause different from apathy's. When you notice the symptoms, try to discover the cause. Is it boredom? If so, the clients are growing too slowly; the work is too easy. Is it apathy? If so, your clients are questioning the point of what it is they are doing.

Apathy: A lack of interest and enthusiasm caused by a sense that an activity has little or no purpose. Apathy leads to a loss of energy and poor motivation.

Boredom. A lack of desire to perform an activity because it is not challenging, is perceived as too easy.

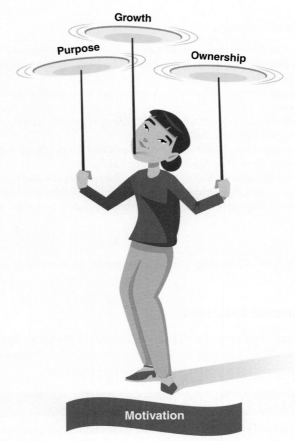

FIGURE 10-4 Motivational Balance. Purpose, growth, and ownership must be balanced to maintain motivation.

Clinician: Anna, we have been progressing nicely up until now. But in the past couple of sessions, you have seemed listless. Now you tell me you didn't have time to do your daily exercises. You seem to be lacking the enthusiasm you've had in the past.

Anna: Well, we haven't changed the exercises for a couple of sessions. I think I'm very good at them now; doing them is a drudge, frankly.

The clinician has reason to believe the issue is boredom.

Clinician: Are you bored? Would you like more of a challenge?

Anna: Yes.

Clinician: So, you're still committed to the goals.

Anna: Definitely. I think we can progress faster, that's all.

Clinician: OK. Let's figure out how we can increase the pace and difficulty, get you charged up again.

The clinician hit on the problem. In our terminology, Anna is out of balance on the growth connection. She needs the opportunity to grow more quickly. You may address Anna's lack of energy by requiring accuracy at a particular level of competence before having your her proceed to the next level. A guideline like this is an acknowledgment of the need to balance the growth connection. Anna and her clinician will have to figure out how to move more quickly from level to level or add more variety within each level.

Anna's lack of enthusiasm, however, may not be a result of boredom. Her behaviors may be pointing to a more difficult condition, a lack of emotion. This is called apathy.

Clinician: Anna, we have been progressing nicely up until now. But in the past couple of sessions, you have seemed listless. Now you tell me you didn't have time to do your daily exercises. You seem to be lacking the enthusiasm you've had in the past.

Anna: Frankly, I don't see the point. These exercises just seem silly, and I don't see how they are going to make my voice last longer when I'm teaching.

The clinician now suspects the issue is apathy, a problem with the purpose connection.

Clinician: You don't see the connection between these exercises and our longer-term goals.

Anna: No. I don't.

Clinician: Would it help if we went over the steps from this exercise to the goal? There are about four intermediate exercises and this one is the first. We did discuss these at the outset, but I am happy to review them again, if you want.

At this point Anna might agree to review the steps, and that review might resolve the issue and restore Anna's motivation. If Anna still balks, the clinician must be prepared to dig deeper and question the process as it has been set up. It is very important to reestablish the purpose connection, even if a change of direction is required. If Anna does not believe what she is doing is worthwhile, success in therapy will be put at risk.

A graver situation arises when clients start to question the value of therapy itself. This can result in apathy at its deepest level. The loss of purpose in therapy is devastating, so you want to address the very first signs of it. Review the long-term goal or goals on a continual basis. Check to make sure, explicitly, that your clients are still enthused about their goals, still believe the goals are worth striving for.

Addressing Resistance

Apathy and boredom show themselves in a lack of energy, a lessening of involvement, withdrawing, or tiring. Resistance is more active. Resisting clients exhibit opposition and pushback when you try to gain their cooperation. Resistance has intensity. The motivation model can help pinpoint the reason for the resistance, but you should look at some other possible causes before you consider the model.

Once you have eliminated lack of clarity, lack of a sense of progress, and outside causes, look for motivational imbalance. Three of the most common (Tellis, Barone, &

> Resistance: Opposition and pushback when cooperation is sought. Resistance has intensity and focus.

Some Causes of Resistance

- Sometimes clients get confused or forget aspects of what therapy is trying to accomplish, and they express resistance because of that lack of clarity. Make sure goals and processes are clear.
- Resistance can be the result of a lack of encouraging signs of positive results. Make sure clients know how they are doing, that they are making progress.
- Sometimes resistance has nothing to do with what is happening in therapy; it is coming from a crisis in a totally different area. Check occurrences in clients' lives that may be impinging on their ability to focus or spend time on their goals.

Barone, 2014) sources of resistance are (1) being obsessed, (2) being overwhelmed, and (3) being frustrated (**Figure 10-5**).

Being obsessed with improvement may seem a positive thing, but it must be perceived as a form of resistance. Ibrahim, a 12-year-old middle school student, is a highly willing client working on the correction of a speech disorder that involves several different types of exercises. His clinician has begun to notice an excessive intensity in the way Ibrahim is going about performing his regimen of exercises.

Clinician: So, in the past two weeks, you have been practicing tongue placement on all the sounds? All of these?

Ibrahim: Yes. I work at them constantly.

Clinician: I thought our understanding was that you would start with tongue placement only on /s/ and /z/. We haven't even addressed some of your other sound issues.

Ibrahim: I know, but this is everything in the world to me. I don't think of anything else. I just want to improve.

Clinician: I can see that you are dedicated, but you have other important things in your life: homework, soccer…

Ibrahim: I'm thinking of quitting soccer. This really is taking up all my time.

Clinician: Ibrahim, you love soccer.

Ibrahim: It doesn't matter. I'm completely committed to my therapy.

Clinician: Let's discuss what that commitment means. I think it means incorporating therapy into your total life, not replacing your life with therapy.

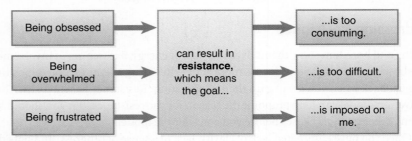

FIGURE 10-5 Reasons for Resistance. There are three possible emotional states that result in resistance. Assessment of the goal is needed to minimize resistance.

Ibrahim: Why shouldn't I?

Clinician: Because we will be integrating your improved speech into your everyday life, and I want you to have an everyday life. Also, my experience tells me that when you go at this practice with this level of intensity, you run the risk of burning out and giving up.

Although it is most often the case that the more one practices the better the production, situations like Ibrahim's do exist. The clinician must get Ibrahim to agree to moderate his regimen of practice so that he also has time to enjoy other aspects of his life. You should be on the alert for signs of this kind of obsession. As soon as you begin to address it, you may likely detect the pushback that signals resistance, not cooperation. Work with clients on a regimen that is acceptable to them. Have clients create a practice schedule and make sure to include time for other activities.

A common form of obsession can come, not from your clients, but from client advocates, parents or spouses, perhaps, who go all out and put undue pressure on clients with no letup. You may hear about this from clients themselves, or you may observe it directly. If you suspect obsession from someone in the clients' Circle of Power, investigate it, and, if appropriate, discuss the issue with the advocate. Your objective is to get the advocate to ease up and to validate a more restrained approach to therapy and practice. Provide advocates with time frames for practice: "This week, spend five to ten minutes a day working on Jane's /r/ words. The rest of the day I don't want you to mention it to her again. This plan will give Jane the practice she needs but will not overwhelm her with constant reminders. I think she'll work harder during those practice times. Let's try it for this week. I definitely want to hear how it worked out when I see you next week."

Resistance may be caused by the fact that clients have become overwhelmed. They are trying to accomplish too much in too short a space of time. Two ways of being overwhelmed can present themselves: (1) clients may not have the skills yet to engage in a specific exercise or practice, or (2) clients may be trying to do too many things at once. If lack of skill is the problem, the solution is to backtrack and hone the relevant skills and competencies before assigning the exercise or practice. If clients are being asked to do too much, you should find ways to trim your expectations. Do this in dialogue with clients, and approach the change as a redefinition of goals.

Being overwhelmed can result from lack of skill or lack of time, but being frustrated comes from a lack of control. You know that ownership is central to motivation and to the solution-focused approach. The sense that ownership is slipping away is the sense of frustration. Clients feel backed into a corner, stripped of options, forced into whatever they are being asked to do. Resistance is expressed as a loss of personal power. Listen for statements depicting that loss.

"I don't feel like this is my goal, that this goal is mine anymore."

"I've lost control…"

"So, I don't have a choice, right?"

"I'm just so helpless."

"I feel like you're making me do this."

Increasing the Sense of Ownership

- Restore choice, the conviction that your clients have options.
- Emphasize that this is their process and these are their goals.
- Brainstorm their options to show explicitly what their choices are.
- Identify what they think is "forcing" them, even if it is something you are doing; plan to remove those elements.

If you worked with your clients to establish the ownership connection, you have an advantage when they experience frustration. You have the language to discuss their resistance and to reempower them. You want their frustration to decrease and ownership to increase.

One of the least pleasant aspects of being frustrated and being overwhelmed is the potential for clients to exhibit sudden high emotion, such as crying or losing their temper. You may be among the minority of clinicians who do not experience discomfort at outbursts of emotion from clients, but you should always be prepared to effectively manage high emotion. A good idea is to have a number of strategies at hand for dealing with these charged situations so you yourself do not become frustrated or overwhelmed.

Of the strategies listed here, make sure you select ones that fit your own temperament and personality. The emotion of your client is already a source of uneasiness; employing an unsuitable technique for dealing with the emotion could lead to real distress and undesirable outcomes.

When clients get emotional, that is a strong signal to you to stay calm. In many cases mirroring clients' attitude is a good tactic, but in these instances mirroring is usually counterproductive because it is rarely a good idea to increase the sum total of emotion being displayed. Allow clients some room to "vent" their feelings. Tears may be involved, so have a box of tissues handy.

Let clients tell you what is bothering them; listen. Do not simply say, "Calm down." Use the "attending behaviors," such as maintaining eye contact, leaning forward, and adopting an open, relaxed posture. Provide an empathetic response such as, "This really upsets you, doesn't it?" or "That makes you very angry" to reflect clients' emotions and let them know you consider what they are feeling and why they are feeling it.

Listen, too, for the informational content accompanying the emotion. Perhaps the client is overwhelmed with many emotions and the reason why she is crying is because she is finally facing the reality of the situation. An advocate may exhibit high emotion and share that he somehow feels responsible for his daughter's communication disorder. A client's anger could also signal a difficult week dealing with her hearing loss in a communication situation the client had not encountered previously. Gather the relevant information from these moments of high emotion. You may not use the information immediately, but it may be useful in a future session to probe feelings about these situations or issues, demonstrate clients' ability to cope with deficits and difficulties, or even provide an example of how therapy has improved issues that previously caused high emotion.

Akiko: [*Crying.*] My daughter did not stutter when she was very young. I think it happened when I would correct her pronunciation. Pronouncing words correctly was always very important to me. I am to blame for her stuttering.

Clinician: You feel responsible for Hikaru's stuttering?

Akiko: Yes.

Clinician: You know, a great deal of study has been done on this, Akiko. I can tell you there is no evidence that your daughter's stuttering was brought on by having her pronounce words correctly.

The clinician reflects Akiko's emotion and her apparent reason for it. In the real world, this portion of the conversation may go on for a while. Throughout the exchange, the clinician should maintain open, engaged body language, good eye contact, and a positive demeanor. The clinician should avoid folded arms, crossed legs, or downcast eyes. When Akiko is able to receive the counter evidence, the clinician gently informs her of data that can correct her misperception.

Clients may be frustrated and overwhelmed at the pace or difficulty of the exercises they are assigned. In that case, an outburst of anger may result. Again, you should listen, reflect their feeling with empathy, and allow for the emotion to take its course. When clients calm down enough to hear you, make very clear that you are open to altering goals and changing the pace as well as the exercises.

On those occasions when clients become too distraught or angry, you may have to cut the session short. This occurrence is rare, but you should be prepared for it. Avoid negative statements like, "You're in no condition to proceed…" or "I don't think it's a good idea to continue." These statements might exacerbate the emotion or lead to self-blaming. Prefer a more positive phrasing, like, "Let's start fresh next session…" or "I think we should discuss this when you are feeling up to it." The clinic is a safe space. Emotion is acceptable. No one is to blame. You can always continue at a later time. Make sure that clients are able to compose themselves before they leave.

On very infrequent occasions, a client will get so emotional that you are best advised to stop immediately. The client might threaten you or make a threatening move. In these extreme circumstances no effective counseling strategies are available. You will have to take steps to secure the client's safety or your own safety. Your action depends on a number of factors: the age and size of a client, the type of intense emotion being displayed, your level of training in dealing with these crises, and your previous history with a particular client. You might leave the room or call for assistance. Events like these are quite extraordinary, but they are not unheard of. In some settings, written guidelines or protocols are in effect to address these situations, and you should of course follow these when applicable.

Except for the most extreme situations, you will find that high or sudden emotion is a challenge like others you face. It requires effective counseling techniques and a willingness to endure the discomfort. You need patience, calmness, and, of course, empathy. Many clinicians report accelerated progress after a difficult emotional event has been handled successfully.

Discouragement:
Loss of heart,
a dwindling of
passion and desire.
It is marked by
a general lack
of energy and
enthusiasm about
progressing in
therapy, similar
to the symptoms
of apathy and
boredom but
displaying a
noticeable sadness,
a sense not that it is
worthless to achieve
the goal but that it is
useless to try.

Addressing Discouragement

Along the way, you may avert boredom and resistance, deal with strong emotions, yet still confront the specter of discouragement. The Latin root of the word *discouragement* is "heart." Discouraged clients have lost heart; their innermost passion and desire have dwindled, at least temporarily. Your task in this situation is to encourage, to "en-hearten" your clients. Discouragement is something many clients face at one point or another in therapy. Sometimes discouragement can be a transient emotion, but you should be aware that discouragement can be an effect of depression.

Discouragement is marked by a general lack of energy and enthusiasm about progressing in therapy, similar to the symptoms of apathy and boredom. Discouraged clients, however, give evidence of a noticeable sadness, a sense not that it is worthless to achieve the goal but that it is useless to try. This impulse is the urge to give up, and clients succumb to it for a variety of reasons, from depression to more specific grounds—being too old to change now, not being supported by family, or always failing no matter how hard they try.

When clients are discouraged, they sometimes respond to the same techniques and strategies that are effective when they are frustrated, overwhelmed, apathetic, or bored. Look to these strategies for ways to address discouragement. Often, though, discouraged clients suffer a form of ego impedance where clients' self-concept dooms them to failure. They feel that it is just not in them to succeed in therapy. If this feeling turns into a conviction, clients cannot progress because they will not progress. Their responses to your efforts will be a shrug or an expression of self-pity. They may tell you to stop wasting your time. You can try a number of steps to remove this ego impedance, and you should avoid measures that could be detrimental.

The way back from discouragement may be long and slow, or clients may just "snap out of it." Some clients regress into discouragement more than once during therapy. Your task is to help them recover their "heart," the perception that they are indeed the kind of person who can and will achieve the goals they and you have set.

Steps to Avoid with Discouraged Clients

- Avoid reverting to slogans, telling them, "Don't worry, be happy," or "It's always darkest before the dawn." Discouraged clients tend to be cynical about such bromides, which rarely have a positive effect.
- Avoid cheerleading, saying things like, "I know you can do it," if that has not been working. They do not believe you, and repeating it does not make it more believable.
- Avoid the impulse to tell them they are wrong to feel discouraged. They don't feel wrong right now, and you have to take that position as your starting point.
- Avoid telling clients it is all up to them. This assertion is not empowering, because discouraged clients already feel alone.
- Avoid scolding clients for feeling sorry for themselves. They will probably agree that they deserve scolding and feel worse as a result.

Measures to Try with Discouraged Clients

- Put the stress on what you know they accept: that the goal is worthwhile, that they have made progress, that the exercises will lead to goal attainment, and so forth.
- Make sure they know you believe in them, no matter what. You should say, "I have faith in you," rather than, "I know you can do it."
- Keep them aware that members of their Circle of Power are rooting for them; they are not alone.
- Stay in touch with clients' Circle of Power and seek their help in looking for positive indicators.
- Maintain the dialogue about how it felt when they were making progress, and discuss how they think they might get that feeling back. Keep looking for the spark of motivation.

Addressing Denial

Discouragement is the feeling that the problem or disorder is so cataclysmic that there is no use trying to improve. Denial seems to occupy a point at the other end of the spectrum from discouragement. Clients in denial often appear to be quite casual about the problem they are facing. After all, the problem is not really there!

The function of denial is to avoid facing a problem or issue by pretending and even thinking it is not real. As the first of the stages of grief, denial can be useful in coping with a trauma when a person needs time to process and accept what has happened, but it is not a long-term solution to a problem that requires correction.

Clients in denial often occupy Q2 on the CI Matrix, high impact on quality of life and a low willingness to change, although they often do not admit the impact on their quality of life. Rational emotive behavior therapy (REBT) is an approach that focuses on addressing and changing irrational thinking, and denial clearly falls into the category of irrational beliefs. REBT posits three steps to getting clients in denial on track. (1) Clients must be able to observe that their evaluations are irrational and are harmful to them. (2) They must become convinced that they are capable of thinking differently. (3) They must use REBT strategies to make progress in changing their thinking in a more rational direction.

One of the most difficult obstacles clients in denial face is their ability to see that their beliefs are irrational. Sometimes a seemingly insurmountable task, your job is to help clients see that their evaluation of themselves is unreasonable and ultimately harmful to them and their quality of life. To create this change in thinking, you can try a number of techniques. Begin by defining the terms *rational* and *irrational*. Always ask clients to identify their beliefs about their situation and categorize each belief as one or the other.

Ask clients what they are afraid of when discussing their disorder or issue. Suggest that they be totally honest. Provide a comfortable environment to allow clients to express their fears and emotions openly. Have clients enumerate the things that will happen if they take no action on dealing with the irrational belief. If they say that nothing will happen, accept that as an answer and have them attempt to brainstorm other possible answers. Use members of your client's Circle of Power to deal with denial.

Sometimes group therapy can be used to help them see different ways of thinking about communication disorders.

After a stroke or other trauma, clients might experience anosognosia, a condition of physiological origin that often sounds like denial (Heilman, 1991). Because anosognosia may be a symptom of brain damage, counseling will have a limited effect. Coordinate with the medical and psychiatric team working with these clients; do not be surprised if the clients seem unaware of their communication disorder. Your main focus with them is to help them increase their awareness of the existence and nature of their communication disorder. This awareness may be the first step in treatment.

Forms of denial other than anosognosia are more amenable to the approaches recommended. If clients in denial are in Q2 of the CI Matrix, your task is to move them toward Q1. That means making them more fully aware of the negative impact of their disorder on their quality of life. Even if they remain skeptical, you have made progress if they admit that you "may have a point" or they "will give therapy a try." If you have an opportunity to help them make observable progress, they may move out of denial and into a more realistic perspective on their situation.

Other Factors That Hinder Progress

Bullying

As we have discussed in the previous section, emotions can be triggered by many experiences. In some cases, a specific experience evokes particular emotions, but it is not always an emotion that directly hinders progress in therapy. The experience itself can be the overwhelming deterring obstacle. Bullying is one of these experiences. Clients with communication disorders are often targets of bullying because they sound, talk, act, understand, and hear differently.

The U.S. government defines bullying as "unwanted, aggressive behavior among school aged children that involves a real or perceived power imbalance." The behavior may be repeated day after day and can involve such intimidating behavior as "making threats, spreading rumors, attacking someone physically or verbally, and excluding someone from a group on purpose" (U.S. Department of Health and Human Services, 2015).

Bullying is one of the worst cases of adversarial behavior. Bullies can thwart your efforts and waylay the carefully constructed plans you have made for improvement. With school-age clients, you will want to ascertain whether any level of bullying is going on, what effects it is having on your clients, and how you can get the bullying to stop.

Researchers typically look at bullying from three perspectives, that of the bully, the victim, and the bystander or witness (Cheng, Chen, Liu, & Chen, 2011). The types of bullying usually fall into four categories. *Physical* bullying is the use of force to intimidate or to get a victim to do the bully's bidding. *Verbal* bullying uses words to put down, shame, threaten, and ostracize. *Relational* bullying attempts to damage the victim's self-esteem, relationships, or social life by, for example, excluding the victim from events or spreading vicious rumors about the victim's alleged conduct in specific settings. *Cyberbullying*, a more recent form, is the use of social media to do all the things bullies do.

Bullying:
Unwanted, aggressive behavior that involves a real or perceived power imbalance. The behavior may be repeated day after day and can involve such intimidating behavior as making threats, spreading rumors, attacking someone physically or verbally, and excluding someone from a group on purpose.

Detecting bullying is not always easy. Most counseling educators recommend open-ended discussions that look for signs that bullying is happening. You will want to work with your Circle of Power, the allies around your clients, to find out whether clients are experiencing bullying. Parents, of course, are a key resource, and you should not hesitate to contact them if you suspect bullying.

An excellent time to get a read on this issue is at the beginning of sessions. Ask open-ended questions. "What is it like on the school bus?" "How are things between classes or during lunch?" "When other kids mention your [disorder], what do they say?" "How does this make you feel?" Probe with a view to uncovering signs of bullying.

If your suspicions are aroused, get more specific. "What does Jonette say to you that makes you feel bad?" "What do they put on Instagram?" Always ask, "How often does this happen?" "When does it happen?" "How do you feel when this is happening?" Obviously, be on the lookout for signs of physical threat or endangerment, which must be met with swift action to secure the safety of your clients.

If you find that bullying is going on, counseling is almost certainly indicated. Rational emotive behavior therapy, the cognitive behavioral therapy approach, was mentioned earlier in reference to the issue of denial. Some psychologists find CBT well suited to helping bullying victims (Lohmann, Taylor, & Kilpatrick, 2013). CBT examines the connection between the negative thoughts and feelings engendered by bullying and the sometimes detrimental behavior victims can exhibit.

CBT moves clients away from illogical and harmful thoughts that can stem from being bullied and toward rational and empowering notions that result in healthy, helpful behaviors—such as achieving the goals you set in therapy.

Murphy, Quesal, Reardon-Reeves, and Yaruss (2013) provide helpful strategies in their program to minimize bullying in children who stutter. Many of aspects of their program can be applied to any type of bullying related to communication disorders. The basic framework of their approach consists of four steps:

Step 1: Get the facts. Know the facts about the communication disorder and aspects of the disorder that are targets of bullying. These facts teach clients that the disorder and the bullying are not their fault, bullying should never be accepted as the right course of action, and clients can take actions to stop bullying.

Step 2: Give the facts. In this step, clients are encouraged to acknowledge to bullies that clients know they in fact have a communication disorder: "Yes, you're right, I do stutter." And then they can educate bullies on the communication disorder: "Let me tell you about stuttering" or " I can show you how to stutter."

Step 3: Help yourself. Clients in this step are advised to keep trying different strategies to stop the bullying and to always remember that they are in charge, not the bully. Clients should feel ownership of the choices they make to help themselves deal with and stop the bullying.

Step 4: You are not alone and you can do it. Clients' Circle of Power, including family, friends, teachers, and other advocates, should work to provide a safe network for the clients so that clients do not feel alone against bullying. Clients should also seek out others who will be helpful and provide support.

Practices That Are Not Helpful in Dealing with Bullying

- Do not look for the "upside" of bullying by suggesting that the bully can motivate your client to improve so as to "remove the cause" of the bullying. This is just a form of blaming the victim and is potentially damaging.
- Do not advise a physical response to the bully.
- Do not work directly or independently on the bullying. It is inappropriate for you to contact bullies, their teachers, or their parents. Use the Circle of Power.
- Do not assume that the bullying has stopped just because the client is no longer mentioning it or is seemingly casual about it.

In summary, when working with clients be on the lookout for signs that bullying is taking place. Once you detect bullying, address it immediately. Collaborate with parents and other authority figures to make the issue visible and see that it is taken seriously and addressed. Every effort should be expended to get the bullying to cease. Keep updated on the effects of bullying, how severe it is, and how effectively your client is dealing with it. This awareness helps you choose the best counseling strategies.

Facing Crisis

If you are a clinician in a nursing home, hospital, or other medical facility, you will work with clients who are facing serious, even life-threatening challenges. These challenges can include surgery affecting the vocal mechanism or auditory system, dementia, brain injury, trauma, and, finally, the approach of life's end. In these severe circumstances you may be called upon to counsel clients and their advocates, family members, and others close to them. The clients' capacity to improve may be greatly impaired, and their emotional states may vary significantly within and between sessions. You may be daunted as you try to maintain empathy without becoming despondent.

Take advantage of your clients' network of support, which may include clinical staff, psychologists, physical therapists, home nurses, hospice, and other caretakers. As much as feasible coordinate your planning with them and stay in communication so you can update your knowledge of what is happening to the clients and develop ideas to make therapy as useful as it can be. Your counseling challenges with your clients and their Circle of Power will differ greatly depending on the age of your clients, onset of the disorder, or progression of the disorder.

Catastrophic Loss

Catastrophic loss: A devastating life change due to physical or cognitive damage to oneself or a loved one.

Clients who have suffered a catastrophic loss have experienced a devastating life change. Examples include individuals who have had complete or partial laryngectomies, global cerebral vascular accidents, lung or esophageal surgery, transition to late-stage dementia, diagnosis of a progressive neurological disorder, deafness, or events of similar gravity. When you enter into the therapy process with such clients, you gather information, listen, set goals, plan, and counsel as advised throughout this book.

Those common aspects of therapy are often appropriate in instances of catastrophic loss. What is different is the gravity of your clients' overall state and the implications of that difference. Listed below are some of the conditions you should anticipate in the case of clients who have suffered catastrophic loss. Not all of these are true of all clients in this category, but they are common enough to merit mention.

- Clients may be depressed or unmotivated, especially soon after the loss.
- Clients will usually have a network of professionals playing various roles in recuperation or amelioration.
- Clients may have serious limitations in possible improvement or recovery.
- Clients may have diminished capacity to communicate or understand.
- Clients will usually be contending with difficulties or medical conditions over and above the communication disorder you are treating.

Techniques and strategies have already been proposed for creating motivational balance and responding to loss of enthusiasm. The stages of grief are also relevant, because these clients may be the ones most likely to pass through the stages. With clients suffering great loss, you may be called upon to exercise considerable patience and perhaps to allot more time than usual to counseling. Although you and your clients seek improvement where possible, your goals must be realistic and responsive to change as the clients' condition changes.

Some conditions, such as dementia, are progressive and worsen with time. As your clients' abilities diminish, their goals change. In cases like these, your task may be to slow down the decline in quality of life rather than improve quality of life. This objective is every bit as worthy as the restoration of a function or ability.

In some clinical settings you coordinate with other caregivers in your clients' life. You may be required to cooperate formally with reports or periodic meetings. These formal responsibilities are serious obligations; meet them conscientiously and fully. Even if you have few of these requirements, make use of the insight of other caregivers by keeping open lines of communication, welcoming advice, and, when possible, adjusting the schedule of sessions to give clients the optimum overall treatment experience.

End of Life

The ultimate loss, of course, is the loss of life itself. You are in a profession that has a role with clients at every point in life, from very early days to the final days. You may treat clients with a relatively minor hearing or speech-language disorder. You may treat clients desirous of communicating with loved ones during their last hours on earth.

These clients may be in a special care unit of a medical center, in their nursing home, or in their private home with family and friends nearby. Nurses, doctors, clergy, and hospice may be in attendance. Medications are usually involved, and these may be powerful and may affect your interactions with these clients. You are their speech-language pathologist or their audiologist, and as such you are helping them with their communication disorder.

You are, however, more than that. You are part of your clients' end-of-life process. You are gently, patiently, and professionally helping them in their preparations for that passage. They have things to say and hear, moments to pass in communication with those dear to them. You may be their ultimate link with the world they are leaving. You may provide them with assistive technology to express their wants and needs. Your job is difficult and probably stressful, but it is important to your clients and those around them. Do that job with courage, caring, and compassion.

The topic of this chapter is "creating the preferred future." You now see that the preferred future can encompass the restoration of a speaking voice in an elementary school teacher and the passing of a patient's final days in communication with loved ones. The future you and your clients imagine is one that your clients find purposeful, one that challenges them to grow, one they can possess and call their own. The counseling you do on the road to that future removes obstacles that otherwise would overwhelm. Your counseling breaks through the insecurities, disappointments, and discouragements your clients experience so they can stand strong and continue the journey to a future they and you have found worth all the time and all the effort.

Review of Key Points

- To create the preferred future, your clients need motivation. You and your clients must address emotions that can stand in the way of success; effective counseling can manage those emotions.
- Clients often move through five stages or attitudes toward their condition: denial, anger, bargaining, depression, and acceptance.
- A major reason to counsel is to create and sustain the motivation to succeed and to achieve the therapy goals. Motivation creates enthusiasm and energy, the willingness to spend time working on the goals, and connects your clients with their goals in a focused manner.
- It is not enough to have a goal. The goal must become a purpose; it must be seen as worthwhile, that is, worth the investment of time and hard work to achieve it. A purpose is a reason to act, an explanation of why a particular goal is important or meaningful.
- Change is a critical component of the therapy process. Therapy is literally senseless without it. Clients are committing to growth, improvement. They are not just becoming different in some way, they are becoming better in some way.
- As soon as you use the purpose connection to clarify the importance of the goal, you should use the growth connection to clarify the challenge of achieving the goal.
- Clients need to own the process, make it truly theirs. The solution-focused approach emphasizes this critical connection.
- The steps to determining the emotions present in your clients are always the same. Generally, it is a good idea to follow these steps in order and to use the resulting information when adopting your counseling strategies. Monitor all these steps on a continuing basis and adapt your counseling activity to respond assertively when potentially detrimental changes occur. Emotions can hinder progress in therapy, and counseling can address the encumbrance.
- Your clients can become "unbalanced" motivationally when something goes wrong with the purpose, growth, or ownership connections. Counseling is often a process of maintaining or reestablishing balance in purpose, growth, or ownership.
- When your clients become apathetic, they are out of balance in the purpose connection. Apathy is the sense that the goal or task is worthless, not worthwhile. Clients get deenergized, less willing to make an effort.
- Boredom can look like apathy and result in all the same behaviors, but boredom denotes a lack of balance in the growth connection, so it has a different cause from apathy. If clients are bored, they are growing too slowly; the work is too easy.
- Resistance is more active than apathy or boredom. Resisting clients exhibit opposition and pushback when you try to gain their cooperation. Resistance has intensity. The motivation model can help pinpoint the reason for the resistance, but you should look at some other possible causes before you consider the model.

- Resistance can be caused by a number of things: unclear goals and processes, lack of information about the progress they are making, a lack of encouraging signs of positive results, or occurrences in their clients' lives that may be impinging on their ability to focus or spend time on their goals. Three common sources of resistance are (1) being obsessed, (2) being overwhelmed, and (3) being frustrated.
- If you worked with your clients to establish the ownership connection, you will have the language to discuss their resistance and to reempower them. You want their frustration to decrease and ownership to increase.
- Sudden high emotion, such as crying or losing their temper, can be difficult to manage effectively. Have a number of strategies at hand for dealing with these charged situations. Make sure you select ones that fit your own temperament and personality.
- When clients get emotional, stay calm. Allow clients some room to "vent" their feelings. Let clients tell you what is bothering them. Use attending behaviors. Calmly presenting relevant data may be effective, provided the client is in a condition to take it in.
- Discouragement is marked by a general lack of energy and enthusiasm coupled with a noticeable sadness, a sense that it is useless to try. This impulse is the urge to give up.
- With discouraged clients, avoid sloganeering and saying, "I know you can do it." Don't tell them they are wrong. Don't tell them it is all up to them. Don't scold. Stress what you know they accept, and make sure they know you believe in them. Keep them aware that their Circle of Power is rooting for them; they are not alone. Maintain the dialogue about how it felt when they were making progress. Keep looking for the spark of motivation.
- In severe circumstances you may be called upon to counsel clients and their advocates, family members, and those close to them. The clients' capacity to improve may be greatly impaired, and their emotional states may vary significantly. Take advantage of your clients' network of support, coordinate your planning with them, and stay in communication.
- The four different types of bullying, physical, verbal, relational, and cyberbullying, often create unforeseen obstacles in therapy and should be addressed accordingly. Follow the steps provided and enlist the appropriate allies to help your clients.
- Clients who have suffered a catastrophic loss may be depressed or unmotivated but will usually have a network of professionals playing a role in recuperation or amelioration. They may have serious limitations in possible improvement or recovery and may have diminished capacity to communicate or understand. They will usually have difficulties or medical conditions beyond the speech-language or hearing disorders you are treating.

- You may treat clients desirous of communicating with loved ones during their last hours on earth. You are part of your clients' end-of-life process. You are gently, patiently, and professionally helping them in their preparations for that passage. Your job is difficult and probably stressful, but it is important to your clients and those around them. Do that job with courage, caring, and compassion.

Practical Exercises

For this assignment, read each scenario and determine which stage of grief best fits each client, which stage best fits each client's caregiver, and explain why you chose those stages. Identify three emotions each individual is likely to exhibit.

1. John is a 33-year-old man who recently suffered a left-hemisphere stroke, which resulted in focal damage to Broca's area, significantly hindering his expressive language and ability to find his words. He often gets frustrated when trying to communicate and is beginning to demonstrate aggressive behaviors when he is frustrated. John's wife, Emily, pleaded with John's speech-language pathologist and told her that she would give anything to help her husband get better.

2. Juliette, a 9-year-old girl, has started isolating herself at school and frequently cries when asked to read aloud to her class. When her teacher asked her what was wrong, Juliette reported that she is very sad because her peers have started calling her "J-J-J-Juliette" because of her "bumpy" speech, and it makes her not want to talk at school. Juliette's teacher contacted her father, Jason, to discuss the possibility of a speech-language evaluation to assess the severity of her stuttering. He refused the evaluation and told the teacher that Juliette is fine and does not stutter.

3. Eleanor is a 77-year-old woman who was diagnosed with amyotrophic lateral sclerosis (ALS) 2 years ago. Eleanor communicates minimally using an augmentative and alternative communication (AAC) device that is activated by her eye movements. When her medical team recommended her family begin the process of transferring her to hospice care, they protested, insisting that their mother had much more time to live. Using her AAC device, Eleanor indicated that she was "ready."

REFERENCES

Bonanno, G. (2010). *The other side of sadness: What the new science of bereavement tells us about life after a loss.* New York, NY: Basic Books.

Cheng, Y., Chen, L., Liu, K., & Chen, Y. (2011). Development and psychometric evaluation of the school bullying scales: A Rasch measurement approach. *Educational and Psychological Measurement, 71*(1), 200–216.

Heilman, K. M. (1991). Anosognosia: Possible neuropsychological mechanisms. In G. P. Prigatano & D. L. Schacter (Eds.), *Awareness of deficit after brain injury: Clinical and theoretical issues* (pp. 53–55). Oxford, England: Oxford University Press.

Konigsberg, R. D. (2011). *The truth about grief: The myth of its five stages and the new science of loss.* New York, NY: Simon & Schuster.

Kübler-Ross, E. (1969). *On death and dying.* New York, NY: Macmillan.

Lohmann, R. C., Taylor, J. V., & Kilpatrick, H. (2013). *The bullying workbook for teens: Activities to help you deal with social aggression and cyberbullying.* Oakland, CA: New Harbinger Publications.

Murphy, W. P., Quesal, R. W., Reardon-Reeves, N., & Yaruss, J. S. (2013). *Minimizing bullying for children who stutter: A guide for SLPs.* McKinney, TX: Stuttering Therapy Resources.

Tellis, C. M., Barone, N. A., & Barone, O. R. (2014). Counseling. In M. H. Manasco (Ed.), *Introduction to neurogenic communication disorders* (pp. 239–259). Burlington, MA: Jones & Bartlett Learning.

U.S. Department of Health and Human Services. (2015). What is bullying. Retrieved from http://www.stopbullying.gov/what-is-bullying/

CHAPTER 11

Goal Attainment: Tools and Strategies

KEY TERMS

- Deterring forces
- Enhancing forces
- Hunch
- Leverage
- Planning Process Model
- Probes
- Quit option
- Reluctance
- Silence

LEARNING OBJECTIVES

After reading this chapter, you will be able to:

- Define the stages of the Planning Process Model
- Explain how deterring and enhancing forces affect goal attainment
- Describe advanced communication skills

The tale of *The Wizard of Oz* illustrates four important concepts that encompass what a client needs to be successful in therapy and what a speech-language pathologist or audiologist requires to be an effective clinician. These needs are epitomized in the four desires pursued by the main characters. The Scarecrow wanted a brain, just as you, the clinician, need an intelligent procedure that clients can follow to reach their goals. The Tin Man needed a heart, and in the same way your clients need an emotional connection with their goals and with you. The Cowardly Lion desired courage. Clients too require a courageous determination. Dorothy's quest for home is the last of the four, and this quest represents the therapy journey itself. For your client and for you, too, home is the end point of the journey. Home is the goal, the achievement of success; the attainment of what is called the "preferred future."

As a speech-language pathologist or audiologist conducting therapy, your ultimate success depends on two outcomes: (1) the degree to which the goals you set with your clients are achieved and (2) the permanence of the resulting changes in your clients' quality of life related to their communication disorder. These desirable outcomes are a result of a therapy process that could take weeks or months or even years.

Planning Process Model: A seven-step process for formulating and achieving therapy goals.

Reluctance: Hesitancy.

Leverage: In therapy, knowledge of what is important to clients, their desires, wants, and needs, utilized to encourage clients to work through obstacles, roadblocks, and blind spots they may face throughout the therapy process. Leverage gives the clinician the positional advantage.

The beginning of the chapter is devoted to reviewing some now familiar concepts that are incorporated into a Planning Process Model. You will learn to help your clients take action toward their preferred future by explicitly stating their problem, deciding on potential strategies, creating and evaluating goals, and then committing to those goals.

Clients may display resistance or reluctance to moving decisively toward their goals. As their clinician, you help your clients decide to take action by identifying and addressing obstacles to action as well as assessing the forces that help or hinder the process. Elements of the process are depicted in the dialogues presented throughout this text. The dialogues represent clients or members of a client's Circle of Power as they engage in therapy. Each of the clients has a speech, language, or hearing issue that the therapy is addressing.

Basic communication skills such as attending behaviors and restatement can be used to respond to clients during treatment sessions. This chapter explores the more advanced communication skills used in dealing with clients' attitudes and emotions. It addresses how finding leverage and challenging clients appropriately help to overcome roadblocks and maintain progress in therapy.

Although this chapter focuses on the successful completion of therapy, sometimes you or your clients decide that therapy is no longer productive even though your clients' goals have not yet been achieved. Whatever the reasons for this decision, your relationship with your clients will end. If you believe that your clients have reached their potential in therapy, then you will encourage your clients and their Circle of Power to continue to maintain the progress they have made. If your clients decide that they no longer need therapy or are no longer invested in therapy, then you will likely want to keep the door open for them to return if and when they are ready to continue the pursuit of their goals.

If therapy is successful, then, in a sense, therapy does not end. True, no more regularly scheduled sessions will take place; no more goals will be attained in partnership with you. You are no longer in the picture in the same way. Still, clients should be highly motivated to maintain and generalize their gains. The repatterning you and they have accomplished should now be a permanent change. Your clients become their own clinicians.

Action and the Preferred Future: The Planning Process

When you do an initial evaluation, you get the client's story, you set goals, and you make a plan. As therapy progresses you continue to monitor that plan and make adjustments when necessary. In the scenario below, the clinician is noticing that Laura is inconsistent about coming to therapy.

Clinician: Laura, you have only come for three therapy sessions in the past six weeks. I'm wondering why you have missed the last couple of sessions.

Laura: Things are really busy at school right now. I have midterms coming up, and I had two papers due last week.

Clinician: So, you are feeling a little overwhelmed?

Laura: Yes, I guess so.

Clinician: Last session you were having trouble with the exercises we were doing. Remember we were working on producing /r/ in the beginning of words. I sensed you were frustrated at the end of the session, and then when you didn't come back last week...

Laura: No, I wasn't frustrated. I knew this would be difficult. I worked on this a few years ago, but I just didn't feel like my speech pathologist knew what she was doing. Now I need to get this /r/ correct or I'm worried I won't get an internship at the local radio station this summer. No one will hire me if I say my /r/s like this.

On the surface it seems as though Laura is motivated to work on her /r/ because she wants to get her internship. The clinician, however, is also sensing that Laura is resistant to making the changes necessary to produce the /r/ phoneme correctly. The next few sections of this chapter explore a Planning Process Model (**Figure 11-1**). This model can be used at any point in therapy to evaluate your clients and help provide them with an action orientation toward their preferred future.

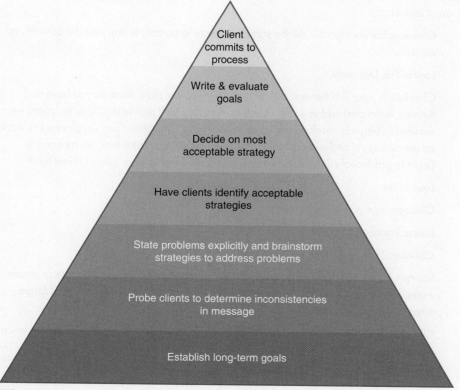

FIGURE 11-1 The Planning Process Model. This model provides guidelines for evaluating and establishing goals to help clients commit to the therapy process and achieve their preferred future.

Identifying the Challenge: Frame the Problem

In the scenario with Laura, the speech-language pathologist should evaluate the present situation and determine whether a new plan needs to be established. Assessing whether the clients still perceive their goals in the same way is the first step in the Planning Process Model.

> **Laura:** No, I wasn't frustrated. I knew this would be difficult. I worked on this a few years ago, but I just didn't feel like my speech pathologist knew what she was doing. Now I need to get this /r/ correct or I'm worried I won't get an internship at the local radio station this summer. No one will hire me if I say my /r/s like this.
>
> **Clinician:** So, your goal is still the same: you want to be able to say your /r/ correctly all the time.
>
> **Laura:** Yes. Definitely.

Probes: Questions or statements clinicians can use to dig deeper into what clients say to clarify clients' intentions or emotions.

Once Laura's long-term goals are confirmed, then the clinician needs to gather more information to determine whether the original plan created to achieve those goals is still acceptable to her. Probing clients to determine the acceptability of the plan is the second step in the Planning Process Model. Probes are questions or statements you can use to dig deeper into what your client is saying to clarify your client's intention or emotion.

> **Clinician:** So, your goal is still the same: you want to be able to say your /r/ correctly all the time.
>
> **Laura:** Yes. Definitely.
>
> **Clinician:** In your first therapy session, we reviewed our plan. Because you have had therapy in the past and you seem to be doing pretty well producing /r/ in isolation, we decided to begin by working on /r/ at the beginning of words. Then we planned to work on producing /r/ at the end of short words. Once you mastered that, we planned to begin to produce /r/ in other word positions. Do you remember talking about that?
>
> **Laura:** Yes.
>
> **Clinician:** Are you still okay with this plan?
>
> **Laura:** I guess so. I mean, yes.
>
> **Clinician:** That doesn't sound convincing.
>
> **Laura:** I just thought it might be easier this time. Sometimes I can get it and it's so simple, especially when you're around. But then other times, when I get home, it's like I forget what I'm supposed to do.
>
> **Clinician:** So, sometimes you have a hard time figuring out how to produce the /r/ when you don't have me to model it for you.
>
> **Laura:** Yes, then I get frustrated with myself and I don't want to practice.
>
> **Clinician:** Maybe we need determine ways for you to have the auditory model accessible to you or make sure you feel comfortable knowing how to make the sound on your own.

Guidelines for Using the Planning Process Model

- Evaluate the current situation for inconsistencies in what the clients say or in their actions.
- Confirm that clients agree with the long-term goals and plans.
- Review the plan with clients.
- Probe clients to determine whether the plan is clear, purposeful, and acceptable.
- Identify challenges or issues.
- State each problem explicitly and confirm accuracy with your clients.
- If there is more than one problem, prioritize by importance. Do not forget to return to the other issues.

After only a few probes the clinician was able to determine at least one of the challenges Laura is facing as well as the need to modify the therapy plan to address this issue. Your clients may have many issues or layers of issues; attacking one at a time is best. Begin with what your clients and you agree is the priority and follow that issue through the Planning Process Model. Do not forget the other roadblocks or concerns your clients may have. The following are some guidelines that may help you during this phase of the Planning Process Model.

Brainstorming Possibilities: Decide How to Decide

Once you have explicitly stated a problem, you and your clients can begin to determine the range of possible approaches available to remediate the problem. In many instances clients do not have the ability to see past a roadblock. They often feel that they have tried everything and keep producing the same outcome. Clients may also believe that they just "can't do it." In the brainstorming phase of the Planning Process Model, your job is to open up the range of possibilities. First, you show clients that there is more than one way to approach an issue, and, second, you allow clients to feel more ownership of the process. They are, in fact, proposing possibilities with you.

When brainstorming with clients, encourage them to suspend judgment on any possible strategies. Ask clients to allow themselves to come up with their wildest possibilities, even if they would never consider actually enacting them. Write all of their ideas on a piece of paper so they can see them. When clients have completed the brainstorming exercise, evaluate the possibilities. Have clients circle the strategies they believe are realistic and acceptable to them and cross off the ones they do not believe they will use. Of the ones circled, order them according to acceptability.

Clinician: So, sometimes you have a hard time figuring out how to produce the /r/ when you don't have me to model it for you.

Laura: Yes, then I get frustrated with myself and I don't want to practice.

Clinician: Maybe we need determine ways for you to have the auditory model accessible to you or make sure you feel comfortable knowing how to make the sound on your own.

Laura: Do you really think that will help?

Clinician: Let's find out. Presently, something in the way we are approaching therapy is not working for you. You are ending up frustrated, and then you are not motivated to practice. We need to find a way for you to feel like you know how to produce /r/ all of the time, even when I'm not around.

Laura: OK. How do we do that?

Clinician: Well, let's brainstorm some possible ways we could get you to feel like you know how to produce /r/. Can you think of any?

Laura: I really don't see what else we can do.

Clinician: Mm-hm. [*Maintains eye contact and remains silent.*]

Laura: I guess we could continue practicing /r/ in the beginning of words as we've been doing in the therapy sessions.

Clinician: OK, good. What we are already doing is definitely one possible strategy.

Silence: Often a powerful tool that can be used during treatment sessions to encourage clients to think of ideas on their own. Silence is an actual response. Sometimes not saying anything at all provides the client with time to formulate an idea, ask a question, or find the courage to say something.

In this scenario Laura starts by saying that she does not think there is any other way to approach therapy. The clinician responds with an attending behavior (eye contact) to indicate that she is with the client and remains silent, allowing Laura time to think before providing any input. Silence is often a powerful tool that can be used during treatment sessions to encourage clients to think of ideas on their own. Many novice clinicians fear silence in therapy sessions. They believe that if the client is not talking, they should be talking. A strategy for becoming more comfortable with silence is to realize that silence is an actual response. Sometimes not saying anything at all provides the client with time to formulate an idea, ask a question, or get the courage to speak up. Count slowly to five in your head while maintaining gentle eye contact. Do not extend silence so that it becomes awkward. If the client does not provide a response within the five seconds, you can say something like, "OK, maybe you'll come up with something later. Make sure to let me know if you do," or "Sometimes it's difficult to come up ideas on the fly. Here's one I thought of." In the case with Laura, silence was effective and provided time for Laura to offer an idea.

Laura: I guess we could continue practicing at the beginning of words as we've been doing in the therapy sessions.

Clinician: OK, good. What we are already doing is definitely one possible strategy. How about trying to come up with another possibility? At this stage, try not to make a judgment about whether strategies are right or wrong. Let's just see what we can come up with.

Laura: Well, I could stop therapy all together. I mean, I'm not going to do that, but it is a possibility.

Clinician: Yes it is, and a good one to mention even if you won't consider it a real option.

Laura: I seem to have an easier time producing /r/ after a vowel especially /i/, like in the word *ear*. What if we tried working with /r/ in words like that?

Clinician: Sure, that's a great idea. Are there other times you find making your /r/ is easier?

Brainstorming Options

- Restate the problem.
- Urge clients to think of possible approaches to remediate the problem without making judgments about the acceptability of the approach.
- Reinforce good thinking when clients offer a possibility.
- Probe clients to encourage them to think of possibilities on their own.
- Write down possibilities for clients.

Laura: Making the /r/ sound is easier when I spread my lips, like when I say /i/. Maybe I could practice the /r/ sound with my lips more spread. My tongue seems to get higher in my mouth. We could check that I'm producing /r/ correctly without words at the beginning of each session, just to make sure I have it before moving on.

Clinician: Yes, that's also a possibility.

At this point in the process Laura is able to generate some options on her own with little input from the clinician. Allow clients to take ownership of the ideas they offer even if they provide strategies that you have already been working on with them. Their belief that the strategies are their own ideas will more likely foster their use in therapy.

Depending on the age, cognitive ability, and willingness of your clients, you may need to take a more active role in the brainstorming process. Providing cues may help. Cues include questions like, "When do you find it easiest to produce [your technique]" and "Which activities are most difficult?" You may also take turns providing possibilities. Ask clients directly first regardless of age and cognitive status. Even clients as young as 2 can provide at least one possible idea or strategy. If caregivers and advocates are present, you might use them as resources when clients have difficulty communicating possibilities or do not provide any.

In the dialogue above Laura proposes the possibility of stopping therapy altogether. This proposition is called the quit option. Although this may not be the option you would like your clients to propose, it is a real one and one that should be noted. Clients who are frustrated with therapy may feel empowered by the realization that quitting is a possibility. Allow clients to entertain the option. If they decide for themselves that quitting is not an option, they usually feel more ownership of the process. Productive discussions about clients' feelings and attitudes toward therapy can be generated by the suggestion of quitting. If clients do in fact decide to quit, then they have at least made an informed choice.

> **Quit option:** The decision to end therapy.

Creating Goals: Determine Acceptability and Choose

After the brainstorming activity is complete, you have a list of possible approaches that you can employ to write potential intermediate goals. In this next stage of the Planning Process Model, your clients indicate the acceptability of each approach to determine which ones will be formulated as goals. Simply read out or have your clients read the possibilities from your worksheet. They can circle the approaches they feel are acceptable and cross out the ones that are not acceptable. At this point you should try to encourage clients to make their judgments based only on whether they view the goal as acceptable or not. Their willingness to commit to the goal involves other factors such as time, criteria, and doability. Your knowledge of therapy is important at this goal-writing stage. If your clients determine that an approach is acceptable but you know a more effective way to address the goal, you may need to tweak the wording when writing the goal.

> **Laura:** That's about all I can think of.
>
> **Clinician:** You really thought of a lot of possibilities. Now what I want you to do is circle the ones you think are acceptable and cross out the ones you definitely do not think you will do in therapy.
>
> **Laura:** OK, I think "working on /r/ in words with the /i/ vowel" is acceptable to me. So is "producing /r/ with my lips spread." I'll circle them. I definitely won't quit, so I'll cross that one out.
>
> **Clinician:** Those seem like appropriate choices. One of your goals, then, would be, "Laura will produce postvocalic /r/ correctly at the word level with clinician cue with ninety percent accuracy." Once you meet that criterion, I will drop my cueing. That will assure us that you are able to do it without my help.

In this phase of the Planning Process Model, the clinician had Laura look through the options she brainstormed and choose ones that were acceptable to her. The clinician then developed the structure of the goals based on Laura's choices. When working with your clients through this process, it is important to evaluate your goals based on the criteria.

Review Goals with MUSTDO Criteria

When evaluating your goals using the MUSTDO criteria (**Figure 11-2**), it is important to remember that your goals should meet all six criteria, but you do not have to evaluate them in the specified order. The acronym provides you with a mechanism to remember each criterion: measurable, understood, solution focused, time

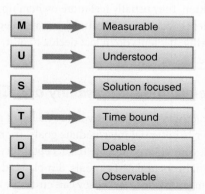

FIGURE 11-2 MUSTDO. A well-constructed therapy goal should meet the six MUSTDO criteria.

bound, doable, and observable. Make sure to involve your clients, to the extent they can be involved, when assessing their goals using these criteria. As you become a more seasoned clinician, you will be able to more quickly write your goals keeping the MUSTDO criteria in mind. You may then use the MUSTDO criteria mainly as a method to help your clients assess the goals with you and, in turn, gain more ownership of their goals and the therapy process.

Strategies within MUSTDO

When you review goals with clients, you may adopt strategies within each criterion of the MUSTDO acronym that can help you determine your clients' acceptance of each criterion. Keep in mind that you do not have to go in order.

> **Clinician:** Those seem like appropriate choices. One of your goals, then, would be, "Laura will produce postvocalic /r/ correctly at the word level with clinician cue with ninety percent accuracy." Once you meet that criterion I will drop my cueing. That will assure us that you are able to do it without my help. Do you feel that this goal is working toward your long-term goal of producing /r/ correctly all the time?

> **Laura:** Yes, I definitely see this intermediate goal as a way to achieve my long-term goal.

> **Clinician:** All right, you had an issue concerning the change in our treatment plan to help you determine whether you are producing /r/ correctly without my help. Do you see these goals as solving that issue?

> **Laura:** Yes.

The clinician decided to start with the solution-focused criterion (S in MUSTDO). The clinician began by asking Laura whether the goals will achieve her long-term objectives as well as address her frustration with not knowing whether she is producing /r/ correctly without help. At that point the clinician was better able to determine whether the entire goal needed to be changed before addressing the other MUSTDO criteria. In this situation, Laura agrees that the goal is acceptable, and the clinician knows that for the time being the goal can remain as it is.

When you consider whether the goal is solution focused, you are, of course, establishing the relevance of the goal and ensuring that an intermediate goal aligns with a long-term goal. For these reasons clinicians often consider the solution-focus criterion early in the discussion of MUSTDO.

> **Clinician:** OK, good. I explained to you that I will drop my cue for /r/ once you are able to produce /r/ correctly ninety percent of the time with my cue. This is how we'll measure your ability to produce /r/.

> **Laura:** OK, and when I can produce /r/ at the ends of words without your model, then I know I will be able to move on from that goal.

> **Clinician:** That's right.

In this exchange, the clinician reviewed with Laura how the goals will be measured (M in MUSTDO). Most clinicians also make sure the goal is measurable before considering the rest of the criteria, because the measure or measures establish that you and your clients can tell when the goal is achieved.

Depending on their age and cognitive ability, clients will know to some extent that they are being evaluated. If they are part of the process of setting how the goals will be measured, then they know the target they need to work toward. Clients also have a chance to determine whether they believe the measure, and therefore the goal, is doable or not.

Assessing whether clients believe their goals are doable (D in MUSTDO) is a critically important process. Doability signals readiness and willingness on the part of your clients, and the counseling component will be strong. You can create as many goals as you want, but if your clients do not believe that they will be able to "do" your goals, then there will be a decreased willingness to participate in therapy. The clinician experienced this with Laura at the beginning of the dialogue. Even if Laura felt she could produce /r/ at the beginning of words during the session, she was unsure when she got home whether she was producing /r/ correctly or not. Laura started to get frustrated, would not practice, and stopped coming to therapy. The clinician knew something needed to change. If the clinician does not check the doability of the new goals, then Laura could become frustrated again. Initial assessment of doability is essential; continued monitoring may be critical.

One way to determine whether clients believe their goals are doable is to ask them.

Laura: OK, and when I can produce /r/ at the ends of words without your model, then I know I will be able to move on from that goal.

Clinician: That's right. Do you think you will be able to perform the activities needed to work toward these goals?

Laura: Yes, I think so.

Clinician: Do you think the measurement we set for each goal is acceptable?

Laura: Yes.

Laura is very amenable. Not all of your clients' goals, however, will meet the doability criterion so easily. Let's consider an example with Laura questioning her ability to perform the activities within the goal.

Clinician: That's right. Do you think you will be able to perform the activities needed to work toward these goals?

Laura: I'm not sure. I think I will be able to do the activities when I'm with you, but practicing at home still seems like a problem for me. How will I know I'm producing /r/ correctly when you're not around?

You may opt to brainstorm with your clients to determine strategies with them. You also may offer information and suggestions about how they can transfer what they have learned in clinic to home. In Laura's case a recorded example may help her if she is having trouble remembering what to do. Writing down cues and enlisting allies may also be helpful. Depending on your clients' learning style, knowledge, and experience, you will decide on a method to increase their willingness to participate.

Laura: I'm not sure. I think I will be able to do the activities when I'm with you, but practicing at home still seems like a problem for me. How will I know I'm producing /r/ correctly when you're not around.

Clinician: I could provide you with a recorded version of my model as well as a recording of you producing /r/ correctly so you can refer to it when you get stuck.

Laura: That sounds like a great idea. I told you, too, that I'm busy right now at school. What if I can't find the time to practice?

Time is also a factor in assessing doability. You may want to consider the amount of physical time you have in therapy with your clients, how many times an insurance company will pay for a client to come to therapy, or how much time clients have to practice outside of therapy. Clients find it useful when clinicians provide strategies to manage time.

Help clients to identify what time of day is best for them to practice. Make a schedule and see that they stick to it. Remember, changing a habit is hard. Not only are you asking them to make changes to their speech, language, voice, hearing, or swallowing but you are also asking them to change their daily schedule to incorporate practice. Be a good role model; make the best use of your time during each session. Clients want to see that you are organized and that you follow an agenda.

Incorporate time into your goals. Make your goals time bound (T in MUSTDO). This step provides clients and caregivers with guideposts for how long you will work on a goal before reassessing the criteria. Time-bounding also makes it more difficult for resistant clients to procrastinate or avoid therapy. Clients have a time line that they know they need to follow.

Laura: That sounds like a great idea. I told you, too, that I'm busy right now at school. What if I can't find the time practice?

Clinician: Let's give you two weeks to work with these new goals. You'll have your recorded examples when you go home, and we'll set up a schedule for you to follow at home. If you haven't made improvements in two weeks, then we'll reassess the goals.

Laura: How will you know if I've practiced?

Clinician: Good question. I hope to see improvement session to session. I also want you to record yourself when you practice at home so I can make sure you are producing /r/ correctly.

Remember that your goals need to be observable (O in MUSTDO). As a clinician you will develop strategies to determine whether and how your clients are practicing outside of sessions. Journaling, using recording devices, tracking data, and asking allies to help are some techniques you can use to make data observable. Progress on goals also needs to be observable to the clients. Charting that progress is one way to show clients how they are performing. Making sure goals are observable is one way to help clients monitor their own improvement and keep them motivated.

The remaining MUSTDO criterion that the clinician needs to review with Laura is U, Understood. As a clinician you will want to check whether your clients understand each criterion in MUSTDO. By establishing that each criterion is understood, you confirm that your clients' understanding of the goals is the same as yours. Communication is, in fact, receiving the package of information from the listener in the same way it was intended by the speaker. The client demonstrates understanding when information is received correctly.

Laura: How will you know if I've practiced?

Clinician: Good question. I hope to see improvement session to session. I also want you to record yourself when you practice at home so I can make sure you are producing /r/ correctly. How does that sound to you?

Laura: I think that will work.

Clinician: Do you understand the goals we have set so far?

Laura: Yes.

Making a Decision

Once the goals have been set, evaluated, and understood, you have to confirm that your clients are willing to make the decision to continue with the process. Understanding the goals is part of the process; making the decision to act is another. As willingness is part of assessing the doability of a goal, readiness is inherent in making the decision to proceed with the goal. If clients are ready, implementation of the plan will be seamless from creation to action. With clients who are hesitant, obstacles will arise in predictable places. These obstacles may manifest in unproductive behaviors such as procrastination and resistance. After you determine where the obstacle is, your task is to uncover forces that facilitate progress and those that hinder progress.

Let us say you now understand the obstacle. Your clients have an unhelpful belief or a doubt about which you have been unable to persuade them to believe differently. In discussion with your clients, you need to pinpoint the factors that might help persuade and those that are making the new belief unpersuasive. Enhancing forces include clients' prior experiences that tend to make the new belief seem reasonable, and deterring forces include past experiences that reinforce the unhelpful belief (**Figure 11-3**).

Existing needs may become enhancing or deterring forces. Laura had the need to speak well so she could obtain an internship. This need was a strong enhancing force for her clinician in the clinician's efforts to get Laura to practice.

Earlier therapy might also have occasioned enhancing and deterring forces. In the example of Laura, she resisted returning to therapy for her /r/ because of a past negative experience with another clinician. That past negative experience has become a deterring force in her current therapy.

Once you identify deterring forces, you should plan to dispel them. If a client has an unhelpful belief that is driven by earlier experiences in therapy, emphasize how matters are different now: you are a different clinician; the methods may be different; clients have matured and are no longer in the same situation they were in previously.

If you are successful, you might actually change a deterring force into an enhancing force. If prior therapy starts as a deterring force, the differences between that

Enhancing forces: Clients' prior experiences that tend to make a new belief seem reasonable, when clients have an unhelpful belief and the therapist is proposing a different way of thinking.

Deterring forces: Past experiences that reinforce an unhelpful belief.

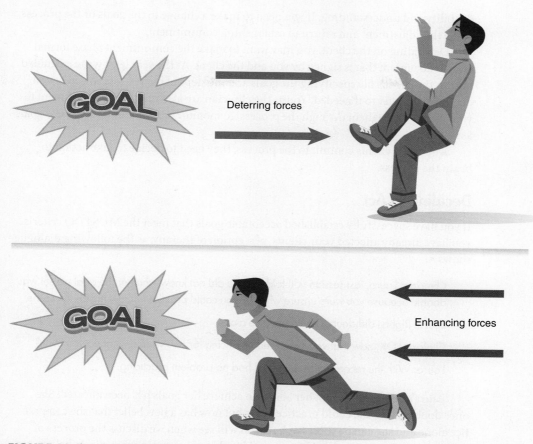

FIGURE 11-3 Impact of Enhancing and Deterring Forces. Enhancing forces help clients progress toward their goals, and deterring forces create obstacles to progress.

therapy and the current therapy might come to serve as enhancing forces. Of course, you have to identify those differences with clients and help them see that things are more positive now.

Committing to the Process

In the business world, when a deal is made, the two parties shake hands to show good will and a commitment to follow through on their part of the process. In therapy for speech-language pathology and audiology, it may not be necessary to shake hands, but a commitment to the process should be established. By committing to the process, your clients explicitly indicate their willingness and readiness to embark on their journey. If clients are hesitant in committing to the process, then there was probably a breakdown in communication when you evaluated their goals. Check back to see where the breakdown occurred. Confirm their long-term goals, state the intermediate goals identified by your clients, validate each of the MUSTDO criteria stressing doability and understanding. If you need to make a change to the goals or the process, make the adjustment and return to establishing commitment.

Depending on the client, you may want to make the commitment phase formal. Draft a document that is signed by you and the client. At the very least write a detailed note in the client's file specifying the goals and the steps of the process so you have a document to refer to if needed. You as the clinician are also making a commitment to your clients to see them through the process, to monitor progress, and to reassess goals as needed.

After your clients commit to the process, they need to decide to take action to begin the process.

Deciding to Act

If you have successfully established acceptable goals that meet the MUSTDO criteria, you have already affected your clients' perception of therapy, as the following dialogue shows.

Clinician: Laura, last session you told me you did not know whether the goal we set was doable because you were unsure whether you could practice without me on the scene.

Laura: Right. I did doubt I could practice alone.

Clinician: OK, now that you have tried practicing for two weeks, what do you think?

Laura: With the recording as a guide, I had no problem practicing.

Laura's perception about her ability to achieve her goals has been affected. She once doubted that she could practice alone but now has a new belief that she can practice alone and she can be successful. As you will see when we discuss the process of challenging clients, you should try to avoid making changes in what clients believe are certainties. These are areas of the clients' beliefs that they feel very strongly about; they are difficult, often impossible to change. In most cases, these aspects of clients' beliefs should be respected and not altered.

As you deal with clients' belief systems, make sure you follow the guidelines below.

As you make progress in therapy, an important task is to use counseling to uncover what you need to know to move clients to act. Laura, in the previous dialogue, altered a belief she held: that she was unable to practice without her clinician. If the

Ways to Deal with Clients' Belief Systems

- Determine as precisely as possible clients' perceptions about their diagnosis, current situation, goals, and therapy. Assess how they relate to the actions you want clients to take.
- Make sure you are not trying to change what your clients believe are certainties.
- If a change is necessary, clarify for yourself and your clients just what that change is.
- Clearly lay out the steps you and your clients will take to make the change.
- Guide and monitor your clients through the process of change.

issue is not beliefs or certainties, a different approach is indicated, as in the following dialogue.

Clinician: You have not managed to practice a half hour each day?

Laura: I don't have the time.

Clinician: You are finished with classes each day by three, right?

Laura: Three thirty.

Clinician: OK, what do you do then?

Laura: I hit the gym for an hour and get back to my apartment, usually by five.

Clinician: Mm-hm.

Laura: Then I decompress with a little TV; I record shows to watch them when I have time.

Clinician: How long do you watch TV?

Laura: I don't know. We eat at six thirty, so I guess maybe an hour and a half.

Clinician: Let's say you cut down your TV time and free up a half hour to practice.

Laura: I guess I could do that.

Clinician: Will you?

Laura: Yes. Sure. I'll take a half hour from five to five thirty for practice.

The clinician worked on Laura's wants. Whenever you get clients to examine their priorities, you are dealing with their wants or needs. Even though Laura and the clinician were discussing her belief that she did not have time, the clinician rightly shifted the topic to Laura's wants. Yes, she wanted to "decompress" with TV, but she was able to be convinced that she did not really want a full hour and a half of viewing more than she wanted a half hour of practice.

Laura's perceived needs can constitute a powerful incentive. At the beginning of the chapter Laura revealed a definite need when she said, "Now I need to get this /r/ correct or I'm worried I won't get an internship at the local radio station this summer. No one will hire me if I say my /r/s like this." Clearly, she does not merely "want" to produce the /r/ phoneme correctly; she needs to do so, or she will not obtain the coveted internship.

Sometimes, appealing to your clients' moral convictions can help you make your case.

Clinician: Practicing between sessions is absolutely essential to therapy.

Laura: I know. I take this very seriously.

Clinician: Why, Laura?

Laura: Because my Dad has paid a lot to get me into speech therapy. He isn't rich; he and Mom are really sacrificing to get me an education and to provide this therapy.

Clinician: So, you have an obligation to them.

Laura: Yes. It would be wrong for me to take this lightly. I owe it to them to do the best I can.

Clinician: Does that include the practice we've been talking about?

Laura: Yes. Sure it does.

Clinician: So?

Laura: So, I better practice if I want to do the right thing.

Laura's sense of right and wrong, her convictions, became a motivator or an incentive to practice between sessions. In this case nothing was imposed on Laura; her existing convictions about justice and rightness served the clinician's purpose. The clinician gently guided Laura to make the connection between those convictions and the proper attitude toward practice.

Laura's belief system will not always require changing. Her conviction about honoring her parents' sacrifices for her and her need to speak correctly to obtain an internship were both beliefs of hers all along. Remember, she came to therapy with her attitudes, beliefs, and feelings intact. These beliefs can be used to complement therapy, but the clinician must first be aware of them and then be willing to work with them to begin and advance the process. Sometimes clinicians need to utilize techniques beyond basic communication skills when dealing with clients' beliefs, attitudes, and feelings. The next section offers advanced communication skills for clinicians to consider when working with clients.

Utilizing Advanced Communication Skills

There are five intentions of communication: information, small talk, self-affirmation, persuasion, and feeling. Each of them is important to counseling throughout the Solution Cycle. Although specific intentions are appropriate to individual stages in the Solution Cycle, you and your clients will utilize all of these five intentions throughout therapy. As the clinician, you must always keep in mind your clients' communication intention to help you determine your reaction or response to what your clients are saying.

When counseling clients, it is also important for you to identify your own communication intention or assess the clients' need for you to adopt a specific intention. For example, your client may express the need for more clarification of the purpose of therapy. If you misunderstand your client's information intention, you might respond defensively because you feel as if the client is expressing a dislike of your therapy approach. When you misunderstand in this way, your analysis of the situation and subsequent choice of communication intention are incorrect and could be detrimental to the therapy process. If you assess your clients' comment accurately as a need for clarification of the purpose, that is, an information intention, you will correctly respond by providing the information requested.

There are two phases of listening: (1) understand and (2) assess. During the understand phase, you use basic communication skills like attending behaviors (e.g., head nods) and vocalizations (e.g., "mm-hmm" and "uh-huh") to show that you are "with" your clients. You also use basic responses such as echoing, parroting, summarizing, and restating to help clients continue to tell their story. Once you have received the message and understood it, then you need to assess the message and respond. In formulating your response you are required to use logic and critical thinking skills. You have to weigh options and make judgments based on the facts.

The assess phase of listening requires you to use more advanced communication skills like finding the message within the message, relying on your intuition to extract meaning from the message, and challenging clients when needed. This section addresses these skills.

Themes within the Message

Clients may have difficulty explicitly stating a fear, a feeling, or a reason for behaving a certain way. They may embed the meaning of their message within language they feel safe sharing. Your job as the clinician is to identify themes within the message to extract the truth from the message.

In the dialogue with Laura, the clinician heard her indicate that she "needed" to say /r/ correctly because those potentially hiring her as an intern would require it. People use the word *need* in different ways. Laura certainly could mean that she needs to produce the /r/ phoneme correctly and is therefore firmly committed to that goal and the actions necessary to attain it. Possibly, however, she could be saying that she needs to make the correction, sure, but the commitment and determination to change are not really very strong.

In fact, clients sometimes use phrases like "I need to," "I have to," "I must," "I should," and "I'll try" as a way of avoiding statements like "I will." When you hear a "need-must-try" type of statement, you will often find it useful to respond with a question like, "Yes, I understand; now, what are you going to do?"

Commitment should be expressed in an affirmative will to act. If clients are committed, they invest the time, energy, and focus on the action they are committed to taking, no matter what they need to do, ought to do, or are "trying" to do. If you get your clients to say "I will do it," you are not guaranteeing that they will be committed. You are simply requiring them to use the language of commitment. That is a good place to start.

Trusting Your Intuition

When clients do not explicitly state portions of their message, it is important for you to tune into their actions and behaviors. Clients may momentarily avert their eyes, strum their fingers on the table, and fidget in their seat. Their voice may crack a bit or tremble. They may pause too long or quickly change the subject. All of these behaviors are cues that maybe what your clients are saying is not really what they mean. As the clinician, you should trust your instinct, go with your gut. If something does not seem right, it may be a signal that you need to take time to investigate the true meaning behind the message.

Hunch: An intuitive guess about how to proceed in a given situation. Experienced therapists know how to value their hunches and make appropriate use of them.

You can couch your suspicions as a hunch. This advanced communication skill is less direct and provides your clients with an opportunity to view what they are saying in a different light. The hunch takes the basic communication skill restatement to the next level. Instead of restating what clients are saying, you are taking a stab at another way to interpret what they are saying.

Back in the beginning of the chapter, the clinician indicated that Laura seemed frustrated. The clinician posited that this might be the reason why Laura missed a few therapy sessions. Laura refuted the idea that she was frustrated, stating that she "knew this would be difficult." She then reinforced her "need" to correct her production of /r/ because of the internship. We already discussed how to pick up on themes within the message. Just looking at words from the dialogue, you may get the impression that Laura means more than what she is saying.

Clinician: Last session you were having trouble with the exercises we were doing. Remember we were working on producing /r/ in the beginning of words. I sensed you were frustrated at the end of the session, and then when you didn't come back last week…

Laura: No, I wasn't frustrated. I knew this would be difficult. I worked on this a few years ago, but I just didn't feel like my speech pathologist knew what she was doing. Now I need to get this /r/ correct or I'm worried I won't get an internship at the local radio station this summer. No one will hire me if I say my /r/s like this.

Some questions may go through your mind as Laura is explaining herself, such as, "Why didn't therapy really work the last time?" "Was the speech-language pathologist really to blame?" "Laura feels like she needs to correct her production of /r/, but does she really want to invest the effort it takes to accomplish that goal?" "Is Laura just resisting change?" When you invest time in your suspicions, you may not always be welcomed with acceptance. Because Laura has already missed several sessions and has indicated that she did not succeed at therapy before, it seems like the risk of upsetting Laura is worth the cost. The hunch provides you with the opportunity to address your concerns while treading lightly.

Laura: No, I wasn't frustrated. I knew this would be difficult. I worked on this a few years ago, but I just didn't feel like my speech pathologist knew what she was doing. Now I need to get this /r/ correct or I'm worried I won't get an internship at the local radio station this summer. No one will hire me if I say my /r/s like this.

Clinician: I hear you say that you need to correct your /r/ because you aren't sure you'll be hired for the internship if you don't say /r/ correctly.

Laura: Yes, that's right.

Clinician: I get the feeling, though, that the investment in time and effort that you need to really change how you produce /r/ is harder to commit to than you are saying.

You can state your hunch in many different ways. In this example, the clinician first used a basic communication skill, summarizing, to clarify that the clinician received Laura's message correctly. The clinician then stated her hunch as "I get the feeling…" You could also use "I have a hunch," "It seems to me," "I get the impression," or "I'll take an educated guess."

Clinician: I get the feeling, though, that the investment in time and effort that you need to really change how you produce /r/ is harder to commit to than you are saying.

Laura: It is hard to find the time to practice.

Clinician: Putting all outside sources aside, is this something you really want to change?

Laura: Yes, I want to change how I say my /r/s.

Sometimes the hunch does not work. When that happens you may need to be more direct with your clients. Challenging is another advanced communication skill you can use when your clients do not seem to be saying what they mean.

Challenging Clients

When you challenge your clients, you are taking a further step. You are pushing them to rethink or reimagine some aspect of their world. You should therefore be acutely attuned to exactly what you are challenging. There are three major areas of challenge, all of them part of the total set of perceptions held by your client. These areas are beliefs, norms, and wants.

You may need to challenge some of your clients' beliefs so you and your clients can move forward in the therapy process. Clients may believe, for instance, that their disorder cannot be adequately addressed because they are physically incapable of correcting it. If you do not effectively challenge that belief, progress will be close to impossible.

Norms are behaviors your clients exhibit consistently under a particular set of social conditions. Sometimes it is necessary to challenge a norm. For example, it may be a norm for some clients to check their text messages whenever their phone beeps. You do not want them to check their text messages in the middle of a therapy session. You will have to challenge the norm.

Wants are what your clients desire. Clients may want you to show them an easier, less time-consuming path to the correction of their disorder. You may need to challenge that want so they will adopt a more realistic perspective on the attainment of their therapy goals.

When you challenge your clients' perceptions in one of these areas, for example, a belief, you can expect a pretty specific response. If your challenge targets a different area, for example, a norm, the expected response will be different. Knowing these different expectations is important for you if you want to be well prepared to issue the challenge effectively.

If you challenge a belief held by clients, they will feel disoriented or seem to be floundering. Something they thought was so is being questioned. If, for instance, clients feel they are physically incapable of producing a particular phoneme, you might use a strategy to have them do an exercise that results in their producing the phoneme without realizing it. Imagine their turmoil when you play the exercise back on an audio recording device, and they hear themselves doing what they thought they could not do. Disoriented and floundering would likely describe their state, at least for a while.

If you challenge a norm, clients might feel embarrassed or awkward because you are alerting them that they are acting in a socially inappropriate way. Let's say your clients are unaware that they are required to practice between therapy sessions. When they show up for their following session, you ask them to demonstrate the improvement they made since the previous session. They look at you sheepishly and claim they "just didn't know they were supposed to work on this." They are embarrassed. It is an awkward moment.

If you challenge a want, clients might feel less powerful because you are telling them they will not be obtaining something they desire. Clients may want to progress more quickly, skip steps, and achieve their goal with less effort. They will experience a degree of frustration when you stand firm on the importance of staying the course, seeing through the process. Despite the momentary decrease in ownership, if you believe standing firm in the process will ultimately lead to client success then ownership will be reestablished when clients see improvement and growth.

Exercise care when challenging clients. You are always creating discomfort, and that may be an acceptable price to move clients to a better place as therapy progresses. When your challenge creates disdain or severe disapproval in your clients, however, the price is too high. To effectively challenge your clients' beliefs, attitudes, or feelings, you must be aware of their limits. A challenge must appear, just that way, challenging, but not unattainable or one that cannot be denied as being important. Offering a challenge while relating it to what is important to the client helps to offset any extreme discomfort associated with the challenge. If clients ultimately see that addressing a misconception or irrational belief can help them to reach their desired goal, they may be more inclined to at least entertain the idea that there may be another way to think about things.

Finding Leverage

By knowing what is important to clients, understanding their desires, wants, and needs, you can encourage clients to work through obstacles, roadblocks, and blind spots they may face throughout the therapy process. Astute clinicians who invest the time in studying and knowing their clients find these points of leverage that can be used when clients become frustrated, doubtful, and unsure about continuing with any or all aspects of therapy.

Leverage gives the clinician the positional advantage. In the example of Laura, the clinician took note of Laura's belief that she needs to be able to say her /r/ correctly to be in a position to get an internship. This belief can be used to remind Laura of the goals she is working toward if she gets frustrated with therapy. Building credibility also helps the clinician establish leverage. Clients are more inclined to participate in exercises and activities, even difficult ones, when they trust and believe in the clinician. Clients who commit to change and continue along the process of change eventually reach the stage where they no longer need to be in therapy and can maintain the behavior on their own.

Review of Key Points

- As the clinician, you must always keep in mind your clients' and your own communication intentions to help you determine your reaction or response to what your clients are saying.
- As therapy progresses you need to monitor your original plan and make adjustments when necessary. You can use the Planning Process Model at any point in therapy to evaluate your clients and help provide them with an action orientation toward their preferred future.
- The first step in this reevaluation of the plan is to assess whether the clients still perceive their goals in the same way.
- Probing clients to determine the acceptability of the plan is the second step in the Planning Process Model.
- In the brainstorming phase of the Planning Process Model, your job is to open up the range of possibilities. You show clients that there is more than one way to approach an issue, and you allow clients to feel more ownership of the process. They are proposing possibilities with you.
- After the brainstorming activity is complete, your clients indicate the acceptability of each approach to determine which ones will be formulated as goals. Their willingness to commit to the goal involves factors such as time, criteria, and doability.
- When evaluating your goals, use the MUSTDO criteria. There are strategies you may adopt within each criterion that can help you determine your clients' acceptance of each criterion.
- Once the goals have been set, evaluated, and understood, you have to confirm that your clients are willing to make the decision to continue with the process. A commitment to the process should be established.
- Clients' belief system can complement the therapy process, but the clinician must first be aware of these beliefs and then be willing to work with clients to begin and advance progress.
- Enhancing forces are forces that can serve or propel progress in therapy; deterring forces tend to hinder or obstruct progress.
- The assess phase of listening requires you to use more advanced communication skills like finding the message within the message, relying on your intuition to extract meaning from the message, and challenging clients when needed.
- Commitment is expressed in an affirmative will to act. Clients invest the time, energy, and focus on the action they are committed to taking, no matter what they need to do, ought to do, or are "trying" to do.
- When clients do not explicitly state their message, tune into their actions and behaviors for cues that what your clients are saying is not really what they mean. Trust your instinct. You may need to investigate the true meaning behind the message.
- A hunch is an advanced communication skill that takes the basic skill of restatement to the next level, to investigate the message within the message.

- Challenging is another advanced communication skill you can use when your clients do not seem to be saying what they mean. When you challenge your clients, you are pushing them to rethink or reimagine some aspect of their world.
- Exercise care when challenging clients. You are always creating discomfort, and that may be an acceptable price to move clients to a better place as therapy progresses.
- Leverage gives the clinician the positional advantage to help clients address roadblocks, blind spots, and obstacles to therapy.

Practical Exercises

1. A 62-year-old man retired early from his job right before he had a right hemisphere stroke. He is being seen in an inpatient rehabilitation center by his speech-language pathologist. In one of his sessions, he has begun talking about how his stroke has affected his life. In particular, he has been dealing over and over with the issues of loss. He says: "I don't get to see my grandchildren much anymore. I love when they come to visit. But now I … well, I can't work. My wife said to retire. We had plans. Now, I just sit here and do nothing. I suppose I should just stop … going to therapy … trying to get better … what's the use? I'm not going to need those skills anymore anyway."

   Provide three emotions that this client is feeling.

   What is your hunch and your reason for it?

   Provide an advanced communication response using your hunch.

2. Olivia reported to her audiologist that her hearing impairment has been causing her problems at her university. She finds that, despite wearing hearing aids, many of her classmates often have to repeat themselves when sharing information with her or asking her to complete a task. When sharing this information with her audiologist, Olivia said, "I was the only person in my class who was left without a group. For the biggest project of the semester." She broke eye contact and shifted uncomfortably in her seat. She continued, "It doesn't bother me much, though. I work better by myself, anyway."

   Provide three emotions that this client is feeling.

   What is your hunch and your reason for it?

   Provide an advanced communication response using your hunch.

CHAPTER 12

Becoming One's Own Clinician

KEY TERMS

- Compromise
- Confidence
- Confidence zone
- Five Intentions of Communication
- Incremental independence
- Motivational interviewing
- Relapse
- Solution Cycle
- Undeclared adversary

LEARNING OBJECTIVES

After reading this chapter, you will be able to:

- Define a solution-focused approach to counseling
- Explain the importance of a client building confidence prior to dismissal from therapy
- Describe the types of limitations that might arise throughout the therapy process

Finding Solutions

Counseling was defined throughout this textbook as caring support in the form of information, guidance, and assistance provided to clients, families, caretakers, and advocates. Clients can use such support and insight to pursue realistic and clearly understood goals and attain a more fulfilling quality of life. A solution-focused approach to counseling is recommended because the pursuit and accomplishment of productive goals emerge as the point of counseling.

In speech-language pathology and audiology, counseling is distinguished from disorder-specific treatment not as a semantic exercise but as a way to clarify and practice specific skills and techniques defined by the activity of counseling. Treatment addresses actions, strategies, and techniques that can result in remediation, improvement, or maintenance of hearing, speech, language, voice, and swallowing abilities; counseling tackles barriers that stand in the way of successful treatment.

Barriers amenable to counseling may include lack of motivation, poor self-image, or a misunderstanding about the purpose, time line, or structure of clients' goals. Counseling might not remove the barriers, but, if effective, it renders the barriers surmountable, meaning they are able to be overcome. Lack of motivation is addressed and transformed into sufficient motivation. Poor self-image becomes healthier self-image, and misunderstandings are discussed and corrected.

Because your approach is solution focused, you are free to use the insights of a wide variety of counseling strategies, including behavior management, cognitive therapy, and the humanistic approach. More recently developed methods, particularly motivational interviewing (Behrman, 2006; McFarlane, 2012; Miller & Rollnick, 1991), tend to be client centered and goal oriented and therefore compatible with the solution-focused approach.

> **Motivational interviewing:** A client-centered and goal-oriented technique, compatible with the solution-focused approach

Solution-focused counseling shines a bright, unwavering light on what you and your clients are out to accomplish. You are strongly biased in favor of clarity, of figuring out what has fallen below the bar of acceptability, where that bar actually is, and how your clients can reach the bar.

If you are solution focused, you are inherently optimistic. A problem exists, yes, but the task you and your clients are working on is to develop a solution to the problem. *Problem* is not a bad word, not a term to be avoided or downplayed. Problems are meant to be solved, and solution focus insists that together you and your clients can solve them.

You and your clients define the problem when you ask, "What's going on?" "What's wrong?" "How is this making things difficult?" "How is this affecting quality of life?" You are developing a solution when you ask, "What has to change?" "What would make things better?" "How will I know when the client has improved?" "What would a more robust quality of life look like?"

Of course, when your clients reach a counseling goal, they have not met a disorder-specific target. What counseling can do is pave the way for clients to accomplish the goals of therapy. Solution focus in one area enables solution focus in the other.

Clients Are Not All the Same

Counseling takes dramatically different forms depending on several client-related factors. Clients' age, cognitive functioning, previous experience in therapy, and cultural differences are some factors that dictate how you approach counseling.

You do not counsel 5-year-olds like 13-year-olds. Young children have different needs from adolescents, and adolescents have different needs from adults. Similarly, older adults are in important ways unlike those in their 30s. In fact, from one age group to another, you may find few parallels in tactics, language, or the problems you are likely to encounter.

Some rules apply across the board regardless of age. Always demonstrate respect for your clients. Be realistic about your client's abilities, but never underestimate what your clients are able to achieve. Address your clients first before seeking information from caregivers, significant others, or friends. Allow your clients to communicate to you their wants and needs to the extent that they can. With permission from your clients, you can ask caregivers and significant others to help fill in the gaps. Remember that in most cases you will get the most accurate information from your clients themselves.

Always assume a communicative intent. Do not judge the intent without verifying it first, but always assume meaning from clients' action or inaction. An outburst from a toddler or a nonverbal client may indicate frustration, boredom, tiredness, or hunger. Do not assume that your client is just "acting out." They are always acting out for a reason. It is your job to figure out that reason and then deal with it accordingly. You will be surprised at the response you get when you simply ask, "What's wrong?"

Sometimes clients are just done, fed up, or too tired to carry on for the day. Know your clients' limits. You should be aware of how far you can push clients past their breaking point. You may want a preschool client to complete three more repetitions of a task before the client is allowed to end the session. Be clear about what you are asking your clients to do, and be consistent. If you state that a particular client has to complete three repetitions before the client is allowed to leave, make sure you figure out a way to determine that three repetitions are completed. In being consistent, you maintain credibility and you stay in charge. Compromise is often a good option when you are approaching a client's limits.

> **Clinician:** How many more are you willing to do today, Jack, before you are done?
>
> [Jack puts his head down on the table.]
>
> **Clinician:** I would like you to do three more, but because I can see you're tired, I'll let you go if you do just one more. What do you think?
>
> [Jack lifts up his head to proceed.]

Compromise provides the client with the opportunity to take ownership of the situation. In this example the clinician offered a suggestion that Jack determined was doable. If the clinician had required the three repetitions knowing that Jack would not budge, a battle of wills may have ensued. Allowing Jack to leave without completing what was required may have set up a potential problem for future sessions.

Culture, too, affects counseling choices. Consider such notions as stigma, self-image, and acceptability. Cultural variations can affect the impact stigma and self-image may have on the way you counsel clients. Deafness and stuttering, for example, are often perceived differently in different cultural contexts.

Beliefs about making eye contact, shaking hands, observing personal space, deferring to authority, involving family members in therapy, and being on time also vary by culture. When considering culture, always remember that, although individuals may identify themselves as members of a particular culture, they do not necessarily subscribe to the stereotypes of that culture. Take time to get to know the relevant thoughts and beliefs of each of your clients. Do not assume that their beliefs or cultural norms are the same as yours, but also do not assume that their beliefs and actions align exactly with those of the culture to whom they identify

Cognitive functioning is another area that requires the clinician to assess counseling methods and techniques as well as the development and implementation of goals.

Compromise: An agreement reached when both sides make some concessions; useful in therapy to avoid making demands that will strain a client's limits.

Your language and word choice will differ based on your clients' cognitive status. Simple sentences and commands are more effective for individuals with lower cognitive functioning. Use only the words necessary to convey your message or instruction with these clients. Do not adopt a patronizing tone or prosody when speaking to clients with cognitive deficits. Remember to maintain respect for your clients. When dealing with individuals with typical and higher-level cognitive status, you need to adjust your tone and syntax accordingly.

All these variations—age, culture, and cognitive functioning—may require you to assess and alter your counseling strategy. You need not acquire the expertise of a psychologist, psychiatrist, or clinical social worker to counsel effectively. Your scope of practice as an audiologist or speech-language pathologist encompasses communication issues, and counseling is geared to achieving goals within this scope.

The Core Process

Solution cycle: A four-stage, nonlinear leadership model designed to be a guide through the often complex integration of counseling with treatment. Phase One is the learning stage; Phase Two is the development of an alliance base or Circle of Power; Phase Three is the description of a vision of success and associated goals; Phase Four encompasses the achievement of the goals.

Appropriate models and strategies, beginning with a solution focus, can guide your counseling decisions and procedures. The first of these models is the Solution Cycle itself. The Solution Cycle provides you with a four-stage sequence that keeps the counseling process on track and rolling.

Phase One, learning, is always the starting point. You review documentary information on the client. Through interviewing, observation, discussion, and, primarily, listening, you find out what you need to know to get started in treatment and counseling. Once engaged, learning never ceases. It is the lifeblood of counseling effectiveness.

As you learn, you soon enter the second phase of the Solution Cycle. You begin networking, building a Circle of Power comprising the allies who will support the efforts you and your clients expend to achieve your goals. Anyone who might help can join the circle—family, friends, coaches, coworkers, and other professionals.

With a growing support network and an expanding knowledge base, you and your clients can progress to the third phase, the establishment of your mission. At this point you envision the preferred future, what the world will look like when goals are achieved. You commit to those goals, and devise your plan for improvement. Solution focus means you always work from goals you set together with your clients.

The Solution Cycle culminates in the execution of the plan, the effort clinicians and clients put forth to achieve the goals. The payoff is a distinct improvement in the clients' quality of life. You actually bring the preferred future into the present.

The Reasons Communication Happens

Five Intentions of Communication: Reasons people send and receive messages. They include self-affirmation, small talk, information, persuasion, and feeling.

Throughout the therapy process, you constantly communicate with your clients. You should always maintain awareness of your communication intention at any given moment. The Five Intentions of Communication guide the counseling process from one moment to the next. These are the reasons you communicate: to share information, to affect attitudes and behavior, to affirm yourself, to influence or express emotions, or to engage in small talk. These are also your clients' possible communication intentions.

Is it important to know, for example, when you have an information intention and when your intention is to change behavior? The answer is a definite yes, because your entire mode of communication can be affected by what you want to achieve.

The Solution Cycle and the Five Intentions form the underpinnings of your counseling efforts. They provide a structure in which you can ascertain where you are in the counseling process and how you are communicating to achieve your goals.

Armed with a reliable and workable therapy process, along with an astute and timely use of counseling, you and your clients achieve your goals. You never lose sight of why you are engaging in therapy. Your destination is what we call the preferred future. Your clients are pursuing specific improvements in their quality of life, improvements cast as solutions and framed as goals.

Goals and solutions define the preferred future, but goals and solutions also populate the road to the preferred future. Shorter-term, intermediate goals mark the milestones to the ultimate objective. They can be counseling or treatment-related goals. They are called MUSTDO goals, because they have to be achieved for progress to be made. MUSTDO is also an acronym specifying the distinguishing characteristics of intermediate goals.

For goals to follow the MUSTDO criteria, they can be measured and understood by all parties. They solve problems and are completed within a specific time frame. They can be done here and now. Their accomplishment is real and visible. They propel your clients to the preferred future.

The Confidence Zone

Inevitably, the therapy process comes to an end. If all goes well, the ultimate goals are reached; the preferred future is realized. If the therapy process has been inadequate, clients may regress, fail to maintain the gains they made, or find that their newly acquired skills begin to deteriorate. If the preferred future is reached, your clients are ready to proceed on their own. If you and they have prepared well, the improvements they have achieved will be lasting. In some cases, for instance, improvement was never a target and more realistic goals such as decreasing the rate at which a symptom worsens, maintaining current abilities for as long as possible, or preparing for end of life was achieved.

Your task, as the culmination of therapy draws near, is to keep your clients in the confidence zone, where they possess a strong trust in the skills, powers, and abilities they have worked hard to acquire. You have no airtight guarantee that clients will remain in their confidence zone once they leave therapy, but you have a number of ways to increase the probability that results will be long-lasting.

This dialogue with Laura illustrates a situation in which Laura was lacking in confidence, was out of the confidence zone, when it came to demonstrating her new skill between therapy sessions.

Confidence zone: An inner state where clients possess a strong trust in the skills, powers, and abilities they have worked hard to acquire.

Clinician: So, sometimes you have a hard time figuring out how to produce the /r/ when you don't have me to model it for you.

Laura: Yes, then I get frustrated with myself and I don't want to practice.

Clinician: Maybe we need to change the way we are approaching therapy then.

Laura: Do you really think that will help?

Clinician: Let's find out. Presently, there is something in the way we are approaching therapy that's not working for you. You are ending up frustrated, and then you are not motivated to practice. We need to find a way for you to feel like you know how to produce /r/ all of the time, even when I'm not around.

Laura: OK. How do we do that?

This type of exchange could take place at any point in the therapy process. The clinician should continually monitor whether Laura is achieving ownership at each stage. As a clinician, you should plan, long before therapy ends, to build client confidence and autonomy. If you have moved through therapy with a solution focus, you will be well positioned to hand ownership over to your clients. After all, ownership is a key component of the counseling you have done throughout the process, so the progressive building of autonomy of your clients has been underway from the very beginning. As the therapy process culminates, the time has arrived to complete the handover in a structured, methodical manner.

The Birth of Confidence: The Land of Yes, I Can

> **Confidence:** A strong trust in the skills, powers, and abilities a person has worked hard to acquire.

Confidence is closely related to the ownership connection, a core feature of motivation. Ownership is possession; confidence is self-possession. The word *confidence* comes from the Latin and means "great faith." Confident clients have great faith in their abilities. They have grown comfortable in demonstrating skills and competencies that may have taken months of therapy to learn. This confidence is essential if clients emerge from the clinical cocoon convinced that the improvements for which they have strived are real and lasting.

You should look for the signs of the birth of confidence as you prepare your clients for life after therapy.

"Yes, I can," then, is not just a slogan or cliché. It is an honest expression of confidence and ownership. Confident clients are not arrogant or cocky; they simply believe that they have learned and practiced enough to exhibit their competencies in their daily life and to exhibit them for the rest of their lives. Repatterning, the achievement of maintenance and generalization, has fully occurred, and clients see little or no prospect of ever reverting to their old patterns.

Signals of Confidence

- In sessions, clients show comfort and lack of hesitation when they demonstrate skills.
- Clients recount credible examples of their use of new skills outside of therapy.
- When discussing the transition to posttherapy life, clients do not express unusual fear of regression or "forgetting" what they have learned.
- Clients speak of their confidence in believable terms, with expressions like "I'm sure I can do it," "This is part of who I am now," and "I'll never go back."

If the emergence of this confidence was sudden or surprising, you would have reason to be suspicious. A person who stutters, for example, sometimes finds success in a technique that quickly results in greater fluency. Because the improvement was rapid, the client might experience a kind of euphoria, a sense that a lifelong breakthrough has happened.

The suddenness of the change, the seeming "miraculous" nature of the improvement, is a warning sign that the transformation may not be permanent. If the person who stutters experiences a relapse, it might be accompanied by severe disappointment. Gradual improvement is a reliable feature of lasting change. Miracles are extremely rare.

Maintenance and Generalization: Reducing the Clinician's Role in Counseling

The gradual acquisition of a competency results in the formation of a new habit, a comfortable and seemingly natural use of the skill whenever appropriate. As clients generalize their new skills outside therapy, the skills become more permanent. This permanent use of a generalized skill is called maintenance, and it is usually one of your primary goals as a clinician.

Maintenance and generalization are established as your influence fades. There are three ways to ensure maintenance after your clients have left therapy (Maas et al., 2008; Schmidt & Lee, 2005). (1) Transfer training is a process that teaches clients, often through behavior modification or behavior management techniques, to apply their new skills in a variety of situations similar to what the clients will meet in the real world. Clients demonstrate the capability to choose to perform the skill or not. (2) Altering the real-world environment usually involves enlisting clients' Circle of Power to assist the clients in maintaining their new skills and competencies. (3) Self-regulation or self-correcting means that your clients learn to "reinforce" their new competencies and avoid permanent regression through methods and techniques they themselves employ.

You can use all three ways with your clients. As you counsel them, you should consider a number of important recommendations.

Lifelong Confidence: The Land of Yes, I Will

Generalization is really adaptation. Clients who are able to generalize can use the new skill not only in the specific setting in which they were trained to use it but also in other settings where the use of the skill is appropriate. Individuals with deficits in

---

Counseling for Generalization

- Frequently ask clients to identify different settings where the use of the skill is appropriate.
- If clients seem confident about a particular application of the skill, encourage them to generalize to that setting and discuss the results with them.
- Note and address any anxiety clients exhibit at the thought of applying their newly learned competencies in other settings.
- Be alert for anxiety about a specific setting, because clients may be apprehensive about only one application of the skill.

pragmatics who use turn-taking skills effectively with their family members are generalizing those learned skills when they are also able to demonstrate the skill with new communication partners.

Like maintenance, generalization is enhanced through transfer training, real-world practice, and self-regulation or self-correction. Generalization requires the additional ability to detect new situations in which the learned skill should be called into service. All of the recommendations used when counseling for maintenance apply equally to counseling for generalization. The next section provides recommendations to use to enhance long-term maintenance and generalization.

Flying Solo

In most cases, your objective as a speech-language pathologist or audiologist is to use the tools and insights of your profession to improve your clients' quality of life. Therapy always comes to an end, but the improvement or maintenance of abilities is meant to be lasting. In treating end-of-life cases or cases of progressively worsening symptoms, the objectives change, but the highest possible quality of life is always foremost.

Incremental Independence

Little by little you guide your clients away from you, like a patient older sister teaching her brother to ride a bicycle. At first she holds both the seat and the handlebars, steering, letting her sibling get the feel of riding a bike. Soon, she is trotting behind holding only the seat to maintain balance. Then, one day, she lets go altogether. Her brother can now ride the bike on his own; he is unlikely to forget how it is done.

Incremental independence does refer to that final break at therapy's end. It is also critical, however, to view incremental independence as a process that goes on throughout therapy. Autonomy, the ability of the clients to act independently of you, is always a key value in clinical work. Seize every opportunity to foster independence, even in very small matters.

A brief dialogue with Robert illustrates a situation in which he was asked to take ownership in an unrealistic manner after losing his voice.

> **Clinician:** Look, Robert, there's no physical problem here. It's up to you to dig down and find out what's going on. I can't do it for you.
>
> **Robert:** I don't know what's causing it. My ENT says it's not physical.
>
> **Clinician:** The ENT can't do it for you either. Surgery won't help you and there are no medications that will get your voice back. It's entirely up to you.

In this dialogue, the clinician gave the reins to Robert a little too early. The clinician told Robert he is pretty much on his own. In a solution-focused approach, Robert is expected to be committed to his goals but also the clinician is expected to be fully engaged and invested in the pursuit of Robert's goals. This scenario does not really transfer ownership to Robert because he is likely to be frustrated when the clinician pushes him prematurely to act on his own. This tactic may, in fact, make ownership far

Incremental independence: A process of increasing client autonomy that goes on throughout therapy and is ideally achieved by the final break at therapy's end. Autonomy, the ability of the clients to act independently of the therapist, is always a key value in clinical work. Information. In therapy, the factual, practical, technical, and developmental knowledge needed to proceed and achieve success.

more difficult for Robert to achieve. The clinician must ease Robert into the process and allow him more and more independence as he is ready.

The Planning Process Model is a model you can use to include your clients in determining their course of therapy at any point in the therapy process. If used at the start of therapy, this model gives clients ownership of the therapy process from the beginning. The model can set the stage for goal development, commitment to the process, and action throughout every phase of the Solution Cycle. Giving ownership to your clients at the beginning of therapy makes it easier for you to hand over gradual control throughout therapy and have your clients ultimately achieve independence. Remember to monitor continually for signs that your clients are overwhelmed or frustrated.

Relapse or Regression

Clients can experience regression or relapse at any point in the therapy process or even when therapy has concluded. You must prepare your clients for this possibility. Astute counseling skills are utilized when a relapse happens. If your clients experience a relapse during therapy, you must take immediate action to discuss what happened and why your clients believe they relapsed. Make sure not to gloss over the fact that your clients are reverting back to old behaviors. Clients often know the exact cause (e.g., breaking up with a significant other, having to give a big speech for a class or for their job, being reminded of how embarrassed they felt about their communication disorder). Sometimes clients relapse because their feelings and emotions about their communication disorder were never fully addressed. Validate their feelings and how difficult it is to experience a relapse. Assess your clients' motivational balance and focus on reestablishing purpose, growth, or ownership. Sometimes a relapse can be the motivation a client needs to move forward.

> **Relapse:** Often sudden deterioration in a skill, technique, or practice after it had apparently been learned, even when repatterning seemed to have taken place.

Relapses can also happen once clients are discharged from therapy. To decrease the possibility of relapse after discharge, make sure your clients are actually ready to be discharged. Often clients have difficulty going from one hour of therapy every week to being completely discharged. You may want to initiate a gradual decrease in the amount of time they come to therapy. Change to a half hour every week or an hour every other week. These are all ways you can monitor whether your clients are ready to maintain their new behaviors without your help.

Once you are sure your clients are ready to end therapy, prepare them for what is to come. Before saying your final goodbyes, set up a date when you will call your clients to check in. Depending on your client, this date could be three weeks or three to six months from the time of discharge. You should also make sure your clients know that they can contact you if a relapse occurs or if they have any questions about their techniques.

This dialogue with Luke provides a potential conversation you may have with your client who is considering being discharged.

Clinician: Luke, that was a great session. I really think you are ready to do this on your own.

Luke: I do too. Sometimes I worry, though, that I'll forget all the techniques you've taught me. I'll just be standing there talking to someone and not know what to do.

Clinician: What situations scare you the most?

Luke: Making presentations in class. I know we've worked on that specifically, and I really do believe I can get up and speak now, way better than I could before. It's just … there are so many people looking at me. Actually, once I'm up there talking … I settle in … I'm fine. It's right before I get up… my stomach feels a little uneasy.

Clinician: I get butterflies in my stomach too almost every time I get up to speak to a group of people. Sometimes when I'm nervous my voice will start to shake or I'll forget what I'm going to say. Are there other speaking situations that make you nervous?

Luke: No, not really. I'm comfortable with my speech now. I know my techniques. They've become part of what I do every day. Even in presentations, I know what to do… it's just getting up there. But I do it.

Clinician: There are days and times that will test you. Most of the time you will get through those days fine, but what happens if you start to get really frustrated and your techniques seem to stop working? Do you remember what we called that?

Luke: Yes, it's called a relapse. I remember having one after my first six weeks of therapy. I thought I was ready to go it alone, but then realized that I wasn't. It was pretty frustrating. I'm definitely better prepared now. I'm okay with the times my speech isn't perfect. I have my support system, too. I know what to do, don't worry.

Clinician: I'm not worried. You are ready. I'm going to check in on you in a month … see how you are doing. You call me before that if there are any problems.

Luke: I will.

The Limits of Progress

In the scenario with Luke, he and his clinician have come full circle. They spent time learning. They enlisted allies for support. They envisioned the future full of possibilities. They created the plan and acted on it. Luke was then ready to go out on his own. Most of the journeys you take with your clients will follow that same path. Sometimes, though, therapy does not go as planned or cannot continue for some reason. As much as you prepare, as motivated as your clients may be, there are limits to progress. You need to be aware of those limits and know what to do when you are up against them. Limits can present themselves within the clinician, a member of the Circle of Power, the clients, and even the disorder itself.

Limitations within the clinician

Sometimes the limits you face are your own limits. As you become a more seasoned clinician, such limitations will arise infrequently, but they will occur. You may face a disorder you have never treated. You remember learning about it in graduate school but never thought you would get that kind of client. For students or even new clinicians, these limits may feel like a daily occurrence. You are still learning. The fact is, though, you are always learning. Continue to expand your mind. Attend continuing education courses and workshops. You need a certain number of credits to maintain your certification, but attend more, attend a variety. Be a consumer of research to keep up-to-date on the latest treatment options. Enlist your own allies to help you when needed, including mentors, colleagues, and other professionals. Learning is not just the first stage in the Solution Cycle. Learning is a lifelong necessity for a successful career in therapy.

Limitations of specific disorders

You may also encounter limits related to specific disorders. These limits can pose roadblocks to the implementation or continuation of the therapy you offer. Although there is no ideal treatment for the voice disorder spasmodic dysphonia, many individuals with this type of dystonia are not effectively treated with behavioral voice therapy alone. Injections of an extremely small amount of botulinum toxin have been shown to decrease the laryngeal muscle spasms in spasmodic dysphonia (Ludlow, 2009; Troung, Rontal, Rolnick, Aronson, & Mistura, 1991). Once that diagnosis is made, attempting to treat the primary spasmodic dysphonia with behavioral voice therapy alone would not be ethically sound. Your counseling should focus on providing information to your clients about the medical management needed to treat the disorder and referring clients to the appropriate physician.

There are also limits related to disorders that feature a progressive decline. In amyotrophic lateral sclerosis, the time will come when clients will not be able to speak, swallow, or control their physical movements. Educate your clients and prepare them for that time. Allow them to make decisions about their care, their preferred way to communicate and obtain nourishment. In individuals with the cognitive decline typical of dementia, inform them that therapy will focus on the maintenance of current function and may transition to helping the Circle of Power communicate with their loved ones in later stages of dementia.

Keep in mind that, although these examples detail the limitations of spasmodic dysphonia, amyotrophic lateral sclerosis, and the decline associated with dementia, you will encounter numerous other disorders or disease processes as a clinician. Remember, no two clients, despite their disorder, are identical. As a result, your approach to counseling varies with each individual client. Often the limits of a disorder are imposed by the client's perception of those limits. Clients may perceive a nondegenerative disorder, such as stuttering or childhood apraxia of speech, as having a limited prospect of progress.

Information about support groups, foundations for specific disorders or diseases, and personal accounts of others facing the same diagnosis are just a few resources that clients might find helpful in coping with perceived limitations of a disorder. **Figure 12-1** lists different types of communication disorders and provides accompanying resources that can be shared with clients or the caregivers of clients to supplement the counseling they receive from you as a clinician.

Limitations imposed by the clients

Clients will also have limits. When you first evaluate clients, you base your prognosis on many factors: clients' motivation, willingness to participate, effect on quality of life,

Disorder	Resources
Autism	• autismspeaks.org • autism-society.org • nea.org
Childhood Apraxia of Speech (CAS)	• asha.org/public/speech/disorders/childhoodapraxia/ • apraxia-kids.org
Child Language	• kidshealth.org/parent/System/ill/speech_therapy.html • asha.org/public/speech/development/chart/ • home-speech-home.com/language-disorder.html
Cleft Lip/Palate	• Operation Smile • cleftline.org • cleftresources.com
Dysphagia	• National Foundation of Swallowing Disorders • American Dysphagia Network • asha.org/public/speech/swallowing/
End of Life	• American Academy of Hospice and Palliative Medicine • Geriatric Mental Health Foundation • compassionatefriends.org/home.aspx
Hearing	• asha.org/public/hearing/Adult-Aural-Rehabilitation/ • asha.org/public/hearing/treatment/child_aur_rehab.htm • nidcd.nih.gov/health/hearing
Neurogenic	• National Parkinson's Foundation (NPF) • National Aphasia Association (NAA) • National Institute of Neurological Disorders and Stroke • asha.org/public/speech/disorders/dysarthria/
Stuttering	• The National Stuttering Association (NSA) • The Stuttering Foundation • stuttertalk.com • stuttersocial.com
Terminal Illness	• American Society of Clinical Oncology • suicidepreventionlifeline.org • cancer.org
Voice	• The Voice Foundation • American Academy of Otolaryngology—Head and Neck Surgery • National Spasmodic Dysphonia Association • International Association of Laryngectomees • asha.org/slp/clinical/voice-disorders/

FIGURE 12-1 Resources for Specific Disorder Types. Counseling differs per disorder as well as per individual client. Online resources can be helpful to clinicians and clients researching information about different disorders.

intellectual capacity, performance on tests, mobility of articulators, and their support system. Take these factors into serious consideration when making your prognosis, and set realistic expectations. Prognoses can give you the inside edge on areas that may need immediate counseling focus, such as winning over an adversary, balancing motivation, and changing a belief.

As a clinician, you never want to tell clients they cannot do something. To make that situation less likely, it is vitally important that you set realistic expectations from the onset of therapy. If your clients exceed your reasonable expectations, you can count that as a great success. If your clients cannot live up to your unreasonable expectations, then you may be setting them up for disappointment and failure. You can use advanced communication skills such as challenging when you do not believe your clients are meeting expectations. Remember, too, that making goals that are too easy sets the stage for clients to become bored. The key to success is motivational balance.

Make sure to set goals that are realistic, to know your clients' limits, and to refer to other professionals when needed. You should also resist making promises you cannot keep. Saying things like, "I can get your voice back exactly as it was," "You will be able to hear completely in all environments with these hearing aids," and "You will be able to do all the things you could do before your stroke" are empty promises that are not likely to produce the outcome you want. Instead, say things like, "We are going to do our best to get as much function back as we can," "Therapy is going to take a lot work; I'll make sure to do my part to help you reach your goals," and "You show a lot of determination and desire to succeed—these qualities will help you achieve your goals."

If you have reached your clients' potential or limits and you believe that you cannot ethically provide services anymore, you first need to determine whether this was a choice made by your clients or by you as clinician. Despite your best attempt to persuade clients to continue, if your clients' priorities shift away from therapy and your clients decide to discontinue therapy sessions with you, then you should let them go. Always make available that olive branch in case your clients change their minds, but giving your clients ownership of their decision to quit puts the responsibility for that decision on them.

If the decision to discontinue therapy is yours and this decision is based on your well-informed professional judgment, then you should explain the decision to your clients and their caregivers. If you are making the decision to end therapy and this decision is partly the result of a personal limitation (e.g., you have taken this particular

Potential Client Limits

- Inability to make the commitment of time to therapy and practice
- Cognitive, intellectual, or physical limitations
- Other medical priorities
- Other life priorities (e.g., care for a child, significant other, parent)
- Conviction that the disorder is too hard to change
- Cultural norms that makes therapy unproductive
- Financial limitations or priorities

client as far as your professional knowledge can take the client), then it is your responsibility to help clients find another speech-language pathologist or audiologist who has more experience or expertise in working with clients like yours.

Limitations imposed by the circle of power

Members of your clients' Circle of Power can also present their own limits to your clients' progress in therapy. Undeclared adversaries can be troublesome to the therapy process because these individuals often believe they are helping clients. The opposite is usually true: their behavior or beliefs hinder clients' progress. An undeclared adversary who insists on making a client practice techniques incessantly at home may contribute to the client's feeling of being overwhelmed. Caregivers who insist on being in the clinic room may also decrease therapy progress because they interrupt clients or clinician during sessions.

Sometimes, members of your clients' Circle of Power may be openly averse to the therapy process. If clients rely on these individuals for rides to therapy sessions, these individuals may not value time. They might arrive late or might just not bring clients to sessions. They may berate clients or make fun of them when they practice techniques. They may fail to attend meetings with you or to help clients practice their techniques at home. These individuals are true adversaries to the therapy process.

Managing adversaries and minimizing the impact of their actions on the clients' therapy are difficult. Always be aware of these individuals. Maintain open lines of communication, and document any interaction or attempted interaction with them. Discuss how their actions affect your clients. As your clients get older, encourage them to have ownership of their goals so you can minimize adversaries' influence on therapy progress. Work to change adversaries into allies.

Remember to keep the preferred future in mind. Your aim is to help your clients acquire the confidence to be their own clinician, to maintain and generalize their gains and thereby improve their quality of life well beyond the present moment. Perfection is not the goal. No one is perfectly fluent. No one has perfect hearing. The point of counseling is to encourage your clients to begin therapy, frame problems you and they can appropriately address, create goals focused on the solutions to those problems, and engage clients in the process of acquiring the skills and competencies required to achieve those goals.

Then, you and they may part company assured that they leave with new, lifelong habits, their futures truly enriched by the experience of therapy.

Undeclared adversary: A person in a client's Circle of Power who believes he or she is helping the client but whose behavior or beliefs hinder the client's progress. An example is a parent who drives a child too hard to practice improvement techniques.

Review of Key Points

- Counseling is caring support in the form of information, guidance, or assistance provided to clients, families, caretakers, and advocates.
- The solution-focused approach uses the insights of counseling strategies such as behavior management, cognitive therapy, the humanistic approach, and more recently developed methods, including motivational interviewing and counseling.
- Counseling takes different forms depending on such client-related factors as age, cognitive functioning, previous experience in therapy, and cultural differences.
- The Solution Cycle provides you with a four-stage sequence that keeps the counseling process on track. Phase One, learning, is always the starting point. Phase Two is networking, building a Circle of Power comprising the allies who will support the efforts you and your clients expend to achieve your goals. In Phase Three you envision and commit to the preferred future, what the world will look like when goals are achieved. Phase Four involves the execution of the plan. The payoff is improvement in the clients' quality of life.
- The Five Intentions of Communication guide the counseling process. These are to share information, to affect attitudes and behavior, to affirm yourself, to influence or express emotions, and to engage in small talk.
- The Solution Cycle and the Five Intentions form the underpinnings of your counseling efforts.
- As a speech-language pathologist or audiologist conducting therapy, your ultimate success depends on two outcomes: (1) the degree to which your therapeutic goals are achieved and (2) the permanence of the resulting changes in your clients' quality of life.
- If therapy is successful, then, in a sense, therapy does not end. The repatterning you and your clients have accomplished should now be a permanent change. Your clients become their own clinicians.
- Your task, as therapy ends, is to keep your clients in the confidence zone, where they possess a strong trust in their skills, powers, and abilities.
- Ownership, a core feature of motivation, is possession; confidence is self-possession. Confident clients have great faith in their abilities. This confidence is essential if improvements are to become real and lasting. Look for signs of confidence.
- The permanent use of a generalized skill is called maintenance, and it is usually one of your primary goals as a clinician. The three ways to ensure maintenance and generalization are achieved are transfer training, altering the real-world environment, and self-regulation or self-correcting.
- *Incremental independence* refers to that final break at therapy's end, but it is a process that goes on throughout therapy. Autonomy, the ability of the clients to act independently of you, is always a key value in clinical work.

- Relapses can happen when clients are discharged from therapy. Make sure your clients are ready to be discharged. You may want to slowly decrease the amount of time they come to therapy. Monitor whether your clients can really maintain their new behaviors without your help.
- At the end of therapy, prepare clients for what is to come. Set up a date when you will call your clients to check in. Make sure your clients know that they can contact you if a relapse occurs or if they have questions.
- Sometimes therapy does not go as planned or cannot continue for some reason. There are limits to progress. Limits can present themselves as within the clinician, with a member of the Circle of Power, with the clients, and even by the disorder itself. Be aware of your clients' limits and limits to specific disorders.
- Remember the big picture. Your aim is to help your clients acquire the confidence to "be their own clinician," to maintain and generalize their gains and thereby to improve their quality of life well beyond the present moment. Improvement, not perfection, is the goal.

Practical Exercises

For this assignment, read each scenario and identify whether the limitation toward progress is imposed by the clinician, the client, a member of the Circle of Power, or a specific disorder. Explain how you would address this limitation.

1. Chrissy is a 44-year-old woman who was diagnosed with a unilateral vocal fold paralysis following her thyroidectomy 2 years ago. This is her fourth time enrolled in voice therapy since her diagnosis. Chrissy's attendance at therapy sessions is inconsistent, and she frequently tells her clinician that she rarely practices her voice exercises.
2. Victor is an 8-year-old boy who stutters. He has been enrolled in speech therapy for 12 weeks but has made minimal progress in therapy. Victor finally reported to his clinician that he is reluctant to practice his fluency strategies at home because his older brother, Steven, makes fun of him.

REFERENCES

Behrman, A. (2006). Facilitating behavioral change in voice therapy: The relevance of motivational interviewing. *American Journal of Speech-Language Pathology, 15*(3), 215–225.

Ludlow, C. L. (2009). Treatment for spasmodic dysphonia: Limitations of current approaches. *Current Opinion in Otolaryngology Head and Neck Surgery, 17*(3), 160–165.

Maas, E., Robin, D. A., Austermann, H., Freedman, S. E., Wulf, G., Ballard, K. J., & Schmidt, R. A. (2008). Principles of motor learning in treatment of motor speech disorders. *American Journal of Speech-Language Pathology, 17*(3), 277–298.

McFarlane, L. (2012). Motivational interviewing: Practical strategies for speech-language pathologists and audiologists. *Canadian Journal of Speech-Language Pathology and Audiology, 36*(1), 8–16.

Miller, W. R., & Rollnick, S. (1991). *Motivational interviewing: Preparing people to change addictive behavior.* New York, NY: Guilford Press.

Schmidt, R. A., & Lee, T. D. (2005). *Motor control and learning: A behavioral emphasis* (4th ed.). Champaign, IL: Human Kinetics.

Troung, D. D., Rontal, M., Rolnick, M., Aronson, A. E., & Mistura, K. (1991). Double-blind controlled study of botulinum toxin in adductor spasmodic dysphonia. *Laryngoscope, 101*(6), 630–634.

GLOSSARY

Acceptance. The fifth stage in the classically framed stages of grief, when a person faces the reality of the situation and chooses to do what can be done about it.

Activity limitation. A problem in performing particular tasks or functions as a result of an impairment.

Adversary. An individual who has a negative influence or who is not supportive of a client's efforts in the therapy process.

Ally (also called, advocates). In therapy, someone who may be invested in or affected by progress in treatment; perceived as someone who actively supports the client's efforts to achieve therapy goals. An ally is usually a member of the client's Circle of Power.

Anger. The second stage in the classically framed stages of grief, when a person experiences fierce emotional rebellion at the terrible event.

Apathy. A lack of interest and enthusiasm caused by a sense that an activity has little or no purpose. Apathy leads to a loss of energy and poor motivation.

Attending behaviors. Actions, including facial expressions, visible movement, gestures, and sounds, that indicate to a speaker that a person is listening with focus and interest.

Bargaining. The third stage in the classically framed stages of grief, when a person looks for hope, a way to reverse what has happened, to negotiate a deal, or to get a reprieve.

Behavior. A discrete action a person does.

Blocks to listening. Elements in the environment, in listeners, and in speakers that obstruct a person's willingness or ability to listen effectively.

Boredom. A lack of desire to perform an activity because it is not challenging, is perceived as too easy.

Bullying. Unwanted, aggressive behavior that involves a real or perceived power imbalance. The behavior may be repeated day after day and can involve such intimidating behavior as making threats, spreading rumors, attacking someone physically or verbally, and excluding someone from a group on purpose.

Case history. The client's case history is the starting point of information gathering; it covers information on the client's speech-language or audiological record, including issues, disorders, and past treatment, as well as background data on family, education, and occupation, medical, social, and related information.

Catastrophic loss. A devastating life change due to physical or cognitive damage to oneself or a loved one.

Challenge. An advanced communication technique that asks clients to take a new direction, rethink, or "refeel" what they have just expressed.

Chief complaint. The chief complaint can be characterized in a number of ways. It is the primary motive, the reason a client comes to a clinician for an evaluation. It is what is bothering the client the most. It is, importantly, what the client wants to begin working on first in treatment.

Circle of power. The people a person depends on or seeks out to enhance that person's effectiveness at whatever task or project the person is doing or contemplating; an alliance base.

Client advocates. People influential in a client's life. They tend to be assertive in their commitment to what they see as beneficial to the client. They can be helpful in the therapy process, but they may, under certain circumstances, become adversarial.

Compromise. An agreement reached when both sides make some concessions; useful in therapy to avoid making demands that will strain a client's limits.

Confidence. A strong trust in the skills, powers, and abilities a person has worked hard to acquire.

Confidence zone. An inner state where clients possess a strong trust in the skills, powers, and abilities they have worked hard to acquire.

Counseling Integration Matrix (CI Matrix). A useful model that encompasses the impact of a disorder on a client's quality of life set against the client's willingness to make the changes recommended through therapy. The CI Matrix reveals four client states: high negative impact on quality of life with high willingness to change (High-High); high negative impact on quality of life with low willingness to change (High-Low); low negative impact on quality of life with low willingness to change (Low-Low); low negative impact on quality of life with high willingness to change (Low-High).

Counseling. Caring support in the form of information, guidance, or assistance provided to clients, families, caretakers, and advocates; clients can use such insight to pursue realistic and clearly understood goals and attain a more fulfilling quality of life. Counseling achieves its purpose when that support either bolsters clients' motivation to succeed in treatment or reduces attitudinal, behavioral, or emotional barriers to progress in treatment.

Cultural awareness. Sensitivity to differing norms for greeting and interacting, based not on stereotypes or assumptions but on actual differences that exist among various cultures.

Cultural literacy. Knowledge and understanding of specific cultural norms and practices. This knowledge enables a person to navigate comfortably within that culture.

Denial. Often seen as the initial reaction to devastating news or trauma. When in denial, the person experiencing the difficulty simply contends that there is no problem, nothing wrong.

Depression. The fourth stage in the classically framed stages of grief, when a person begins dealing with the present moment, the reality of the situation. Many experience an emptiness for what they have lost or for what they believed would be their future. Those in depression exhibit low energy and low motivation and may become purposeless and apathetic. This stage can reach a state known as clinical depression.

Deterring forces. Past experiences that reinforce an unhelpful belief.

Disability. A term that encompasses impairments (negative changes to the body's anatomy and physiology), activity limitations (problems in performing particular tasks or functions as a result of the impairment), and participation restriction (difficulty with or decreased involvement in social and occupational situations).

Discouragement. Loss of heart, a dwindling of passion and desire. It is marked by a general lack of energy and enthusiasm about progressing in therapy, similar to the symptoms of apathy and boredom but displaying a noticeable sadness, a sense not that it is worthless to achieve the goal but that it is useless to try.

Doable goals. Goals that are clearly able to be accomplished, given the client's knowledge, time, resources, and abilities.

Dread. An emotion that can arise when one engages in or contemplates situations with which one is seriously ill prepared to cope. Dread can come about when an activity is seen as far too difficult or dangerous.

Ego impedance. An aspect of clients' self-perception that prevents them from achieving a goal because of a negative attitude about themselves, their skills, or their abilities. Ego impedance is a negative self-perception created by clients about their ability.

Empathy. A process whereby someone feels and reflects another person's emotions or feelings.

Enhancing forces. Clients' prior experiences that tend to make a new belief seem reasonable, when clients have an unhelpful belief and the therapist is proposing a different way of thinking.

Five Intentions of Communication. Reasons people send and receive messages. They include self-affirmation, small talk, information, persuasion, and feeling.

Frustration. The feeling that one is not in control, is without options, is being forced against one's will.

Generalization. A state of affairs where the correct behavior is elicited in a variety of situations.

Goals. Intended end points of actions and plans.

Growth. In a motivational context, the result of the successful acceptance of a challenge.

Habituation. A term frequently used to denote the process of making a new behavioral pattern comfortable and permanent.

Hidden messages. An unexpressed notion or thought that is contained in the words that a person chooses to utter, the person's prosody or tone of voice, facial expressions, gestures, or body language.

Hunch. An intuitive guess about how to proceed in a given situation. Experienced therapists know how to value their hunches and make appropriate use of them.

Ideal self. The person one would like to be, the fulfillment of one's supreme wishes and ambitions, one's desired state.

Impairments. A negative change to the body's anatomy and physiology.

Incremental independence. A process of increasing client autonomy that goes on throughout therapy and is ideally achieved by the final break at therapy's end. Autonomy, the ability of the clients to act independently of the therapist, is always a key value in clinical work.

Information. In therapy, the factual, practical, technical, and developmental knowledge needed to proceed and achieve success.

Intake form. The clients' intake forms constitute the starting point of information gathering. Filling out the forms begins the process of developing the clients' case history. The forms ask for the information associated with the case history.

Interaction process model. A five-step procedure serving as a guide to a successful meeting. The steps are: (1) prepare, (2) present information, (3) listen, (4) prepare to act, and (5) act.

Interviewing. The interview process is an informational give-and-take between therapist and client, client advocates, and adversaries. It is designed to capture relevant client information in a structured manner. During the interview, clients tell their stories, and the clinician provides necessary information to the clients.

Leverage. In therapy, knowledge of what is important to clients, their desires, wants, and needs, utilized to encourage clients to work through obstacles, roadblocks, and blind spots they may face throughout the therapy process. Leverage gives the clinician the positional advantage.

Listening. A two-part process of first understanding and then assessing messages.

Logical argument. A pattern of reasoning that correctly uses accepted rules of logic to support the conclusion being asserted.

Long-term goals. In therapy, the ultimate end points, the desired results, the preferred future.

Maintenance. A state of affairs where a desirable behavior is elicited regularly.

Measurable goals. Goals that meet the following criteria: they describe what it means to reach the goal; they may be quantitative (what things are to be accomplished?) or qualitative (how well will those things be accomplished?); an outside person, properly briefed, can use the measure to the confirm goal attainment with certainty.

Motivation. A connection between a person and an activity that causes the person to be energized and focused when performing that activity.

Motivational interviewing. A client-centered and goal-oriented technique, compatible with the solution-focused approach.

MUSTDO goals. Intermediate goals seen as requirements for meeting longer-term goals. MUSTDO is an acronym describing this type of goal: measurable, understood, solution focused, time bound, doable, and observable.

Nonverbals. Nonverbals enhance the meaning of what someone is expressing. They are not words, and they do not necessarily accompany specific words, phrases, or sentences being uttered at a given moment. There are many nonverbals, including visuals, that accompany a transmission and add meaningful elements to the communication of a message.

Observable goals. Of a goal, able to be seen concretely when achieved.

Observation. A process whereby someone focuses attention on another person and looks for signs of attitudes, emotions, thoughts, and beliefs that may be hiding even from the other's own awareness. These signs can reveal themselves in words, facial expressions, involuntary gestures, and even the posture of the body.

Obsession. In a motivational context, interest that has become extreme to the point of excluding other possible interests. Characterized by high energy and narrow focus.

Obstacle dominance. An aspect of the outer world perceived by clients as creating a barrier so great that access to the goal is unachievable. Obstacle dominance is a negative self-perception the client has that is related to something external to the client.

Ownership. In a motivational context, the sense that one is in control and has options and the resources needed to achieve the desired end.

Paraverbals. Sounds, sights, touches, and even smells that accompany words (*para-*: beside; *verbals*: the words) and possess or alter intended meaning. There is a paraverbal component to every utterance because words are always spoken with inflection, intonation, or prosody. The inflection conveys meaning or modifies the meaning of the words. A vocal sound by itself may be a paraverbal if it is not a word and yet conveys meaning.

Participation restriction. Difficulty with or decreased involvement in social and occupational situations.

Pattern of behavior. A connected series of actions.

Planning Process Model. A seven-step process for formulating and achieving therapy goals.

Preferred future. The mission, the ultimate goal of therapy, expressed in terms of a vision of success. This vision is a depiction of the changed circumstances desired, sought, and achieved by the collaborative efforts of clinician and client. It is a description of the client's world once the mission is accomplished.

Probes. Questions or statements clinicians can use to dig deeper into what clients say to clarify clients' intentions or emotions.

Probing. A listening technique that begins the assessing phase of listening, when the listener makes judgments about what has been heard. Probing seeks the speaker's take or judgment on what the speaker has transmitted.

Professionalism. Style, manner, and behavior consistent with and demonstrating qualifications in a field of study, career, or expertise.

Psychologists, clinical social workers, counselors, and psychotherapists. Individuals with advance degrees and certification in the assessment and treatment of those with diseases of the brain, emotional disturbances, and behavior issues.

Purpose. The motivating sense that an activity is worthwhile and meaningful and that there is a good reason to perform the activity.

Quality of life. A person's assessment concerning how close he or she is to an acceptable level of perceived happiness and satisfaction in his or her day-to-day condition.

Quit option. The decision to end therapy.

Rapport. A feeling of camaraderie, of having something in common with another person. ("Bad rapport" is the opposite.)

Reciprocity. A situation in which beneficial results flow in two directions, for instance, from ally to client as well as from client back to ally. The benefits are mutual.

Reflecting emotion. Using verbals or paraverbals to clarify a feeling that the listener has received from the speaker.

Reflection. A process of turning one's mind back to an event that happened previously, stopping to think about what occurred. As one reflects on this event, one considers its importance and reaches conclusions that will be of help in planning or determining a course of action.

Relapse. Often sudden deterioration in a skill, technique, or practice after it had apparently been learned, even when repatterning seemed to have taken place.

Reluctance. Hesitancy.

Repatterning. The total process of maintenance and generalization.

Reputation. The regard people have for another because of the other's status, moral standing, expertise, education, wisdom, accomplishments, or any combination of these. One's good name.

Resistance. Opposition and pushback when cooperation is sought. Resistance has intensity and focus.

Responsive listening. A communication activity with a specific objective: to comprehend, evaluate, and retain what is being transmitted by a speaker.

Restatement. Repeating what has been heard in words different from those used by the speaker. Ideally, restatement contains only the meaning transmitted, not implications or assessments of what has been said. Restatement can be a word-by-word paraphrase or a summary.

Roadblocks to repatterning. Complications that obstruct the path to maintenance and generalization. Obstructions can arise in efforts to break an old pattern, or difficulties might be encountered in forming an enduring new pattern. A person might slip back toward the older pattern after repatterning has apparently been achieved, a situation known as relapsing.

Self-affirmation. One of the Five Intentions of a speaker. A direct or indirect assertion by a speaker about the way the speaker thinks and feels about himself or herself.

Self-concept. According to Carl Rogers, "The organized, consistent set of perceptions and beliefs about oneself." Self-concept has three features: self-esteem or self-worth, ideal self, and self-image.

Self-esteem. Self-esteem is the value one places on oneself, acceptance or approval of self. Self-esteem is a sense of self-worth. Largely formed during childhood, self-esteem is thought to be learned through experience, and not something that can be taught.

Self-image. How people see themselves, their current state—beautiful or ugly, smart or dumb, good or bad, fat or thin, or something in between. Self-image does not always reflect reality. In effect, self-image depicts how far people think they really are from their ideal self.

Shame. The abject feeling that a person is a disgrace, unworthy to be in the company of those who stigmatize. Self-image takes a direct hit; in the judgment of others the shamed one is found guilty, subject to shunning, name-calling, and worse.

Short-term goals. An intermediate goal determined to be essential to the accomplishment of longer-term goals. Called MUSTDO goals, an acronym signaling that the short-term goal is measurable, understood, solution focused, time bound, doable, and observable.

Silence. Often a powerful tool that can be used during treatment sessions to encourage clients to think of ideas on their own. Silence is an actual response. Sometimes not saying anything at all provides the client with time to formulate an idea, ask a question, or find the courage to say something.

Small talk. "Chitchat." Discussion of relatively minor matters; used to relax, set a climate, or build a relationship.

Solution cycle. A four-stage, nonlinear leadership model designed to be a guide through the often complex integration of counseling with treatment. Phase One is the learning stage; Phase Two is the development of an alliance base or Circle of Power; Phase Three is the description of a vision of success and associated goals; Phase Four encompasses the achievement of the goals.

Solution-focused goals. Of a goal, seen as improving a situation or solving a problem.

Stigma. An impairment labeled not only as a disorder but as a socially undesirable disorder. Unlike mere insensitivity, stigma carries the implication that a person is unwelcome, a detriment to an institution and its people, a potential embarrassment, a blemish on its reputation.

Study. A set of learning activities that take place offline, at times other than during sessions.

Summarizing. Restating the highlights or main points that were expressed by a speaker.

Time-bound goals. Goals scheduled to be achieved at a finite, established point.

Undeclared adversary. A person in a client's Circle of Power who believes he or she is helping the client but whose behavior or beliefs hinder the client's progress. An example is a parent who drives a child too hard to practice improvement techniques.

Understood goals. Of goals formulated by a therapist and client. Fully comprehended by both parties. The goal must not only be understood but also therapist and client must understand it in the same way.

Verbals. Words, phrases, and sentences used by a speaker.

INDEX

Note: Page numbers followed by "f" indicate figure.